Pocket Guide to ECG Diagnosis

Pocket Guide to ECG Diagnosis

Edward K. Chung, MD, FACP, FACC

Professor of Medicine and Director of the Heart Station,
Thomas Jefferson University Hospital, Philadelphia

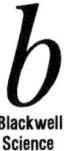

Blackwell
Science

Blackwell Science
Editorial offices:
238 Main Street, Cambridge, Massachusetts 02142, USA
Osney Mead, Oxford OX2 OEL, England
25 John Street, London WClN 2BL, England
23 Ainslie Place, Edinburgh EH3 6AJ, Scotland
54 University Street, Carlton, Victoria 3053, Australia
Arnette Blackwell SA, 224, Boulevard Saint Germain, 75007 Paris, France
Blackwell Wissenschafts-Verlag GmbH
Kurfürstendamm 57, 10707 Berlin, Germany
Zehetnergasse 6, A-1140 Vienna, Austria

Acquisitions: Christopher Davis
Development: Debra Lance
Design and Production: Silverchair Science + Communications
Manufacturing: Karen Feeney

Printed and bound by Braun-Brumfield, Inc.
© 1996 by Blackwell Science, Inc.
Printed in the United States of America
96 97 98 99 5 4 3 2 1

DISTRIBUTORS

North America
    Blackwell Science, Inc.
    238 Main Street
    Cambridge,
    Massachusetts 02142
    (Telephone orders: 800-215-
    1000 or 617-876-7000)

Australia
    Blackwell Science Pty Ltd.
    54 University Street
    Carlton, Victoria 3053
    (Telephone orders: 03-347-
    0300; fax: 03-349-3016)

Outside North America and
Australia
    Blackwell Science, Ltd.
    c/o Marston Book Services, Ltd.
    P.O. Box 269
    Abingdon
    OX14 4YN
    England
    (Telephone orders: 01235-
    465500; fax: 01235-
    465555)

Library of Congress Cataloging-in-Publication Data

Chung, Edward K.
    Pocket guide to ECG diagnosis / Edward K. Chung.
        p.   cm.
    Includes bibliographical references and index.
    ISBN 0-86542-499-3
    1. Electrocardiography--Handbooks, manuals, etc.   2. Heart-
-Diseases--Diagnosis--Handbooks, manuals, etc.   I. Title.
    [DNLM: 1. Electrocardiography--handbooks.   WG 39 C559p 1996]
    RC683.5.E5C4636   1996
    616.1'207547—dc20
    DNLM/DLC
    for Library of Congress   96-3795
                                                              CIP

To my wife, Lisa; my children,
Linda and Christopher;
and my grandson, Nicholas

Contents

Preface

Needless to say, electrocardiography is one of the most important diagnostic tests in medical practice today. Not only various cardiac diseases and related disorders can be diagnosed by electrocardiography, but various noncardiac disorders can be diagnosed by electrocardiography directly or indirectly.

Because of the role of electrocardiography, all physicians, nurses, medical students, and paramedical personnel who are directly or indirectly involved with cardiac care must be fully familiar with common electrocardiographic abnormalities and common cardiac arrhythmias that are frequently encountered in daily practice.

The purpose of this book is not to describe every aspect of electrocardiography. Rather, it is my intention to include only common electrocardiographic abnormalities and common cardiac arrhythmias that all medical students, house officers, cardiac care nurses, and physicians who are not specializing in cardiology should be familiar with. Thus, detailed descriptions regarding electrophysiology, theoretical considerations, and mechanisms are purposely omitted. Relatively new information, such as the diagnostic criteria of right ventricular myocardial infarction and the Q wave myocardial infarction versus non–Q wave myocardial infarction, is included in this book. Because of the nature of this book, the therapeutic aspects are not included.

Pocket Guide to ECG Diagnosis is written in simple language with a concise description and practical approach. The format of the book includes primarily the definition, diagnostic criteria, and diagnostic pearls of each electrocardiographic abnormality. Because of this specific format and the size of the book, it is convenient to carry around in the pocket at all times.

I would like to express my sincere appreciation to Ms. Maureen Gamble, my personal secretary, for her valuable secretarial work to complete this book. In addition, the endless efforts of Elizabeth Willingham at Silverchair Science + Communications and Karen Feeney at Blackwell Science are greatly appreciated.

Lastly, I always owe my deep gratitude and appreciation to my father, Dr. Il-Chun Chung, who had always provided proper guidance and inspiration for me.

EDWARD K. CHUNG, MD
BRYN MAWR, PA

Abbreviations

AF	Atrial fibrillation
APC	Atrial premature contraction
ASD	Atrial septal defect
AT	Atrial tachycardia
AV	Atrioventricular
AV JEB	Atrioventricular junctional escape beat
AV JER	Atrioventricular junctional escape rhythm
AV JPC	Atrioventricular junctional premature contraction
AV JT	Atrioventricular junctional tachycardia
BBBB	Bilateral bundle branch block
BFB	Bifascicular block
BTS	Bradytachyarrhythmia syndrome
CAD	Coronary artery disease
CCU	Coronary care unit
CHF	Congestive heart failure
COPD	Chronic obstructive pulmonary disease
CPR	Cardiopulmonary resuscitation
CSS	Carotid sinus stimulation
DC shock	Direct current shock
DI	Digitalis intoxication
ECG	Electrocardiogram
ERP	Early repolarization pattern
HLVV	High left ventricular voltage
IHSS	Idiopathic hypertrophic subaortic stenosis
JPC	Junctional premature contraction
JTWP	Juvenile T wave pattern
LAHB	Left anterior hemiblock
LPHB	Left posterior hemiblock

LBBB	Left bundle branch block
LGL syndrome	Lown-Ganong-Levine syndrome
LVH	Left ventricular hypertrophy
MAT	Multifocal atrial tachycardia
MI	Myocardial infarction
MVPS	Mitral valve prolapse syndrome
PAT	Paroxysmal atrial tachycardia
PDA	Patent ductus arteriosus
RB	Reciprocal beat
RBBB	Right bundle branch block
RHD	Rheumatic heart disease
RVH	Right ventricular hypertrophy
SA	Sinoatrial
SSS	Sick sinus syndrome
TFB	Trifascicular block
VA	Ventriculoatrial
VEB	Ventricular escape beat
VER	Ventricular escape rhythm
VF	Ventricular fibrillation
VPC	Ventricular premature contraction
VSD	Ventricular septal defect
VT	Ventricular tachycardia
WAP	Wandering atrial pacemaker
WPW syndrome	Wolff-Parkinson-White syndrome

Suggested Readings

Anderson HR, Nielsen D, Flak E. Right ventricular infarction: Diagnostic value of ST elevation in lead III exceeding that of lead II during inferior/posterior infarction and comparison with right-chest leads V_{3R} to V_{7R}. *Am Heart J* 117:82, 1989.

Akhtar M. *Cardiac Arrhythmias and Related Syndromes: Current Diagnosis and Management in Cardiology Clinics.* Philadelphia: Saunders, 1993.

Chakko S, Kessler KM. Recognition and management of cardiac arrhythmias. *Curr Probl Cardiol* 20:53, 1995.

Chung EK. *Cardiac Emergency Care* (4th ed). Philadelphia: Lea & Febiger, 1990.

Chung EK. *Principles of Cardiac Arrhythmias* (4th ed). Baltimore: Williams & Wilkins, 1989.

Chung EK *Electrocardiography: Self Assessment.* Norwalk, CT: Appleton & Lange, 1988.

Chung EK. *Quick Reference to Cardiovascular Disease* (3rd ed). Baltimore: Williams & Wilkins, 1987.

Chung EK. *Cardiac Arrhythmias: Self Assessment.* Vol. 3. Baltimore: Williams & Wilkins, 1987.

Chung EK. *Cardiac Arrhythmias: Self Learning.* Boston: Butterworth, 1986.

Chung EK. *Manual of Cardiac Arrhythmias.* Boston: Butterworth, 1986.

Chung EK. *Electrocardiography: Practical Applications with Vectorial Principles* (3rd ed). Norwalk, CT: Appleton & Lange, 1985.

DiMarco JP, Prystowsky EN. *Atrial Arrhythmias: State of the Art.* Mount Kisco, NY: Futura, 1995.

Falk RH, Podrid PJ. *Atrial Fibrillation: Mechanisms and Management.* New York, Raven, 1992.

Fisch C. *Electrocardiography of Arrhythmias.* Philadelphia: Lea & Febiger, 1990.

Ganz LI, Friedman PL. Supraventricular tachycardia. *N Engl J Med* 332:162, 1995.

Isner JM. Right ventricular myocardial infarction. *JAMA* 259:712, 1988.

Josephson ME. *Clinical Cardiac Electrophysiology: Techniques and Interpretations* (2nd ed). Philadelphia: Lea & Febiger, 1993.

Klein LW, Helfant RH. The Q-wave and non-Q wave myocardial infarction: Differences and similarities. *Prog Cardiovas Dis* 29:205, 1986.

Kulbertus HE, Rigo P, Legrand V. Right ventricular infarction: Pathophysiology, diagnosis, clinical course and treatment. *Mod Conc Cardiovas Dis* 54.1, 1985.

Naccarelli GV. *Cardiac Arrhythmias: A Practical Approach.* Mount Kisco, NY: Futura, 1991.

Podrid PJ, Kowey PR. *Cardiac Arrhythmias: Mechanisms, Diagnosis, and Management.* Baltimore: Williams & Wilkins, 1995.

Prystowsky EN, Klein GJ. *Cardiac Arrhythmias: An Integrated Approach for Clinicians* New York: McGraw-Hill, 1994.

Roberts R. Recognition, pathogenesis, and management of non-Q wave infarction. *Mod Conc Cardiovas Dis* 56:17, 1987.

Wagner GS. *Marriott's Practical Electrocardiography* (9th ed). Baltimore: Williams & Wilkins, 1994.

Yamaki M, Ikeda K, Honma K et al. Diagnosis of right ventricular involvement in chronic inferior myocardial infarction by means of body surface QRS changes. *Circulation* 77:1283, 1988.

Zipes DP, Jalife J. *Cardiac Electrophysiology: From Cell to Bedside.* Philadelphia: Saunders, 1995.

1

Introduction

DEFINITION OF ELECTROCARDIOGRAM

An electrocardiogram (ECG) is a graphic recording of electrical activity generated by the heart.

VALUE OF THE ELECTROCARDIOGRAM

The electrocardiogram is the most important laboratory test in the diagnosis of various heart diseases, particularly myocardial infarction (MI). In addition, the ECG is also extremely useful in helping to diagnose various noncardiac disorders, such as thyroid diseases, renal diseases, and pulmonary diseases, and various electrolyte imbalances (especially hypokalemia, hyperkalemia, hypocalcemia, and hypercalcemia). Furthermore, various abnormalities produced by cardiac as well as noncardiac drugs can be detected by the ECG. One of the essential roles of the ECG is to recognize all types of cardiac arrhythmias. It is obvious that the function and malfunction of artificial pacemakers is difficult to assess without ECG analysis.

In addition, there are many modified forms of the ECG; ambulatory (Holter monitor) ECG and exercise ECG (stress ECG) testing are the two best examples. Continuous ECG monitoring, another example of a modified ECG, is widely used in cardiac care units, emergency departments, operating rooms, postoperative recovery rooms, cardiac catheterization laboratories, and electrophysiologic laboratories.

PRINCIPLES OF ELECTROCARDIOGRAPHIC ANALYSIS

Electrocardiographic analysis should be as precise as possible. The ECG should be interpreted according to all available clinical information, including the patient's age, sex, body build, clinical diagnosis, and drug intake. For example, the electrical axis varies according to the patient's age. A QRS axis of +90 degrees may be normal for a 20-year-old girl, but the same QRS axis is abnormal for a 70-year-old man. Another example is that a very similar, if not identical, ECG finding may be observed in various clinical circumstances. Namely, inverted T waves in leads V_{1-3} may be a normal variant (juvenile T wave pattern), but this finding may be due to various conditions, including anteroseptal myocardial ischemia, pulmonary embolism and/or infarction, myocarditis and/or pericarditis, electrolyte imbalance (especially hypokalemia), and cerebrovascular accident.

One should not overread or depend too much on ECG findings. It should be noted that a normal ECG is not necessarily indicative of a normal heart or vice versa. In addition, the ECG should not be interpreted by a *pattern* method. In other words, the fundamental mechanism responsible for the production of a given ECG abnormality should always be considered. Therefore, the vectorial approach is essential to understanding various ECG findings. Otherwise, an erroneous diagnosis may frequently be made. Furthermore, it is essential to compare ECG tracings with previous tracings if they are available. For instance, an old MI pattern may disappear completely within a few months or years, especially when dealing with diaphragmatic (inferior) or posterior MI.

It is also very important to remember that there are two major types when diagnosing MI. Namely, MI may or may not produce the diagnostic abnormal Q waves. A Q wave MI produces abnormal Q waves, whereas a non-Q wave MI fails to produce the characteristic Q waves (see Chapter 5).

Finally, one should ask the following questions:

Is the ECG tracing normal or abnormal?

If the ECG tracing is abnormal, what is the clinical significance of the abnormality?

Is treatment indicated?

What is the treatment of choice if treatment is indicated?

ORDER OF ELECTROCARDIOGRAPHIC INTERPRETATION

The most important and the first step for the analysis of any ECG tracing is the determination of the mechanism(s) of the cardiac rhythm. In other words, one must determine whether the basic rhythm is sinus or ectopic. It is not uncommon to observe two or more coexisting cardiac rhythms or beats. After determining the mechanism, orders of ECG interpretation should include determining rates (P and QRS complexes), various intervals (P-R, QRS, and Q-T intervals), and the axes of the P, QRS, and T complexes.

A final conclusion will be reached according to the description of each complex (P, P-R, QRS, Q-T, S-T segment, and U wave) in addition to the above-mentioned items.

HISTORY OF ELECTROCARDIOGRAPHY

The presence of an action current associated with the heartbeat was demonstrated for the first time by Kölliker and Müller as early as 1856. Using a frog's nerve-muscle preparation that was contacted to a beating heart, these investigators demonstrated that the twitching of the frog's muscle corresponded to each ventricular contraction. Later, in 1887, a measurable amount of current in the human body corresponding to the cardiac contraction was demonstrated by Waller and Ludwig using a capillary electrometer. The current from the human heartbeat was registered in an accurate and quantitative manner for the first time, however, in 1901 with the introduction of new equipment, the *string galvanometer* designed by Willem Einthoven.

The string galvanometer was initially used to record the heartbeat in experimental studies, but later this instrument was gradually used for the routine clinical evaluation of human heart diseases. The principles of Einthoven's string galvanometer were based on the fact that a magnet and a conductor of current will interact. This equipment consisted of a powerful electromagnet that stretched a fine, metal-covered quartz filament between poles. By connecting the resting subject to the galvanometer string, the electrical potentials generated by the heart were registered as a deflection of the quartz string. The string shadow was photographed on moving film by a system of lenses and a source of illumination. Other types of galvanometer equipment were devised, one of which was the oscillograph, consisting of a small magnet to which a mirror was attached. The magnet was surrounded by coils of wire suspended by a fine thread. The electrical current moved through the coils of wire, deflecting the magnet. A beam of light reflected by the mirror registered this movement.

Later, the direct visualization of the heart's electrical waves with a permanent record became possible with the development of the cathode ray oscillograph. Immediate and direct recordings of the ECG were made possible using vacuum tube amplification equipment with a heated stylus that melted the wax on specially designed ECG paper. At present, there are many newer methods of taking a 12-lead ECG, and various computerized ECG systems are available in most modern teaching hospitals. The computerized ECG system is extremely valuable because of its technical capabilities (e.g., taking ECG tracings, transmitting various information, storage of ECG tracings and necessary information, etc.), but computerized ECG interpretation is far from an ideal situation, especially when dealing with cardiac rhythm analysis.

During the first quarter of the twentieth century, remarkable progress was made in the field of electrocardiography by Sir Thomas Lewis. The unipolar ECG was introduced for the first time by Frank N. Wilson in 1933. At present, the conventional ECG consists of 12 leads: three bipolar limb leads, three unipolar limb leads, and six unipolar precordial leads. In addition, a routine 12-lead ECG often includes additional rhythm strips (e.g., leads II, V_1, and V_5). Right chest leads (leads V_{3R-6R}) may be necessary for certain clinical circumstances (e.g., dextrocardia and other congenital heart diseases, right ventricular MI) as well. The right precordial leads are simply the mirror images of the usual left precordial leads.

In the past three decades, vectorcardiography has become an essential part of electrocardiography. Consequently, the orthogonal lead systems (X, Y, and Z leads) are frequently used in addition to the conventional 12-lead systems. The X lead corresponds to lead I, and the Y lead corresponds to lead aVF of the conventional ECG. The Z lead is a unique lead that is almost the inverted lead of the conventional lead V_1. Even if the actual vectorcardiogram is not taken, the vectorial approach is extremely important to interpret the 12-lead ECG precisely. In other words, full knowledge of vectorcardiography enhances the correct diagnosis of various ECG abnormalities.

In addition to the conventional ECG, the His bundle electrogram has been used recently to locate the precise site of an ectopic focus and the site of a block. In a His bundle electrogram, when the ventricular activity is preceded by a His bundle deflection, the cardiac rhythm is supraventricular in origin. Conversely, in ventricular tachycardia or ventricular escape rhythm, the ventricular deflection is not preceded by the His bundle deflection. The site of a block can thus be identified by the His bundle electrogram. For example, when the block occurs distal to the His bundle, such as in bilateral bundle branch block, the nonconducted P waves are followed by His deflections, and the QRS complexes are not preceded by His deflection. On the other hand, nonconducted P waves are not followed by the His deflections when the block is within the atrioventricular (AV) junction. In addition, the His bundle electrogram enables one to confirm the anomalous conduction pathway in Wolff-Parkinson-White syndrome. In this syndrome, His bundle deflection often occurs after the onset of the QRS complex. In addition, many other sophisticated electrophysiologic studies (EPSs) are now available in most teaching hospitals. By doing so, complex cardiac arrhythmias can be diagnosed and understood more accurately, and the best therapeutic result can be obtained for refractory arrhythmias.

CONDUCTION SYSTEM

It is essential to have a full knowledge of the anatomy of the human heart to understand the fundamental mechanisms responsible for normal ECG tracings as well as for various ECG abnormalities. The human heart consists of four chambers: two atria and two ventricles. Electrophysiologically, these chambers are controlled by the sinus (sinoatrial) node in healthy subjects. Anatomic structures pertinent in relation to various ECG findings include the sinus node, AV node, His bundle, bundle branches, and terminal Purkinje system (Fig. 1-1).

A study of the AV node and its junctional tissue is very important if one intends to accurately interpret various cardiac arrhythmias. The reason for this is that the AV node

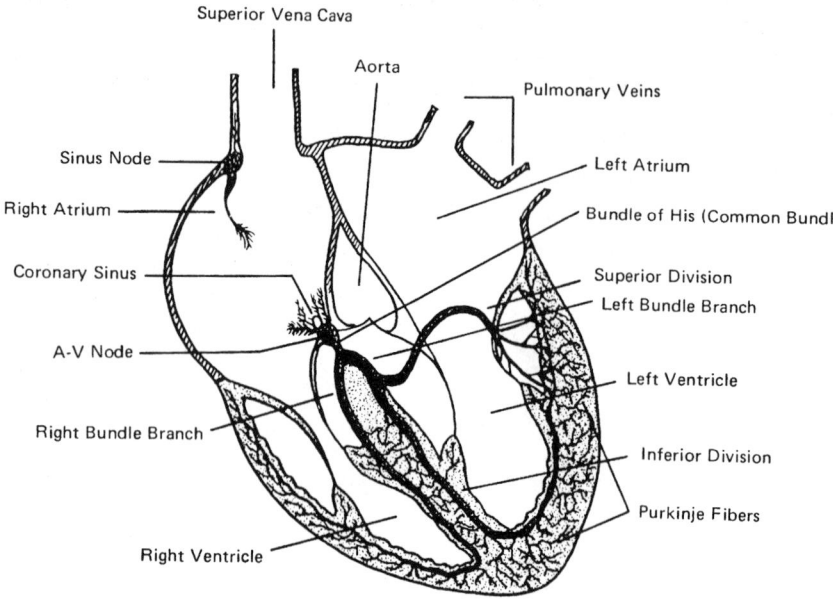

Figure 1-1
The conduction system. In a normal heart, the cardiac impulse arises from the sinus node and is transmitted through the atria. Following activation of the atria, the impulse reaches the atrioventricular junction and is transmitted to the ventricles via the common bundle (bundle of His, or atrioventricular bundle), right and left bundle branches (superior and inferior divisions), and the Purkinje fibers.

(junction) not only functions as a pacemaker (1) when the sinus node fails to produce an impulse (as in sinus arrest), (2) when the sinus node produces an impulse slower than usual (as in sinus bradycardia), or (3) when the sinus impulse is not conducted to the AV node (as in sinoatrial block, AV block, or both), but it also has an important role as a conduction system. Furthermore, most of the complicated rhythm disturbances are almost always related to the function and conductivity of the AV node. For instance, supernormal AV conduction, concealed conduction, unidirectional block, reciprocal beats, and so forth are intimately related to abnormal conductivity of the AV junction.

Because the discovery of the conducting tissue (common bundle, AV bundle) that connects the atria and ventricles was made by His in 1892, it now bears his name (bundle of His).

From the beginning of the AV node to the terminal branches of the Purkinje fibers, the entire conduction system is an anatomically continuous structure. Thus, the AV conduction system and ventricular myocardium are practically one large conduction network. The AV node is connected inferiorly to the common bundle and then to the right and left bundle branches with terminal Purkinje fibers (see Fig. 1-1).

The common bundle, a continuous downward structure from the AV node, penetrates into the central fibrous body. The right bundle branch is the more direct continuation of the AV node and runs along the inferior aspect of the septal band of the crista supraventricularis between the conus and the sinus of the right ventricle.

The left bundle branch is situated beneath the endocardium and divides into an anterior and posterior ramus descending toward the apex of the heart. The main left bundle branch is again divided into two divisions: the anterior and posterior fascicles (see Fig. 1-1). The left bundle branch fibers become progressively larger toward the apex. The terminal fibers end in the anterior and posterior papillary muscles and also course toward the apex of the heart. The left bundle branch is usually larger than the right bundle branch; its width is approximately 3–6 mm.

The terminal conduction system of the heart is a complex of Purkinje fibers, which are continuous structures from the right and left bundle branches (see Fig. 1-1). This terminal conduction network was described as early as 1845 by Purkinje. Purkinje fibers are distributed diffusely in every portion of the ventricles except for the central upper portion of the ventricular septum. This terminal network connects fibers together and leads to countless loops in the ventricular septum. Purkinje fibers are distributed in both the subendocardial and subepicardial myocardium, although they are more abundant in the former.

Beginning with the discovery of the *bundle of Kent* in 1893, various accessory pathways other than the normal AV conduction system have been described by various investigators. Accessory pathways include the *bundle of Kent, Mahaim's fibers, internodal pathways* proposed by James, and preferential pathways responsible for the Wolff-Parkinson-White syndrome and dual AV conduction. It should be pointed out that the anatomic presence of any accessory pathway is not necessarily indicative of physiologic function. These pathways may function under a certain circumstance, particularly when normal AV conduction is impaired.

ELECTROPHYSIOLOGY

EPSs of the heart have been carried out extensively since the late eighteenth century. The use of microelectrodes in the past 30 years has enabled cardiologists to appreciate cardiac arrhythmias more easily. The electrophysiologic properties of the heart include cardiac impulse formation and conduction—namely, rhythmicity (automaticity), excitability, and conductivity. Cardiac arrhythmias may result from the alteration of any of the above properties, which are closely interrelated. Clinically, cardiac arrhythmias are commonly due to an alteration in two or three electrophysiologic properties. Cardiac cells may be divided into two groups: automatic and nonautomatic cells. The former are able to initiate cardiac impulses without extrinsic stimuli, whereas the latter are excited by impulses generated by automatic cells or other stimuli. Most specialized cardiac fibers contain a large number of automatic cells, whereas atrial and ventricular muscle fibers, under normal conditions, are not automatic.

Cardiac arrhythmias may result from an alteration of the automaticity of the sinus node or from an abnormal impulse formation from ectopic automatic tissue (cells). Clinically, an alteration of automaticity is often associated with altered conductivity and excitability.

The conductivity of the heart is intimately related to rhythmicity and excitability. The speed of the conductivity varies markedly in different portions of the normal heart. Alteration of the normal speed of conductivity is one of the important causes of various cardiac arrhythmias. It has been demonstrated that the Purkinje fibers transmit impulses the fastest at a rate of 4000 mm/second, atrial muscle transmits impulses at a rate of 800–1000 mm/second, and the ventricular muscle transmits impulses at a rate of 400 mm/second. The AV node (junction) transmits impulses slowest at a rate of 200 mm/second. The slow conductivity of the AV junctional tissues is an important protective, physiologic property that prevents the conduction of an extremely rapid atrial rhythm, such as atrial fibrillation or atrial flutter. The cardiac impulse may be conducted in a normal fashion; however, it may propagate in an abnormal fashion or it may *not* be conducted, depending on the degree of depressed excitability.

Impairments of conductivity are manifested by a prolongation of the P wave, the P-R interval, and the QRS complex (Fig. 1-2); an unexpected absence of the P wave, QRS interval, or T complexes; or a combination of the above. Impairment of conduction is responsible for the development of various arrhythmias, including intra-atrial block, sinoatrial lock, AV block, intraventricular block, reciprocal beat, concealed conduction, supernormal conduction, dual AV conduction, unidirectional block, and parasystole. Abnormal

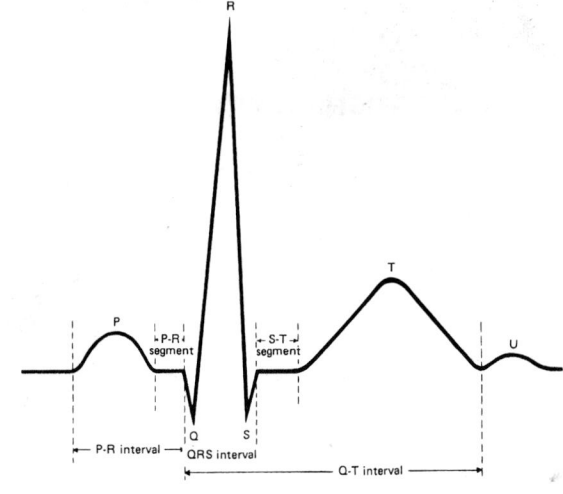

Figure 1-2
Various electrocardiographic complexes and intervals (lead II).

conduction via an accessory pathway is responsible for Wolff-Parkinson-White syndrome.

DEPOLARIZATION AND REPOLARIZATION

Two major electrical processes—depolarization (activation) and repolarization (recovery)—occur during muscular activity. The QRS complex is due to ventricular depolarization; the T wave represents ventricular repolarization (see Fig. 1-2).

During depolarization of a muscle strip, a positive (upright) deflection is recorded when the electrical force is moving toward the electrode (Fig. 1-3). A negative (downward) deflection is recorded when the depolarization process is moving away from the electrode (see Fig. 1-3). In other words, an upright deflection (R wave) is registered when the electrode faces the positive side of the dipole during depolarization. Conversely, a downward deflection (T wave) is registered when the electrode faces the negative side of the dipole during repolarization. Therefore, the directions of the QRS complex and T wave are opposite each other in a muscle strip (Fig. 1-4). Namely, the area that is initially depolarized

undergoes repolarization first, and the final depolarized area is also repolarized last in the muscle strip (see Fig. 1-4).

In contrast to a muscle strip, the direction of repolarization in human ventricular myocardium is reversed. That is, in human ventricles, the direction of depolarization is from endocardium to epicardium, and the direction of repolarization is from the epicardium to endocardium (see Fig. 1-4). In other words, the area that is last depolarized undergoes repolarization first. The exact reason for this phenomenon is still not clearly understood, although sudden pressure changes in the ventricles immediately before the onset of the repolarization process has been considered as a possible explanation. It is of interest that very small numbers of healthy individuals (particularly athletes) may have the same repolarization process as seen in a muscle strip. In these individuals, T waves are inverted in many leads, especially in the precordial leads. In a muscle strip, the T wave deflection is opposite in direction to the QRS complex, and the T wave deflection is in the same direction as the QRS complex in human ventricles (see Fig. 1-4).

During the depolarization or repolarization process, no ECG deflection (or equal amplitude between positive and negative deflection) is produced when the electrode faces perpendicular to the electrical event (see Fig. 1-3). Various locations of the electrodes in relation to the direction of the depolarization process are illustrated in Figure 1-3. The depolarization process is usually faster than the repolarization process.

Atrial depolarization progress occurs in a similar manner to the ventricular depolarization process. However, the repolarization process in the atria occurs in the same manner as that seen in a muscle strip. Namely, the atrial repolarization deflection (T-a wave) is in the opposite direction to the atrial depolarization deflection (P wave) so that, theoretically, the T-a wave is usually inverted in lead II and upright in lead aVR. Nevertheless, in a practical sense, the T-a wave is, as a rule, too small in amplitude to be registered by ordinary ECG equipment. Otherwise, the T-a wave is usually superimposed in the QRS complex, even if the T-a wave is present.

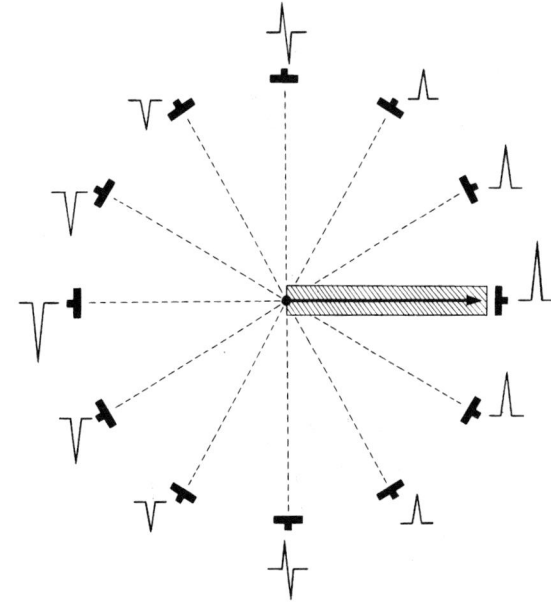

Figure 1-3
Various QRS complexes during the depolarization of a muscle strip plotted in a hexaxial reference frame. This diagram is essential for the understanding of electrical axis determination (see text).

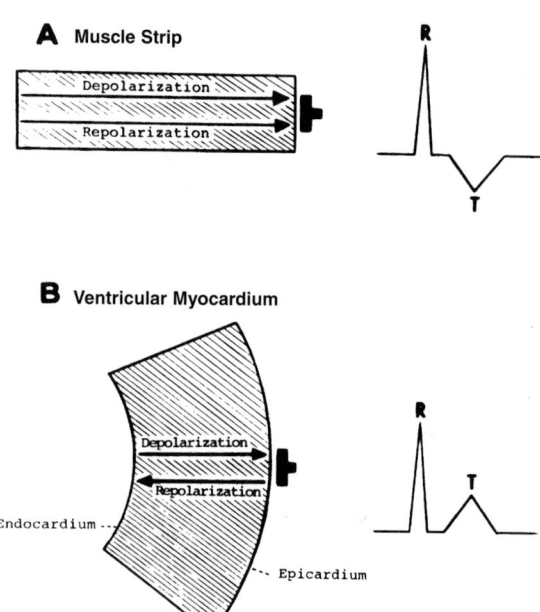

A Muscle Strip

Depolarization

Repolarization

R

T

B Ventricular Myocardium

Depolarization

Repolarization

Endocardium

Epicardium

R

T

ELECTRODES AND ELECTROCARDIOGRAPHIC LEADS

A routine ECG includes 12 leads—namely, six extremity (limb) leads (three bipolar and three unipolar) and six precordial (chest) leads (Figs. 1-5 and 1-6). For certain special purposes, additional leads may be necessary. Before the actual ECG is taken, a full standardization is in order. The full standardization means that 1 mV thrown into the circuit should produce a deflection (standardization marking) of precisely 10 mm on the ECG paper. When a half or double standardization is used, for special purposes, they

Figure 1-4
Depolarization and repolarization of a muscle strip (A) and ventricular myocardium (B). Note that the direction of the depolarization and repolarization processes is the same in a muscle strip. In contrast, depolarization and repolarization processes are opposite in direction in the ventricular myocardium. As a result, the T wave is inverted in a muscle strip, whereas the T wave is upright in the ventricular myocardium.

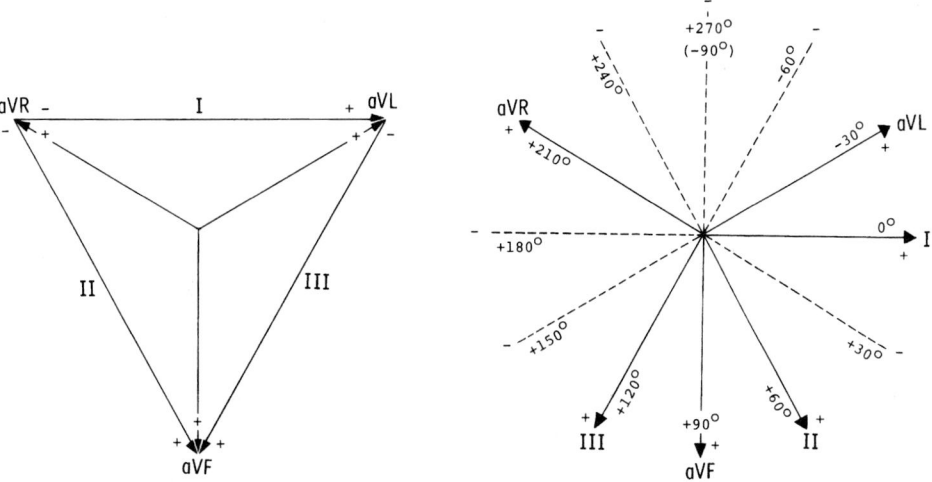

Figure 1-5
Einthoven's triangle and hexaxial reference system. The hexaxial reference system is simply a modified Einthoven's triangle and is much more useful in the determination of the electrical axis than Einthoven's triangle.

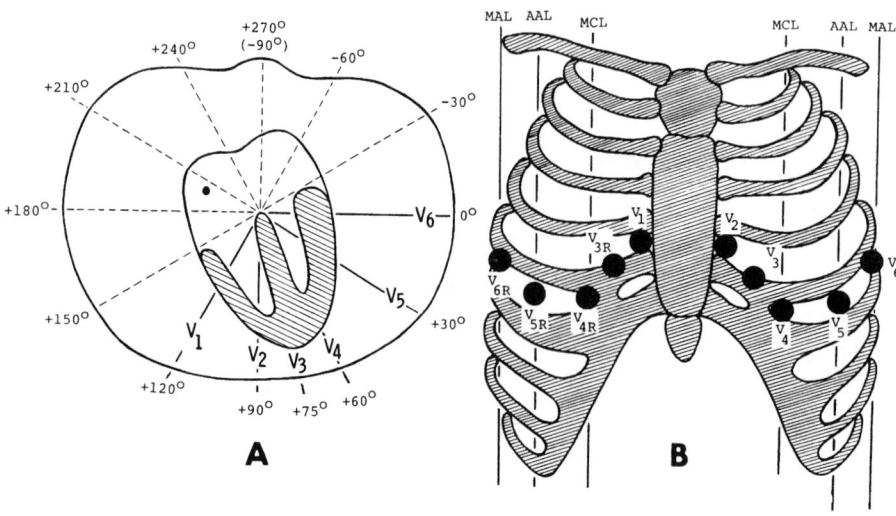

Figure 1-6
Precordial leads system.
(MAL = midaxillary line;
AAL = anterior axillary
line; MCL = midclavicu-
lar line.)

should be so indicated. In addition, placement of the precordial lead electrodes should be as precise as possible according to the standard rule (see Fig. 1-6). Incorrect electrode placement, needless to say, often leads to erroneous ECG interpretation.

1. *Standard lead (bipolar limb lead)*. As the name *standard lead* designates, leads I, II, and III have been the traditional standard leads for more than 60 years. As shown in Figure 1-5, lead I connects the two arms, lead II connects the right arm with the left leg, and lead III connects the left arm with the left leg. Since two electrodes are used in each standard lead, a potential difference between the two connected limbs is recorded. The electrodes are usually placed on the wrists and ankles simply because of convenience. For practical purposes, any electrode location between the wrist and shoulder for the arm electrodes and any location between the ankle and the left groin for the left leg electrode produces the same ECG deflections. In fact, electrode placement on both shoulders and left groin should produce a more accurate ECG tracing, since the heart will be almost in the center of the triangle so formed.

According to Einthoven's law, the ECG complex in lead II is equal to the combination of ECG complexes in leads I and III (II = I + III). This information is useful in ascertaining whether the ECG is mounted correctly.

2. *Unipolar limb leads*. Unipolar limb leads include leads aVR, aVL, and aVF according to the extremity with which the electrode is connected. In this case, since the actual ECG deflections are small, these deflections are augmented (1.5 times). Therefore, the "a" in leads aVR, aVL and aVF signifies this augmentation. The right leg electrode is for grounding.

The following relationship can be obtained between the standard limb leads and the unipolar limb leads: Lead I represents the difference between leads aVR and aVL, lead II represents the difference between leads aVR and aVF, and lead III represents the difference between leads aVL and aVF. Thus, the following formula between the bipolar and the unipolar limb leads can be produced:

Lead I = lead aVL – lead aVR
Lead II = lead aVF – lead aVR
Lead III = lead aVF – lead aVL

By connecting all six limb leads, *Einthoven's triangle* is formed (see Fig. 1-5). In addition, the *hexaxial reference frame (system)* can be produced by rearranging all the limb leads with one center point (see Fig. 1-5). Einthoven's triangle and the hexaxial reference system are essential for determining the electrical axis. It should be noted that the hexaxial reference system (frame) is nothing but a modified Einthoven's triangle.

In summary, the six extremity leads correspond to the frontal plane of the vectorcardiogram. In other words, in this case, electrical events generated by the heart are recorded in the anterior to posterior (A-P) viewpoint. Most necessary ECG information can be obtained from these six limb leads. Among all the limb leads, lead II is the most useful in identifying various cardiac arrhythmias. All electrodes must be placed correctly; otherwise, many unexpected ECG findings will be produced.

3. *Precordial (chest) leads.* Precordial leads consist of six unipolar chest leads (leads V_{1-6}). In 1932, a single precordial lead, which was connected from left leg to the apex beat, was introduced, and it was called lead IV. Soon after, the ordinary six precordial leads became popularized for routine ECGs. As shown in Figure 1-6, lead V_1 is in the fourth intercostal space at the right sternal border, and lead V_2 is in the fourth intercostal space at the left sternal border. Lead V_4 is in the fifth intercostal space along the left midclavicular line. Lead V_3 is halfway between leads V_2 and V_4. Leads V_5 and V_6 are in the fifth intercostal space along the left anterior and midaxillary lines, respectively. For special purposes, additional precordial leads are necessary. For example, additional right precordial leads V_{3R-6R} correspond with the locations of their opposite numbers on the left side of the chest (leads V_{3-6}). These leads are very valuable when dealing with various congenital heart diseases, particularly dextrocardia (see Chapter 15). The right precordial leads are also necessary when right ventricular MI is considered (see Chapter 5). At times, further left and posterior chest leads are necessary. Lead V_7 is in the fifth intercostal space along the posterior axillary line. Leads V_8 and V_9 are at the angle of the scapula and over the spine at the same level as leads V_{4-6}. Occasionally, leads V_{4-6} are taken one intercostal space higher or lower than the usual level. These additional precordial leads

are particularly valuable in diagnosing posterior and lateral MI more accurately.

In summary, the precordial leads correspond to the horizontal or transverse plane of the vectorcardiogram. In other words, electrical events generated by the heart are recorded from the superior to inferior point of view. Since the distance between the electrode and the heart is close in the precordial leads, much more accurate detailed information can be obtained in comparison with limb leads. Various ECG abnormalities such as anterior MI, posterior MI, left or right bundle branch block, and left or right ventricular hypertrophy can be diagnosed accurately from the precordial leads. In particular, anteroseptal MI and posterior MI cannot be diagnosed without precordial leads. In addition, lead V_1 is extremely valuable in identifying P waves even if the P wave is not discernible in lead II.

ELECTRICAL AXIS

The electrical axis of the heart is the vector of the impulses generated by the heart. In conventional ECG tracings, the electrical axis can be determined in the frontal plane (extremity leads) and in the horizontal plane (precordial leads). For practical purposes, however, the electrical axis in the frontal plane is usually determined for routine ECG interpretation. The electrical axes of the P waves, QRS complexes, and T waves should be determined separately. Mostly conveniently, the hexaxial reference system (frame) is used to determine the electrical axis (see Fig. 1-5). As shown in Figure 1-7, the hexaxial reference system is divided into 30-degree segments from 0 to +270 degrees in a clockwise direction and from 0 to −90 degrees in a counterclockwise direction.

1. *Definition of normal and abnormal axis.* Although there is no uniform agreement regarding the definition of normal and abnormal axes, the following criteria are generally accepted: The normal axis is between 0 and +90 degrees, left axis deviation (LAD) is between 0 and −90 degrees, and right axis deviation (RAD) is between +90 and +270 degrees (see Fig. 1-7). It should be noted, however, that the electrical axes of the P, QRS, and T complexes vary markedly due to various factors, particularly the patient's age and body build. Therefore,

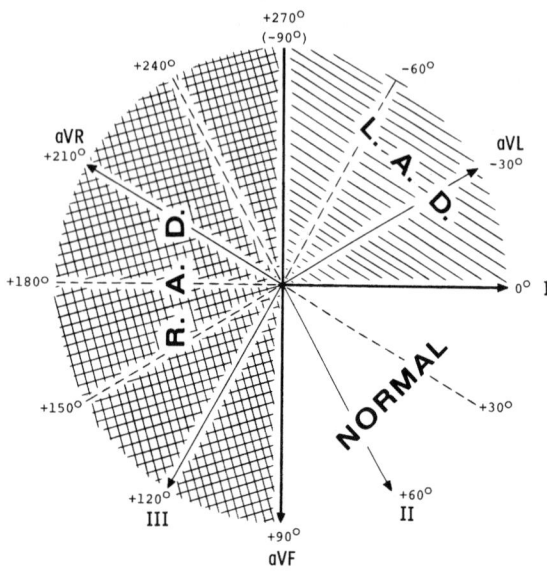

the interpretation of a given axis should be made on an individual basis. The electrical axes between −30 and −90 degrees are often designated as marked LAD. The diagnosis of left anterior hemiblock is made in most cases when the QRS axis ranges from −45 to −90 degrees (see Chapter 4). As can be expected, in extreme cases of given axis such as around −90 degrees, it is difficult to judge whether these figures represent marked LAD or RAD. In these circumstances, the axis should be interpreted in conjunction with the clinical background.

Customarily, the electrical axis in the horizontal plane (precordial leads) is not determined for routine ECG analysis. However, the axis can be easily determined in the horizontal plane by using the precordial

Figure 1-7
Normal and abnormal electrical axes. A normal axis is between 0 and +90 degrees. Right axis deviation (RAD) is from +90 to +270 degrees, and left axis deviation (LAD) is between 0 and −90 degrees.

leads system as shown in Figure 1-6. This frame is also divided into 30-degree segments analogous to the hexaxial reference frame in the frontal plane. In general, the axes between 0 and −30 degrees are considered to be within the normal range. To satisfy these normal ranges, the transitional complex (RS pattern) should be between leads V_2 and V_4. When the electrical axis is between −30 and −90 degrees, the term *posterior axis deviation* should be used. In these circumstances, the transitional zone moves further toward lead V_5 or V_6, and even more posteriorly and to the left. When the transitional zone shifts more anteriorly, the term *anterior axis deviation* can be used. In this case, the R wave in leads V_{1-2} will be tall (or relatively tall); this finding may be due to various factors that are discussed later in this chapter.

It should be noted that the term *posterior axis deviation* has replaced the old term *clockwise rotation* and that the term *anterior axis deviation* has replaced the old term *counterclockwise rotation*. These old terms are erroneous because the heart usually does not rotate anatomically. Rather, the electrical axis changes in these circumstances.

2. *Determination of electrical axis*. In general, there are two methods of determining the electrical axis. One is the conventional method of using two extremity leads; for convenience, leads I and III are commonly used. To determine the QRS axis, the net value of the area under the QRS complex in leads I and III is plotted on the hexaxial reference system. When perpendicular lines from leads I and III axes are dropped, there will be a crossing point between the two lines. The line formed by connecting the center point and the crossing point is the QRS axis in the frontal plane. The identical principle and method are used for the determination of the T wave as well as the P wave axes. In the normal heart, the directions of the QRS axis and the T axis are very similar so that the QRS-T angle (the angle formed between the QRS and T axes) is usually less than 60 degrees. A wide QRS-T angle (≥60 degrees) indicates an abnormal ECG finding or a diseased heart in most cases. Obviously, this conventional method of determining the electrical axis is time-consuming and less practical.

At present, a more practical and perhaps more accurate method is used. The method is a vectorcardiographic approach using all six limb leads. As shown in

Figure 1-3, ECG deflection is directly influenced by the position of the electrode and the direction of the electrical current. Namely, the impulse moving toward the electrode produces a maximum positive (upright) deflection, whereas the impulse moving away from the electrodes produces a maximum negative (downward) deflection. The impulse moving perpendicular to the electrode produces an RS deflection (transitional complex) or isoelectrical line. By using this electrophysiologic principle, the electrical axes of the QRS complexes, T waves, and P waves can be determined readily.

The easiest approach is to look for the lead with the largest upright deflection. This means that the axis is almost the same direction as this lead. Alternatively, the lead with the largest negative (downward) deflection may be detected. This means that the axis is the almost opposite direction to this lead. By doing so, the approximate direction of the axis can be determined. For more accurate determination, the next step is to look for the lead with the smallest deflection (or isoelectrical line) or RS (or QR) deflection. This means that the axis is perpendicular to this lead. As can be expected, the RS deflection may not be present in a given tracing. In such a case, determining the axis is still not difficult using a principle shown in Figure 1-3. With sufficient experience, it becomes very easy to determine the mean axis rather precisely in only a few seconds.

For example, in Figure 1-8, lead II shows a maximum (tallest) upright QRS complex, meaning that the QRS axis is approximately parallel to lead II. Alternatively, lead aVR demonstrates the maximum negative (downward) QRS deflection, indicating that the axis is almost opposite in direction to lead aVR. For accurate determination, however, the RS deflection (smallest complex) is found in lead aVL. Therefore, the mean axis of the QRS complexes is perpendicular to lead aVL, namely, +60 degrees. Using the same principle, the P axis is about +50 degrees, and the T axis is approximately +45 degrees (see Fig. 1-8)

3. *Clinical significance of axis determination.* The most important reason for determining the axis is the diagnosis of sinus rhythm. To conform sinus rhythm, the mean axis of the P waves must be within normal limits (0 to +90 degrees). In addition, many cardiac disorders produce abnormal QRS axes, T axes, or both. As mentioned previously, a wide QRS-T angle almost always

indicates an abnormal ECG or a diseased heart. It should be noted, however, that an axis should be interpreted according to the patient's age and body build. As a rule, individuals who are young and thin tend to produce RAD, whereas individuals who are elderly and obese tend to produce LAD without much clinical significance. In addition, a high diaphragm from pregnancy, ascites, or abdominal tumor may produce LAD.

RAD of the QRS complexes is almost always present in right ventricular hypertrophy (RVH). The sudden appearance of RAD of the QRS complexes often indicates pulmonary embolism, pulmonary infarction, or both. In contrast to RVH, LAD is only present in about 50% of cases of left ventricular hypertrophy (LVH). It must be remembered that pseudo-LAD is commonly due to diaphragmatic (inferior) MI, whereas pseudo-RAD is frequently due to high lateral MI (see Chapter 5). In addition, left anterior hemiblock produces marked LAD, whereas left posterior hemiblock produces marked RAD (see Chapter 4).

In the following circumstances, one should not indicate LAD because LAD is a part of the following ECG abnormalities:

1. Diaphragmatic (inferior) MI
2. LVH
3. Left bundle branch block
4. Left anterior hemiblock
5. Wolff-Parkinson-White syndrome (some cases).

Likewise, one should not indicate RAD in the following circumstances:

1. RVH
2. Left posterior hemiblock
3. High lateral MI
4. Wolff-Parkinson-White syndrome (some cases)
5. Children and young adults

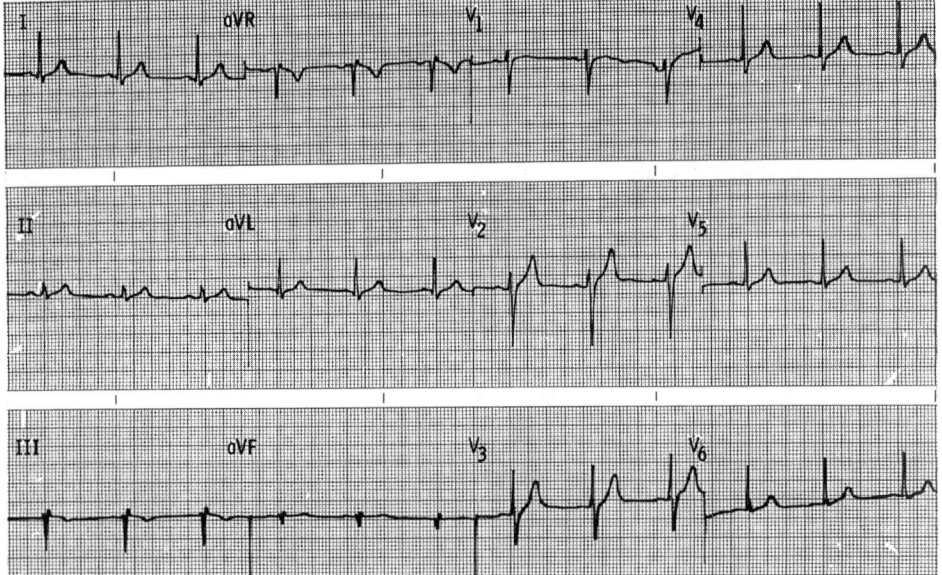

Figure 1-8
Normal electrocardiogram tracing.

2

Normal Electrocardiogram and Normal Variants

NORMAL ELECTROCARDIOGRAM

In the normal heart, the impulse originating from the primary pacemaker (sinus node) passes the sinoatrial (SA) junction and spreads throughout the atria radially as if it were a wave formed on a pond after a stone is thrown into it. During atrial activation, the P wave is inscribed on the electrocardiogram (ECG). The average time required for atrial depolarization in the normal heart varies between 0.08 and 0.10 second (Table 2-1, intra-atrial conduction time). The activation process spreads through the atrial muscle, finally reaches the atrio-A-V nodal junction, and

passes down the AV junctional tissue. In the short stretch of the AV node, with its complex interlacing structure and its slow conductivity, a delay in the activation process permits the atria to complete their systole before transmission of the activation process to the ventricles. The time required for this process is approximately 0.05 second. As the activation process passes from the AV node directly to the AV bundle, the speed of conductivity markedly increases. In fact, the speed of conduction increases to 20 times that of the AV junction on reaching the bundle branches. This rapid conductivity is maintained throughout the entire Purkinje system. It normally takes approximately 0.16 second for the cardiac impulse to travel from the sinus node—via the atria,

Table 2-1. Various normal electrocardiographic intervals

Intervals	Definition	Normal range (sec)
P	Intra-atrial conduction time (atrial depolarization time)	0.06–0.10
P-R	AV conduction time	0.12–0.20
QRS	Intraventricular conduction time (ventricular depolarization time)	0.06–0.10
Q-T	Ventricular depolarization and repolarization time	Varies according to rate

the AV node, the common bundle and bundle branches, the terminal Purkinje network, and the transitional muscle fibers—to the first part of the ventricular myocardium. The time interval from the beginning of atrial depolarization to the beginning of ventricular depolarization is represented by the *P-R interval* on the ECG (AV conduction time); and its average value in normal adults varies from 0.12 to 0.20 second (see Table 2-1). Not uncommonly, however, healthy people, especially healthy young individuals, may have a P-R interval of less than 0.12 second.

It should be noted that in a normal heart the right atrial activation occurs first, and the left atrial activation follows the right atrial activation. Thus, lead V_1 shows biphasic P wave in healthy individuals (see Chapter 3).

The initial activation of the ventricles originates in the septum. The initial septal force (vector) originates from the middle third of the left septal mass. The septal activation vector is directed to the right, anteriorly and either inferiorly or superiorly, depending on the position of the heart. This initial septal vector is responsible for the small (physiologic) q wave in the left precordial leads (leads V_{4-6}) and the initial r wave in the right precordial leads (leads V_{1-2}, Fig. 2-1). After the initial activation of the ventricular septum, the free left ventricular wall undergoes depolarization. This force is directed toward the left—posteriorly and either superiorly or inferiorly. The endocardial surface is activated shortly before the epicardium in each portion of the ventricles because of a certain arrangement of the terminal

Purkinje fibers: The connections of the terminal Purkinje network are such that the papillary muscles are activated earlier than the lateral wall of the ventricles. The activation process in the right ventricle is usually negligible in magnitude as compared to that of the left ventricle, although its activation occurs at the same time. The activation of the left ventricular free wall is responsible for the R wave in the left precordial leads and the S wave in the right precordial leads (see Fig. 2-1).

Following the activation of the free wall of the ventricles, the basal portions of the heart are activated. The basal portions include the superior and posterior portions of the free walls and a part of the ventricular septum that primarily belongs to the right septal mass, including the crista supraventricularis. The vector of this terminal ventricular

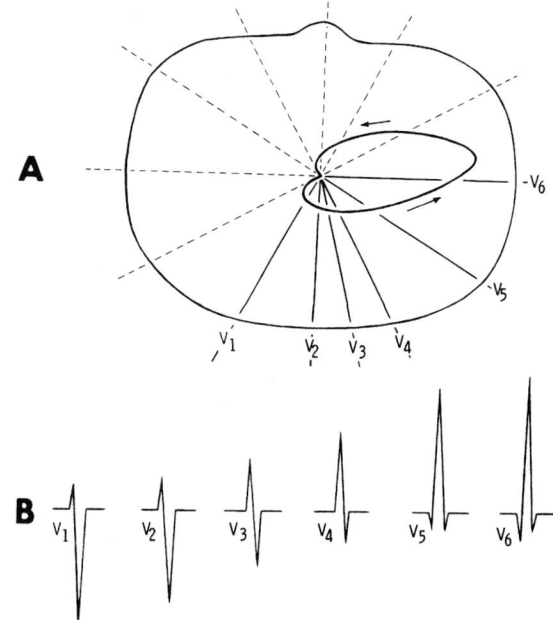

Figure 2-1
A relationship between the vectorcardiographic QRS loop in the horizontal plane (A) and the electrocardiographic QRS complexes in the precordial leads (B).

ation process is directed toward the right, slightly posteriorly and superiorly. This terminal vector is responsible for the terminal s wave in the left precordial leads and the terminal r and r' waves in the right precordial leads or lead aVR (see Fig. 2-1). The interval required for ventricular activation (QRS interval) is usually between 0.06 and 0.10 second in normal hearts (see Table 2-1, intraventricular conduction time). The total duration of the activation process of the entire heart is approximately 0.25 second.

During ventricular depolarization in a normal heart, the amplitude of the R waves in leads V_{1-3} progressively increases until the transitional zone is reached (see Fig. 2-1). When the transitional zone is passed, small septal physiologic q waves begin to appear in leads V_{4-6}, with the development of S waves in these leads (see Fig. 2-1). This ventricular depolarization process is easily understandable from a vectorial approach. The *vectorcardiogram* uses essentially the same principle in registering cardiac electrophysiologic events, but it is recorded from three dimensions: the horizontal (transverse), frontal, and sagittal planes. The horizontal and frontal planes correspond to the precordial and limb leads of the ECG, respectively. The configuration of the QRS complexes in the extremity (limb) leads depends on the QRS axis. By using the same principles described for the precordial leads, the construction of the vectorcardiogram loop from ECG complexes or vice versa can be made without any difficulty (Fig. 2-2). In general, any limb lead facing the right ventricle produces a QRS complex similar to lead V_1, whereas any limb lead facing the left ventricle produces a QRS complex similar to lead V_5 or V_6. Depending on the configuration of the QRS complexes, various terms have been used to describe such findings (Fig. 2-3). *It should be emphasized that both ventricles are activated simultaneously in a normal heart.*

Following completion of ventricular depolarization, the ventricles undergo the repolarization process to produce T waves. As described previously, the direction of the repolarization process in a normal ventricle is from the epicardium to the endocardium, which is in the reverse direction of the repolarization process of a muscle strip (see Fig. 1-4). Therefore, a normal ECG usually shows upright T waves in leads V_{2-6} (see Fig. 1-8). The configuration of the T waves in the limb leads varies depending on the T axis. However, in general, the T wave is inverted in lead aVR and upright in lead II (see Fig. 1-8). The T wave in lead V_1 in a normal heart may be upright, inverted, or biphasic; however, an upright T wave in lead V_1 in older adults is less common.

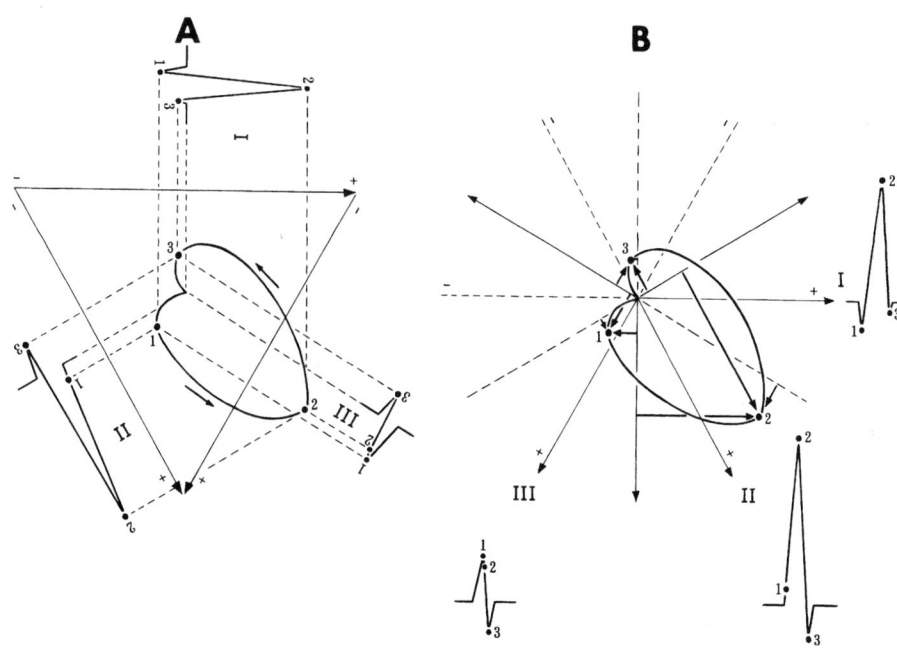

Figure 2-2
A relationship between the QRS complexes in the standard extremity leads and the QRS loop in the frontal plane by using Einthoven's triangle (A) and a hexaxial reference frame (B).

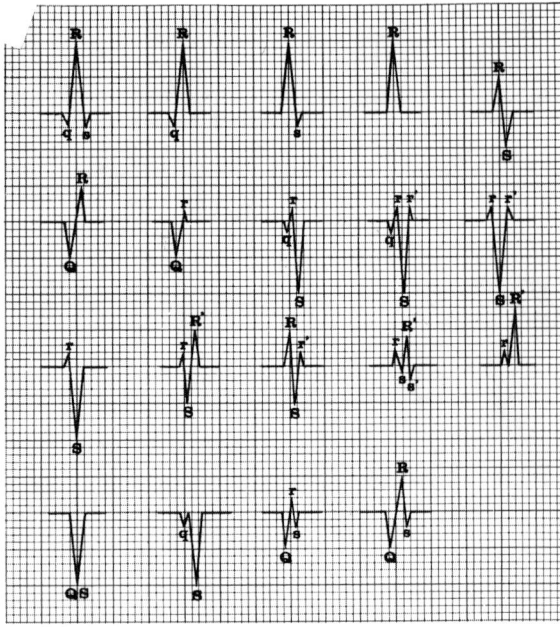

Following the T wave, there is another round, upright wave of small amplitude called the U wave. Not uncommonly, the U wave is superimposed on the last portion of the T wave. The exact mechanism for the production of the U wave is unknown. Nevertheless, the U wave is thought to be produced by potentials elicited by the stretching of ventricular muscle during the period of rapid blood inflow. Alternatively, the U wave is considered to be due to papillary muscle activation by some investigators. The clinical significance of recognizing prominent U waves (U wave ≥ T wave) is extremely important because they almost always indicate hypokalemia. In addition, inverted U waves are usually due to myocardial ischemia.

Normal Intervals

Various intervals on the ECG are usually expressed as *seconds*, but the amplitudes of the various complexes are expressed as *millimeters* (Fig. 2-4).

Figure 2-3
Various configurations of the QRS complexes.

Various intervals in a normal ECG are relatively constant in a given individual unless the heart rate varies markedly from time to time. Various intervals are illustrated in Figure 1-2, and normal ranges of various intervals are described in Table 2-1. All intervals tend to be shorter in children than in adults. For example, the normal P-R interval in children is between 0.12 and 0.18 second, compared with 0.12–0.20 second in adults. The Q-T interval varies much more markedly in all age groups in comparison with other intervals and also according to the heart rate (Table 2-2). Thus, the following formula for determining the Q-T interval may be used in order to determine whether a given Q-T interval is normal or abnormal:

$$\text{Q-T calculation} = \frac{\text{Q-T (measured)}}{\sqrt{\text{R-R interval (second)}}}$$

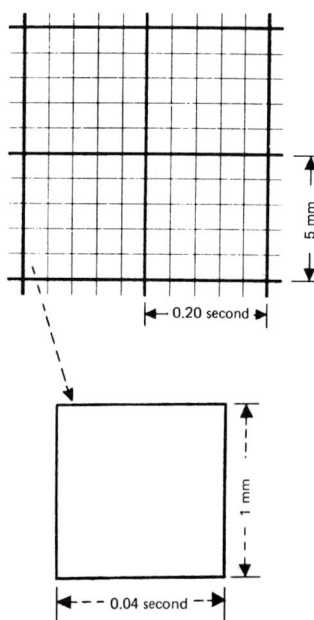

Figure 2-4
The timing and duration of the ECG paper in seconds and millimeters.

e 2-2. Normal Q-T intervals and their upper limits of normal

Heart rate/min	Normal Q-T intervals		Upper limits of normal Q-T intervals	
	Men and children (sec)	Women (sec)	Men and children (sec)	Women (sec)
40.0	0.449	0.461	0.491	0.503
43.0	0.438	0.450	0.479	0.491
46.0	0.426	0.438	0.466	0.478
48.0	0.420	0.432	0.460	0.471
50.0	0.414	0.425	0.453	0.464
52.0	0.407	0.418	0.445	0.456
54.5	0.400	0.411	0.438	0.449
57.0	0.393	0.404	0.430	0.441
60.0	0.386	0.396	0.422	0.432
63.0	0.378	0.388	0.413	0.423
66.5	0.370	0.380	0.404	0.414
70.5	0.361	0.371	0.395	0.405
75.0	0.352	0.362	0.384	0.394
80.0	0.342	0.352	0.374	0.384
86.0	0.332	0.341	0.363	0.372
92.5	0.321	0.330	0.351	0.360
100.0	0.310	0.318	0.338	0.347
109.0	0.297	0.305	0.325	0.333
120.0	0.283	0.291	0.310	0.317

Table 2-2. (continued)

Heart rate/min	Normal Q-T intervals		Upper limits of normal Q-T intervals	
	Men and children (sec)	Women (sec)	Men and children (sec)	Women (sec)
133.0	0.268	0.276	0.294	0.301
150.0	0.252	0.258	0.275	0.282
172.0	0.234	0.240	0.255	0.262

For example, the Q-T calculation will be 0.44 second when the Q-T (measured) interval is 0.40 second and the R-R (measured) interval is 0.81 second.

Example:

$$\text{Q-T calculation} = \frac{0.40}{\sqrt{0.81}}$$

$$= \frac{0.40}{0.9} = 0.44 \text{ second}$$

The Q-T interval is considered to be abnormal if the Q-T calculation is more than 0.42 second.

Determination of Heart Rate

There are several ways to determine heart rate. When the atrial and the ventricular rates are different, such as in a second- or third-degree AV block, both atrial and ventricular rates should be determined separately.

The easiest and the most practical method is to count the cardiac cycles in 6-second intervals and multiply by 10, since most ECG paper conveniently has vertical lines on the top of the paper at 3-second intervals (Fig. 2-5). When such vertical markers are not available or the ECG tracing is cut short, other methods should be used. The ordinary ECG paper speed is 25 mm/second, which

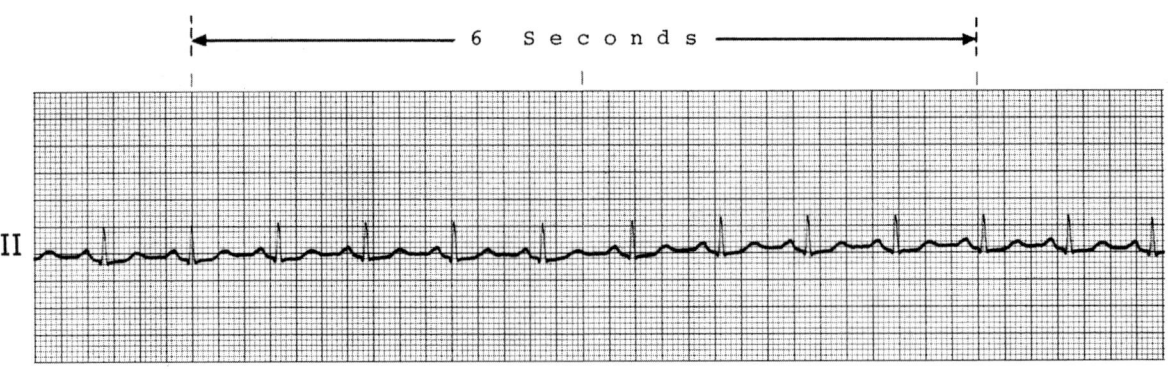

Figure 2-5
A rhythm strip of lead II used for determining heart rate. The heart rate may be obtained by multiplying the numbers of the cardiac cycles within 6 seconds by 10. In this instance, the heart rate is 89 beats/minute.

makes 1500 mm (or 1500 small squares) per minute. Because the interval between two thin lines in the ECG paper is 1 mm, the R-R interval in a given tracing can be easily measured. The ventricular rate can be measured by dividing 1500 by the number of small squares (*rate = 1500 ÷ the number of small squares*). In the same manner, a rough estimation of the heart rate can be made by counting the number of large squares. Each large square (thick line) on the ECG paper consists of five small squares (thin lines). Thus, the ECG paper speed can be expressed as 300 large squares/minute (*1500 ÷ 5 = 300*). The heart rate is determined by dividing 300 by the number of large squares in the R-R interval. For example, when the R-R interval contains two large squares, the rate is 150 beats per minute (bpm). When the R-R interval contains three large squares, the rate is 100 bpm, and so on (Table 2-3). When the heart rate varies markedly from time to time, such as in atrial fibrillation (AF) or sinus arrhythmia, the two extreme values (slowest and fastest rates) should be determined.

Normal Sinus Rhythm

To diagnose a normal ECG, the first step is to confirm normal sinus rhythm.

The cardiac rhythm originating from the primary pacemaker (sinus node) is termed *sinus rhythm*. Most healthy individuals have sinus rhythm, but many patients with cardiac disease also may have sinus rhythm. Therefore, the presence of sinus rhythm does not denote either a normal or diseased heart. The sinus rates in normal subjects differ among age groups. At birth, the rate is between 110 and 150 bpm, and it gradually becomes slower, approaching the rate of the adult population by 6 years of age. The sinus rate at rest is usually between 65 and 85 bpm in the majority of the adult population, but it varies from individual to individual. Nevertheless, a rate between 60 and 100 bpm is arbitrarily considered to be the rate of a *normal sinus rhythm*. A sinus rate faster than 100 bpm is called *sinus tachycardia*, whereas a rate slower than 60 bpm is termed *sinus bradycardia*.

The rate of the sinus rhythm is influenced by various factors, including cardioinhibitory forces (vagal), cardioacceleratory forces (sympathetic), chemical mediators, posture and position, exercise (either emotional or physical), various drugs, cardiac and noncardiac diseases, environmental and body temperatures, and the individual's metabolic and nutritional state. Alteration of the sinus rate is often due to humoral or neurogenic effects rather than to actual anatomic alteration of the sinus node, even in diseased hearts.

When the basic rhythm is sinus, there may be occasional or frequent ectopic beats or even a bout of ectopic tachycardia. In these circumstances, the mechanism of

Table 2-3. Determination of the heart rate by R-R interval

Number of thick-line intervals (large squares)	In seconds	Rate/min
1	0.2	300
2	0.4	150
3	0.6	100
4	0.8	75
5	1.0	60
6	1.2	50
7	1.4	43
8	1.6	37
9	1.8	33
10	2.0	30

the basic rhythm should always be mentioned as the dominant rhythm. Not uncommonly, sinus rhythm and ectopic rhythm may be present independently, as in AV dissociation or parasystole. In these cases, the atrial mechanism should also be mentioned, and a sinus rhythm and an independent ectopic rhythm should be described accordingly.

Diagnostic Criteria

Specifically, normal sinus rhythm is diagnosed only when the following *five criteria* are present (see Fig. 1-8).

1. P wave of sinus origin (normal mean axis of P wave)
2. Constant and normal P-R interval (of 0.12–0.20 sec)

3. Constant P wave configuration in a given lead
4. Rate between 60 and 100 bpm
5. Constant P-P (or R-R) interval

P Wave of Sinus Origin (Normal Mean Axis of P Wave)

Among the five criteria for the diagnosis of *normal sinus rhythm*, the first and the most important step is to prove that the mean axis of the P wave is within normal limits. This is done because a normal mean P wave axis indicates that the P wave is of sinus origin. The mean axis of the P wave may be determined by using *Einthoven's triangle* or the *hexaxial reference frame*.

The P, QRS, and T complexes at birth show marked right and anterior axes deviation and gradually move toward the left and posteriorly during aging. The mean axes of these complexes in most normal adults are between 0 and +90 degrees. Older individuals (older than 60 years of age) may have mean axes between 0 and –30 degrees, even without demonstrable heart disease. For this reason, the mean axis of normal sinus rhythm must lie between 0 and +90 degrees in the adult population. The mean axis in young adults is usually between +60 and +90 degrees,

whereas it is often between +30 and +60 degrees in the older adult population.

To satisfy the criteria for a normal P axis, the P wave must be upright in lead II and inverted in lead aVR. Other extremity leads (I, III, aVL, and aVF) may show different configurations of the P wave, depending on the direction of the P axis. For instance, if the P axis is +90 degrees, the P wave will be isoelectric or biphasic in lead I; inverted in leads aVL and aVR; and upright in leads II, III, and aVF. Another extreme example is a P axis of 0 degrees, which produces an isoelectric or biphasic P wave in lead aVF; inverted P wave in leads III and aVR; and upright P wave in leads I, II, and aVL. Thus, P waves are not necessarily upright in lead I or lead aVF in normal sinus rhythm, although they are upright in most cases. For the same reason, the P wave is frequently inverted in lead aVL in younger adults, whereas it is often inverted in lead III in older adults. From these observations, the most important leads to look for are lead II, which must show an upright P wave, and lead aVR, which must show an inverted P wave. To state that the P wave is upright in leads I, II, III, and aVF and inverted in lead aVR in normal sinus rhythm is erroneous. In the precordial leads V_{1-2}, the P wave of a normal sinus rhythm is usually biphasic and sometimes is predominantly upright or inverted. The remaining precordial leads (V_{3-6}), in general, show an upright P wave in normal sinus rhythm, although this again varies depending on the mean axis of the P wave. By and large, the precordial leads are not recommended to determine normal sinus rhythm.

In addition, it should be noted that the P axis may be altered when there is atrial pathology such as in mitral stenosis or cor pulmonale, just as the QRS axis changes according to alteration in ventricular depolarization due to left ventricular hypertrophy (LVH) or right ventricular hypertrophy (RVH).

Constant and Normal P-R Interval

When the mean axis of the P wave is within normal limits (between 0 and +90 degrees), each P wave should be followed by QRS and T complexes throughout the tracing (see Fig. 1-8). In addition, the P-R interval, which is the AV conduction time (the interval from the beginning of the P wave to the onset of the QRS complex), should be between 0.12 and 0.20 second in the adult population (Table 2-1). In children, the P-R interval tends to be shorter than that of adults, primarily because of the faster heart rate. The P-R

interval is measured in the extremity lead, which shows the longest interval, because the P-R interval is falsely shorter in certain leads. This occurs when the mean axis of a portion of the P wave is perpendicular to that lead.

When the P-R interval is longer than 0.20 second, a *first-degree AV block* is present. Conversely, when the P-R interval is shorter than 0.12 second, it may be due to Wolff-Parkinson-White syndrome, coronary nodal rhythm, or Lown-Ganong-Levine syndrome. It should be noted, however, that some healthy individuals, particularly young people, may have a P-R interval that is shorter than 0.12 second (normal variant). When long and short P-R intervals alternate or occur intermittently, dual AV conduction should be suspected. If the P-R intervals and P wave configuration vary considerably but the P wave and QRS complex are still related, a wandering atrial pacemaker (WAP) should be suspected. Needless to say, complete AV dissociation is present when the P wave and QRS complex are independent (in this case, the term *P-R distance* is substituted for *P-R interval*).

Constant P Wave Configuration in Each Given Lead

To diagnose normal sinus rhythm, the configuration of

the P wave must be constant in each given lead. It should be noted, however, that the P wave configuration may change with respiration in some leads, particularly leads II, III, and aVF. In this circumstance, the configuration of the QRS and T complexes also will be altered to a similar degree. This alteration of configuration due to respiration, needless to say, will be eliminated by momentary breath-holding. When the configuration of the P wave changes from beat to beat or periodically but a normal P axis with a constant or slightly varying P-R interval (between 0.12 and 0.20 sec) is present, a wandering pacemaker is said to be present in the sinus node. Even when the P wave is abnormal in contour, as in mitral stenosis (*P-mitrale*) and cor pulmonale (*P-pulmonale*), normal sinus rhythm can be diagnosed as long as the above-mentioned criteria exist.

Rate Between 60 and 100 Beats Per Minute
As described previously in this chapter, a sinus rate between 60 (P-P interval: 1.00 sec) and 100 (P-P interval: 0.60 sec) beats per minute is arbitrarily considered a *normal sinus rhythm*. Thus, the sinus rate must be 60–100 bpm in a *normal sinus rhythm* (see Fig. 1-8).

Constant P-P (or R-R) Cycle
Although it has been said that a normal sinus rhythm should have a regular rhythm, the P-P (or R-R) cycle is not always precisely regular. In fact, by precise measurement, the cardiac cycle is often slightly irregular in normal sinus rhythm. Therefore, the P-P (or R-R) cycle is considered to be regular when the shortest and longest P-P (or R-R) intervals vary by less than 0.16 second. If the P-P cycle varies more than 0.16 second, *sinus arrhythmia* is present. *Sinus arrest* (pause or standstill) and *SA block* produce marked irregularity or regular irregularity of the P-P cycle, respectively.

NORMAL VARIANTS

Normal variants, which are frequently observed in healthy individuals, are listed in Table 2-4. These normal variants, except for low voltage, are commonly encountered in healthy young adults and children. Rarely, a first-degree or even a Wenckebach AV block (see Chapter 11) may be found in apparently healthy children and young adults (considered to be due to hypervagal tone).

Table 2-4. Normal variants

Juvenile T wave pattern in children and young adults
Early repolarization pattern in young black males
High left ventricular voltage in children and young adults
Short P-R interval
Right axis deviation in children and young adults
Sinus arrhythmia with or without wandering atrial pacemaker
Low voltage in obese individuals
First-degree block or Wenckebach atrioventricular block in children and young adults (rare)

JUVENILE T WAVE PATTERN

Definition

A juvenile T wave pattern (JTWP) is the pattern formed by deformed T waves in leads V_{1-3} (up to leads V_{4-6} in some cases) in healthy children and young adults (Fig. 2-6).

Diagnostic Criteria

- Inverted (not symmetric or deep) or biphasic T waves in leads V_{1-3} (up to leads V_{4-6} in some cases)
- More common in females (usually in women ≤40 years of age) than in males
- Frequently associated with other normal variants (e.g., sinus arrhythmia and high left-ventricular voltage)

Diagnostic Pearls

JTWP should be differentiated from other clinical conditions that produce inverted T waves in the chest leads, including anterior myocardial ischemia, pulmonary embolism, and myocarditis. It should be noted that JTWP does not produce symmetric or deep T wave inversion (see Fig. 2-6).

Figure 2-6
Sinus arrhythmia with juvenile T wave pattern.

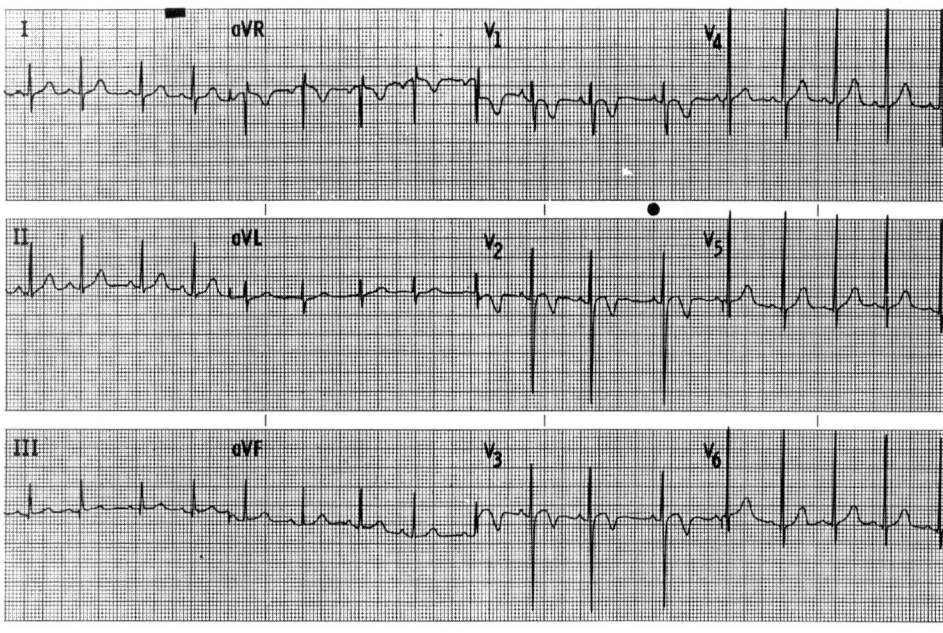

EARLY REPOLARIZATION PATTERN

Definition

An early repolarization pattern (ERP) is the pattern formed by S-T segment elevation (usually J-point elevation) in young healthy individuals, particularly healthy black males (Fig. 2-7).

Diagnostic Criteria

- The J-point S-T segment elevation in leads V_{4-6} (most common)
- Less commonly, the S-T segment elevation in leads V_{1-6}
- Rarely, the S-T segment elevation in leads II, III, and aVF

Diagnostic Pearls

The ERP may superficially resemble acute pericarditis, coronary artery spasm, and an early ECG finding of acute myocardial infarction (MI) (see Chapters 5 and 17). However, the ERP does not produce inverted T waves or abnormal Q waves, and the S-T segment elevation in ERP is always due to J-point elevation (Fig. 2-7).

Figure 2-7
*Early repolarization
pattern.*

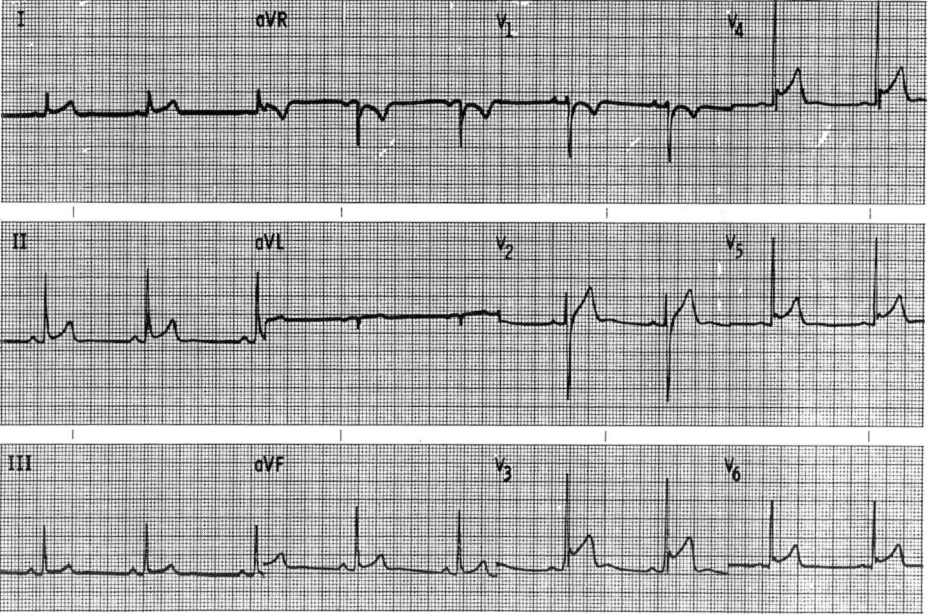

HIGH LEFT-VENTRICULAR VOLTAGE

The term *high left-ventricular voltage* (HLVV) is used when the ECG demonstrates all of the diagnostic criteria for LVH by voltage (see Chapter 3) but the patient is younger than 50 years old. The reason for this is that many young healthy people have HLVV without actual LVH.

OTHER NORMAL VARIANTS

Many healthy children and young adults show short P-R intervals, right axis deviation, and sinus arrhythmia with or without WAP (see Chapter 7). Obese individuals may show LV, and first-degree or even Wenckebach AV block may be observed on rare occasions (see Chapters 11 and 17).

3

Chamber Enlargement

ATRIAL ENLARGEMENT (HYPERTROPHY)

To understand atrial enlargement (hypertrophy), one should be familiar with the P wave configuration in the normal electrocardiogram (ECG). As can be expected, right atrial activation (depolarization) takes place first, since the sinus node is situated in the right atrium (see Fig. 1-1). Soon after the initiation of right atrial depolarization, left atrial activation (depolarization) follows. Since the left atrium begins to be activated before the completion of right atrial depolarization, both atrial activation processes overlap. Consequently, the configuration of the normal P waves in the limb leads, particularly lead II, may show slight notching. The P wave has the largest amplitude in lead II in most normal adults because the P axis is similar to the axis of lead II. However, the P wave configuration varies markedly in different limb leads depending on the P axis of a given ECG tracing. In general, the typical normal P wave demonstrates a small (not more than 2.5 mm in width and depth), round, upright configuration in lead II and an inverted configuration in lead aVR (Fig. 3-1).

In lead V_1, a normal P wave has two components: positive and negative. The reason for this biphasic P wave is that the right atrium is located anteriorly and to the right, whereas the left atrium is located posteriorly and to the left. Thus, in lead V_1, right atrial activation produces the upright (positive) component, and left atrial activation registers the inverted (negative) component (see Fig. 3-1). As described previously, the atrial repolarization process (Ta or Tp wave) is, as a rule, *not* recorded on the ordinary ECG because of its frequent superimposition on the QRS complex. However, on rare occasions, Ta (Tp) waves may be discernible. In this case, the ECG finding may resemble left atrial enlargement.

When right or left atrial enlargement occurs, the configuration of the P wave is altered, with increased amplitude, increased width of the corresponding component of the enlarged (hypertrophied) atrium, or both (see Fig. 3-1).

Figure 3-1
Left atrial hypertrophy (B) and right atrial hypertrophy (C) in comparison with normal atrial size (A) in leads II and V_1.

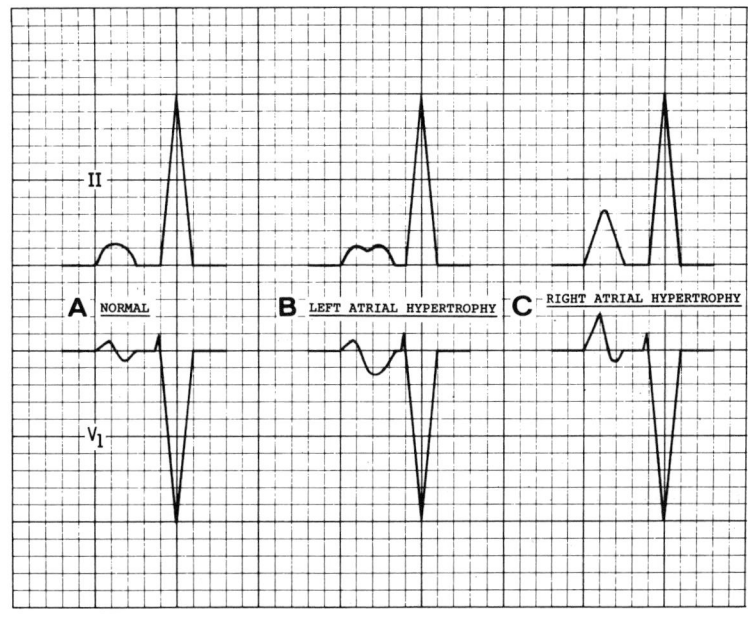

LEFT ATRIAL ENLARGEMENT

Definition

Left atrial enlargement (LAE) is characterized by an increased left atrial electrical force manifested by broad (often notched) P waves in limb leads that are associated with deep and broad P waves of the negative component in leads V_{1-2}.

Diagnostic Criteria (Fig. 3-2)

- Wide (3 mm or more) and notched P waves in leads I, II, and aVL (also in leads III and aVF in some cases)
- A negative (inverted) component of P waves in leads V_{1-2}, with a depth and width of 1 mm or more
- Coarse atrial fibrillation (AF) (fibrillation waves in leads V_1 or V_2 of 1 mm or more)

Diagnostic Pearls

The term *P-mitrale* is often used for marked LAE because mitral valve disease is one of the most common underlying disorders. Any of the above criteria is necessary to diagnose LAE.

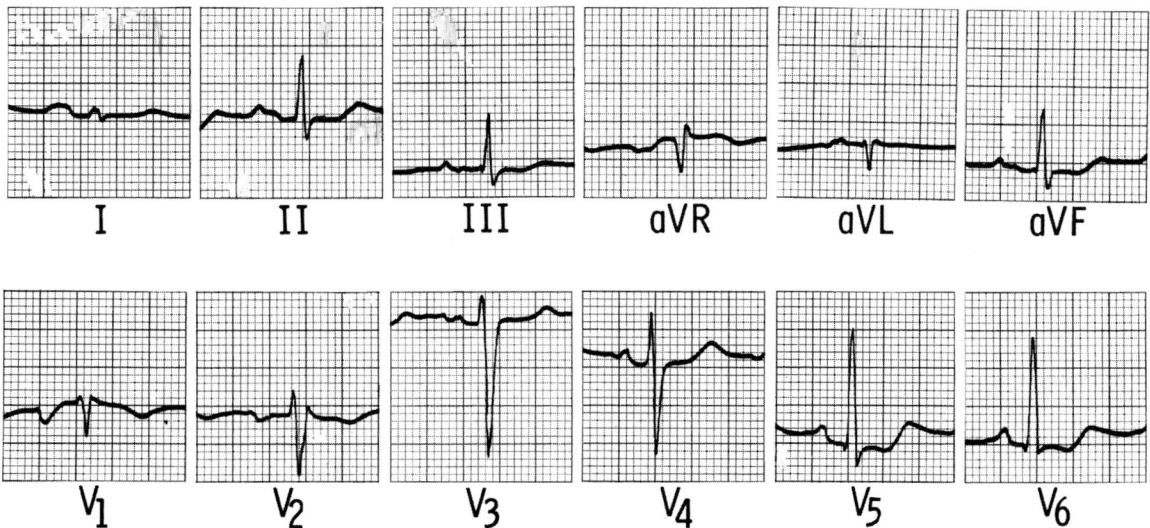

Figure 3-2
Marked left atrial enlargement.

RIGHT ATRIAL ENLARGEMENT

Definition

Right atrial enlargement (RAE) is characterized by an increased right atrial electrical force manifested by tall P waves in leads II, III, and aVF that are associated with tall (lesser degree) P waves in leads V_{1-2}.

Diagnostic Criteria (Fig. 3-3)

- Tent-shaped and tall (3 mm or more) P waves in leads II, III, and aVF
- Less commonly, a positive (upright) component of P waves in leads V_{1-2}, with an amplitude of 2 mm or more

Diagnostic Pearls

The term *P-pulmonale* is often used to designate RAE that is due to various pulmonary diseases, particularly chronic obstructive pulmonary disease (COPD). When RAE is due to various congenital heart diseases, the term *P-congenitale* is used. In severe hypokalemia, the P waves may exhibit peaked and tall configurations that may resemble RAE (see Chapter 16). Any of the above criteria is necessary for the diagnosis.

Figure 3-3
Right atrial enlargement.

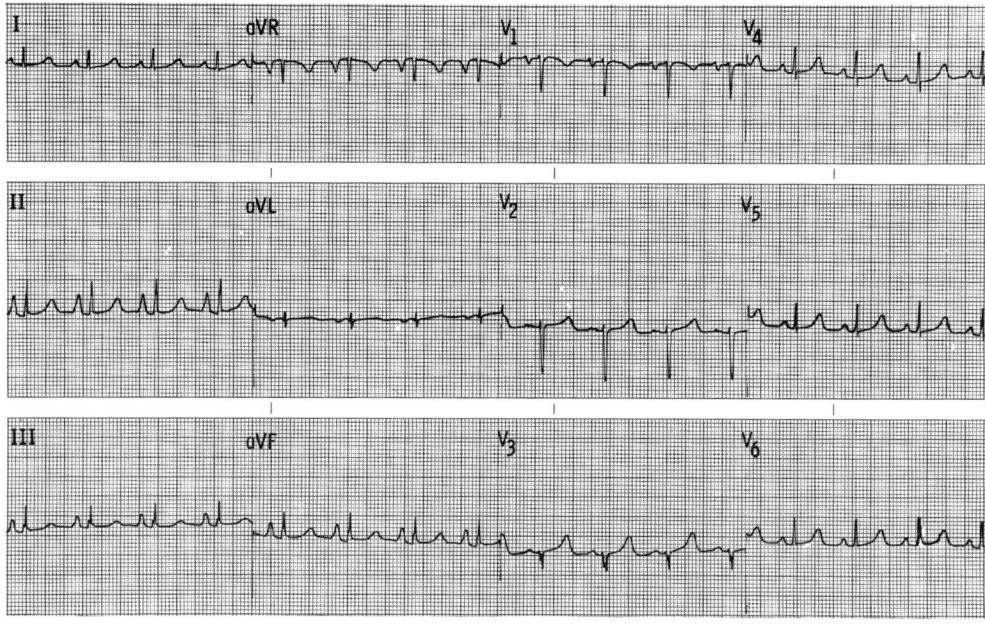

BIATRIAL ENLARGEMENT

Definition

In biatrial enlargement (BAE), the ECG finding is simply a combination of LAE and RAE. Namely, the P waves in many limb leads are tall and wide, and both components (positive and negative) of the P waves in leads V_{1-2} are increased in amplitude and depth (Fig. 3-4).

Diagnostic Criteria (Fig. 3-4)

- Wide (3 mm or more) and tall (3 mm or more) P waves in limb leads
- Positive (upright) component of P waves in leads V_{1-2}, with an amplitude of 2 mm or more, as well as a negative (inverted) component of P waves in leads V_{1-2}, with a depth and width of 1 mm or more

Diagnostic Pearls

The underlying disorders that produce BAE commonly are advanced cardiomyopathy, multivalvular heart disease, and multiple congenital cardiac anomalies. Any of the above criteria is necessary for the diagnosis.

Figure 3-4
Biatrial enlargement with biventricular hypertrophy.

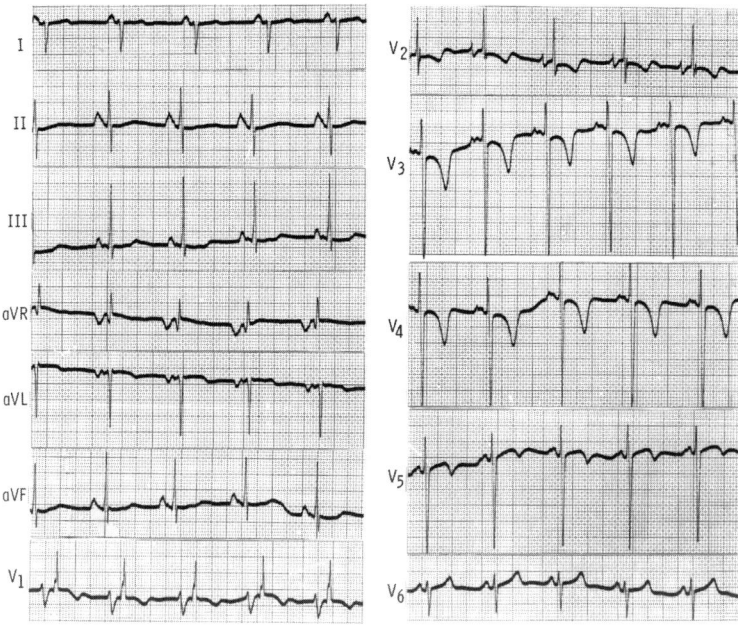

LEFT VENTRICULAR HYPERTROPHY

In left ventricular hypertrophy (LVH), the left ventricle is approximately three times thicker than the right ventricle. In addition, electrophysiologically, the electrical potential of the left ventricle is about 10 times greater than that of the right ventricle. Thus, the configuration of the QRS complex during ventricular depolarization is primarily influenced by left ventricular activation. The six precordial leads give the best information during ventricular activation. Normally, a progressive increment of the R wave amplitude is observed in leads V_{1-6} and small (physiologic) septal q waves begin to appear in leads V_{4-6}. In LVH, this normal relationship between the left and right ventricles is exaggerated. Conversely, right ventricular hypertrophy (RVH) produces a reversed relationship between left and right ventricular depolarization. Diagrammatic representation of LVH and RVH in relation to the normal-sized ventricle in terms of vectorial analysis is shown in Figure 3-5.

Clinically, most patients with left bundle branch block (LBBB) demonstrate LVH. Conversely, there is a poor correlation between right bundle branch block (RBBB) and RVH. The underlying disorder that most commonly produces LVH is, needless to say, systemic hypertension.

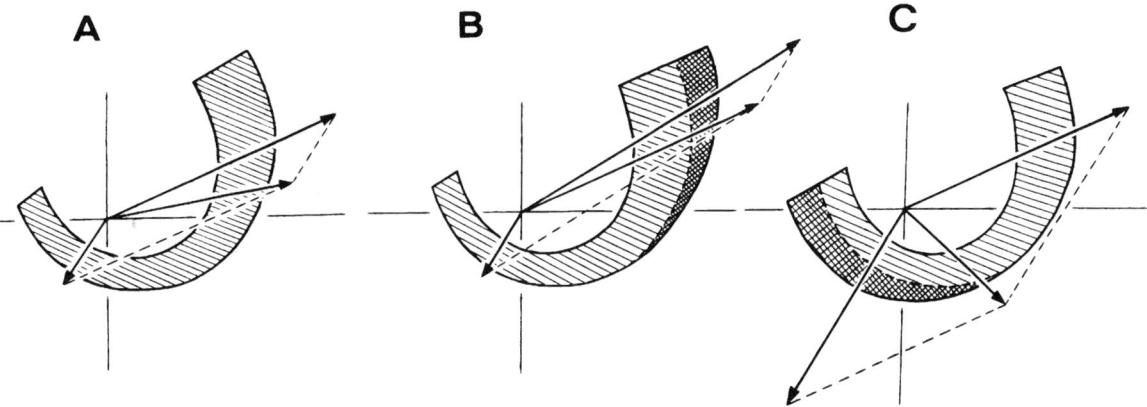

Figure 3-5
Left ventricular hypertrophy (B) and right ventricular hypertrophy (C) in comparison with normal ventricles (A). In left ventricular hypertrophy, there is marked increment of the posterior and leftward forces during depolarization (B). Right ventricular hypertrophy, on the other hand, produces increased forces anteriorly and to the right (C).

LEFT VENTRICULAR HYPERTROPHY
(continued)

Definition

LVH is characterized by an increased left ventricular electrical force manifested by tall R waves in leads V_{5-6} and a deep S wave in lead V_1 that is associated with a secondary T wave change (strain pattern) in leads V_{5-6}.

Diagnostic Criteria (Fig. 3-6)

- An R wave in lead V_5 or V_6 that is 26 mm or more
- An R wave in lead V_5 or V_6 plus an S wave in lead V_1 that is 35 mm or more
- An R wave in lead I that is 15 mm or more
- An R wave in lead I plus an S wave in lead III that is 25 mm or more
- An R wave in lead aVL that is 13 mm or more or an R wave in leads II, III, or aVF that is 20 mm or more
- A secondary T wave change (strain pattern—biphasic to inverted T waves) in leads V_{5-6} (similar finding in leads I and aVL)

Diagnostic Pearls

The most reliable diagnostic criteria of LVH are a secondary T wave change (strain pattern) with a tall R wave in lead V_5 or V_6 (whichever is taller) plus a deep S wave in lead V_1. If there is no strain pattern, the ECG finding should be interpreted as *consider LVH by voltage* for individuals older than 50 years of age. In younger people (age younger than 50 years of age), the term *high left ventricular voltage* (HLVV) is used under this circumstance to signify that the ECG finding is a normal variant (see Chapter 2). It should be noted that leads V_{2-4} are *not* used in the diagnosis of LVH. Left axis deviation (LAD) is observed in approximately 50% of the cases of LVH. Thus, LAD is *not* necessary to diagnose LVH.

Figure 3-6
Left ventricular hypertrophy.

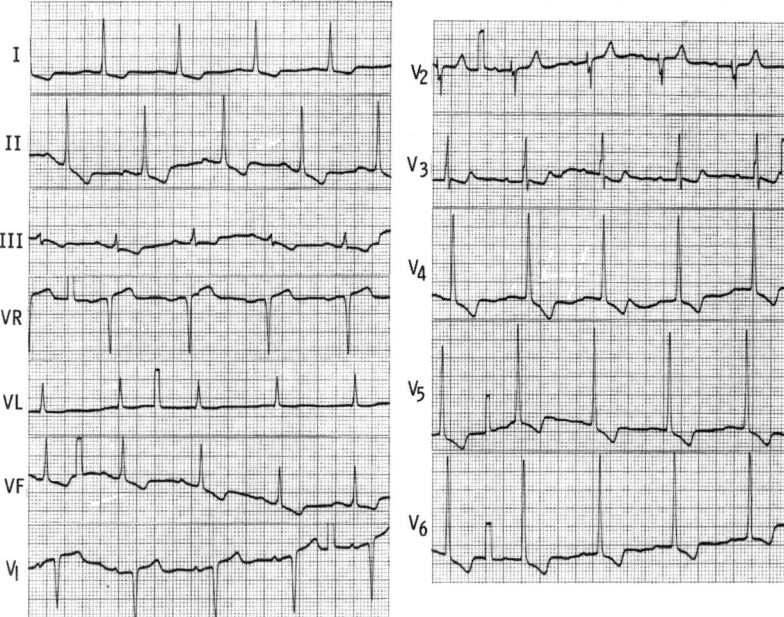

RIGHT VENTRICULAR HYPERTROPHY

Since the thickness and the electrical potential of the right ventricle in a normal heart are approximately one-third and one-tenth of the left ventricle, respectively, slight RVH usually does not produce a significant ECG abnormality. When the right ventricle becomes significantly hypertrophied, however, it eventually becomes the dominant ventricle. As a result, the usual relationship between left and right ventricles is reserved in marked RVH. In a typical and marked RVH, lead V_1 resembles a normal lead V_6, and lead V_6 resembles a normal lead V_1. From a vectorial viewpoint, the major QRS axis moves toward the right and anteriorly in RVH. This is because of the increased force that is produced anteriorly and to the right.

The earliest manifestation of RVH is a progressive QRS axis change in the rightward direction. Therefore, right axis deviation (RAD) is the essential criterion for diagnosing RVH. The next early finding of RVH is a progressive reduction of the depth of the S wave in lead V_1. When the S wave in lead V_1 becomes progressively smaller, the R wave in this lead becomes progressively taller in RVH. As a result, the RS ratio in lead V_1 becomes 1:1 or more (relatively tall R wave in lead V_1).

Not uncommonly, a small q wave may be present in lead V_1 (at times, in leads V_2 and V_3) in pure RVH. The reason for this finding is not fully understood. Nevertheless, this small q wave is considered to be due to the fact that the initial septal force is altered because of the hypertrophied right septal mass in severe RVH. In some cases of RVH, particularly in those due to mitral stenosis or COPD, the QRS complex may show RR' wave (incomplete RBBB pattern) in lead V_1.

RIGHT VENTRICULAR HYPERTROPHY
(continued)

Definition

RVH is characterized by an increased anterior and right-ward force manifested by a tall R wave (sometimes an incomplete RBBB pattern) in lead V_1 that is associated with RAD of the QRS complexes.

Diagnostic Criteria (Fig. 3-7)

- RAD
- Tall (or relatively tall) R wave in lead V_1
- RR' wave (incomplete RBBB pattern) in lead V_1
- Deep S waves in leads I, aVL, and V_{4-6}
- Posterior axis deviation with RAD (some cases)
- Secondary T wave change (strain pattern) in leads V_{1-3}

Diagnostic Pearls

RAD is an essential element to diagnose RVH. Thus, the most reliable criteria of RVH are RAD and a tall R wave or incomplete RBBB pattern in lead V_1. The strain pattern is *not* prominent in RVH in every case. It should be noted, however, that RAD may be due to left posterior hemiblock (LPHB) or pulmonary embolism. By and large, RAD occurs acutely in pulmonary embolism, and the heart rate is usually rapid. LPHB, on the other hand, almost always coexists with RBBB, leading to bifascicular block (a form of bilateral bundle branch block).

Figure 3-7
Right ventricular hypertrophy with diffuse, nonspecific T wave change.

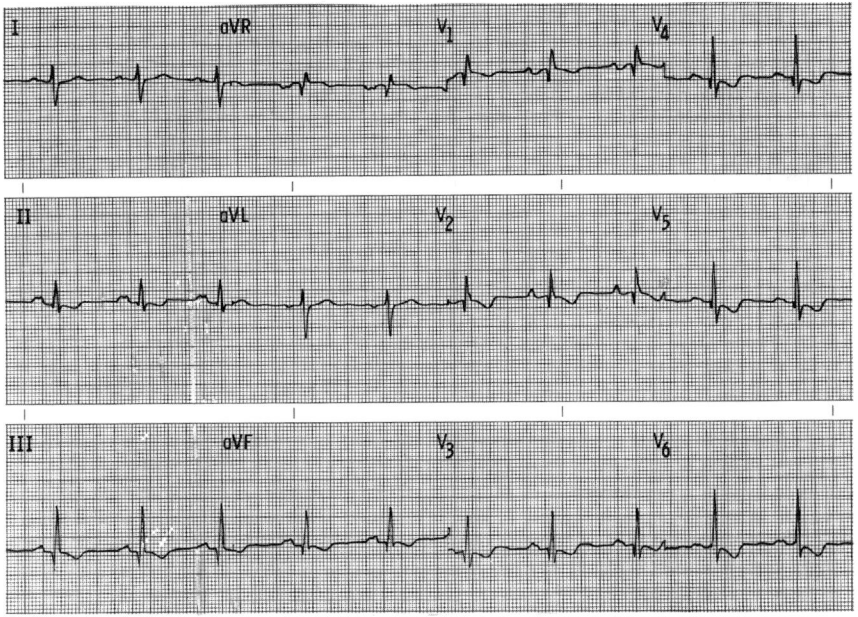

BIVENTRICULAR HYPERTROPHY

The diagnosis of biventricular hypertrophy (BVH) is rather difficult electrocardiographically because increased electrical forces in both ventricles may cancel out each other, at least in part. Theoretically, BVH of exactly equal degree may produce an almost normal ECG. The ECG findings of BVH are greatly influenced by the degree of enlargement in each ventricle.

BVH is frequently due to various advanced congenital heart diseases or cardiomyopathies. Less commonly, BVH occurs in multivalvular lesions. Needless to say, far-advanced heart disease, regardless of the type, may produce BVH.

BIVENTRICULAR HYPERTROPHY
(continued)

Definition

BVH is characterized by increased electrical forces of both ventricles as a result of the ventricular enlargement of both ventricles.

Diagnostic Criteria (Fig. 3-8)

- LVH or LBBB in the precordial leads with RAD in the limb leads
- Tall (or relatively tall) R waves in all precordial leads with RAD in the limb leads (less reliable)
- Katz-Wachtel phenomenon (large amplitude of positive and negative components of the QRS complexes in leads V_{2-4}—usually RS complexes)
- P-pulmonale or P-congenitale in limb leads and LVH in the precordial leads (less reliable)

Diagnostic Pearls

The most reliable diagnostic criteria of BVH are LVH in the precordial leads and RAD in limb leads (see Fig. 3-8). Other findings in BVH are less reliable. It should be noted that RAD may be due to pulmonary embolism or LPHB. In general, RAD develops acutely in pulmonary embolism with various tachyarrhythmias, whereas LPHB almost always coexists with RBBB, leading to bifascicular block (see Chapters 4 and 17).

Figure 3-8
Biventricular hypertrophy.

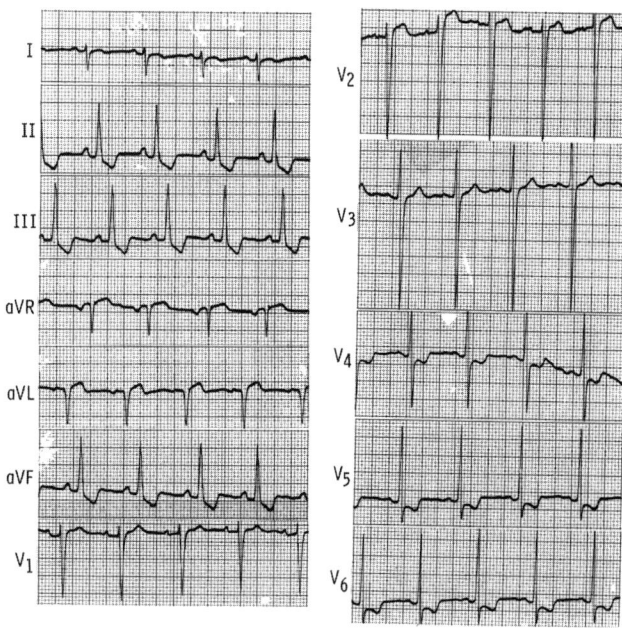

4

Intraventricular Conduction Disturbances

Various forms of intraventricular conduction disturbances (IVCDs) may occur under different clinical circumstances. The most common and well-recognized forms of IVCDs are right and left bundle branch blocks (RBBBs and LBBBs). In a bundle branch block, the impulse is conducted via an intact bundle branch so that the ventricle with a blocked bundle branch is activated later than the ventricle with the intact bundle branch. Therefore, instead of the normal simultaneous activation of both ventricles, a bundle branch block produces asynchronous activation of the two ventricles. The incidence of LBBB and RBBB is considered almost equal. Schematic explanations of RBBB and LBBB are shown in Figures 4-1 and 4-2, respectively.

Although it is less well-recognized, some IVCDs are due to a conduction delay involving both ventricles diffusely. This type of conduction delay is termed *nonspecific* or *diffuse* IVCD. Various factors and clinical circumstances that may cause diffuse (nonspecific) intraventricular block are summarized in Table 4-1. As a rule, IVCDs are recognized by a prolongation of the QRS interval, but some IVCDs produce little or no prolongation of the QRS interval. For example, a block at one of the subdivisions of the left bundle branch system (hemiblock) causes an abnormal QRS axis deviation without significant alteration in the QRS interval.

The left bundle branch consists of two subdivisions: the anterior (superior) and posterior (inferior) fascicles.

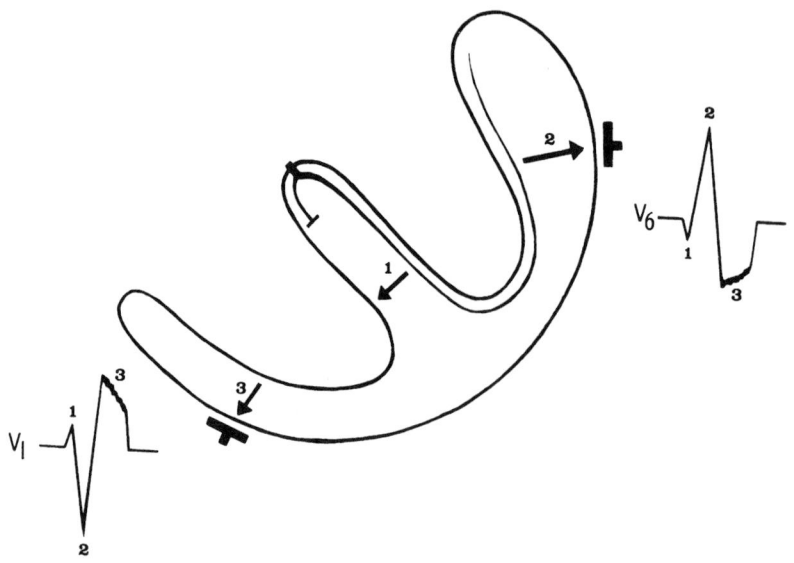

Figure 4-1
Right bundle branch block. The initial septal activation is from left to right and anteriorly, as normal (vector 1). Right ventricular activation (vector 3) occurs following completion of the left ventricular activation (vector 2). Delayed activation of the right ventricle is responsible for the production of the RR' pattern in lead V_1 and the round and deep S wave in lead V_6.

Figure 4-2
Left bundle branch block (LBBB). The most important finding in LBBB is the alteration of the initial septal force, which is directed from right to left and either anteriorly or posteriorly (vector 1). Left ventricular activation (vector 3) occurs after completion of right ventricular activation (vector 2). Delayed left ventricular activation is responsible for the production of the broad S wave in lead V_1 and the broad R wave in lead V_6. In LBBB, physiologic (septal) q waves in leads V_{4-6} are absent because of an abnormal septal activation.

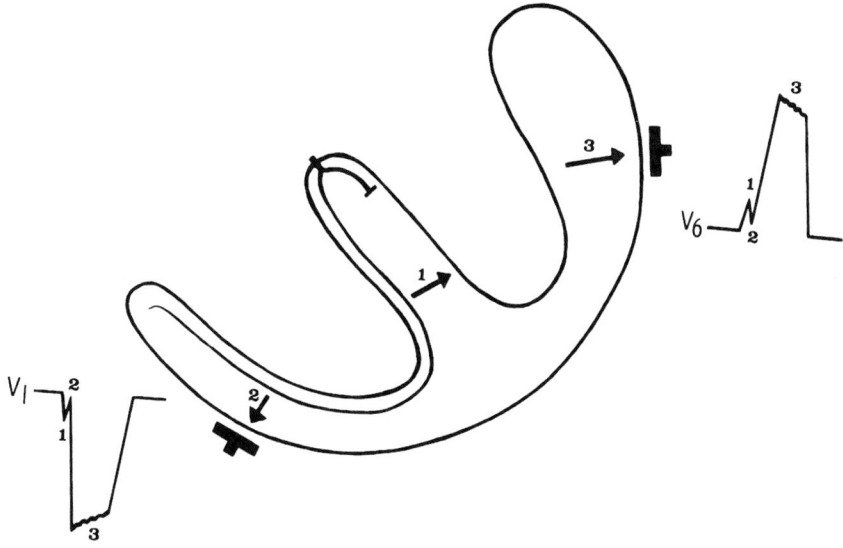

Table 4-1. Factors that may cause diffuse (nonspecific) intraventricular block

Drugs
  Toxic effects of quinidine, procainamide, and other
  similar antiarrhythmic agents
Electrolyte imbalance
  Advanced hyperkalemia
Heart diseases
  Cardiomyopathies
  Myocardial infarction
  Other advanced heart diseases
After cardiac arrest
  Either cardiac or noncardiac in origin
Miscellaneous
  Elderly individuals
  Hypothermia

The anterior division of the left bundle branch traverses the base of the anterior papillary muscle of the left ventricle, whereas the posterior division runs toward the posterior papillary muscle. Anatomically, the anterior division is located superiorly, while the posterior division is situated inferiorly (see Fig. 1-1).

When these two subdivisions are intact, the impulse is transmitted to the left ventricle via anterior and posterior divisions simultaneously (Fig. 4-3). The term *hemiblock* is used when one of the subdivisions of the left bundle branch is blocked. In left anterior (superior) hemiblock (LAHB), the impulse is transmitted through the intact posterior division to activate the left ventricle. Since the impulse conducted via the posterior division is directed superiorly and to the left (see Fig. 4-3), marked left axis deviation (LAD) is observed in LAHB. Conversely, in left posterior hemiblock (LPHB), the left ventricle is activated via an intact anterior division. Since the impulse conducted through the anterior division is directed inferiorly and to the right, right axis deviation (RAD) is produced in LPHB (see Fig. 4-3).

There is usually little (0.01–0.02 sec) or no prolongation of the QRS interval in hemiblocks because the Purkinje fibers in the left anterior and posterior divisions are richly confluent. Hemiblocks may occur intermittently, which is analogous to intermittent bundle branch block.

Bundle branch block has a close relationship to ventricular hypertrophy. This is more so in LBBB because the

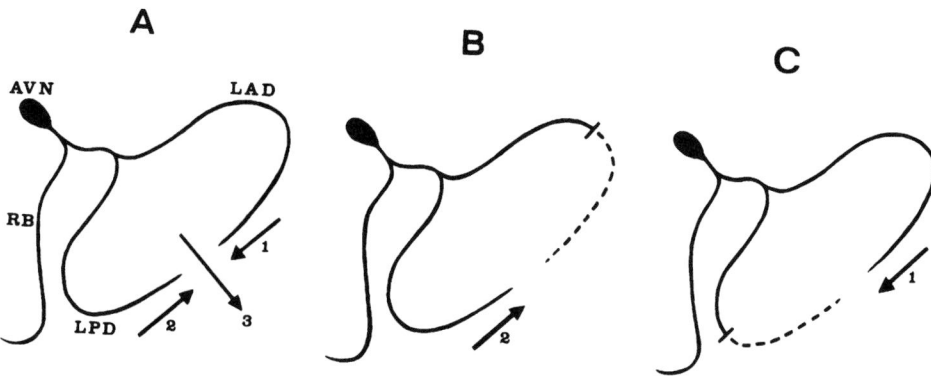

Figure 4-3

Hemiblocks. When both anterior and posterior divisions of the left bundle branch system are intact (A), the left ventricle is activated via both divisions (vectors 1 and 2) so that the resultant forces of vectors 1 and 2 produce vector 3. When one of the two divisions of the left bundle branch system is blocked, however, the impulses must travel through the intact division only—that is, in anterior hemiblock (B), vector 1 is no longer present, and as a result, the left ventricle is activated via intact posterior division (vector 2). In this case, the electrical axis shifts to the left and superiorly (marked left axis deviation). For the same reason, posterior hemiblock (C) produces right axis deviation because the left ventricle is activated via intact anterior division (vector 1). (RB = right bundle branch; AVN = atrioventricular node; LAD = left anterior division; LPD = left posterior division.)

underlying process of LBBB is almost always left ventricular hypertrophy, particularly in adults. In addition, some cardiac lesions, such as an atrial septal defect, are almost always associated with a RBBB pattern.

LBBB tends to produce more widening of the QRS complex than RBBB. A bundle branch block (either right or left) generally is said to be complete when the QRS interval is 0.12 second or wider (in limb leads). Incomplete bundle branch block is diagnosed when the QRS interval is between 0.10 and 0.11 second. Customarily, the term *complete* is omitted for the actual ECG interpretation; thus, bundle branch block without being specified as complete or incomplete automatically means *complete*. The term *incomplete* should always be added in the actual interpretation when applicable. It is not uncommon to observe a relatively narrow QRS interval (<0.10 sec), especially when dealing with incomplete RBBB.

Bundle branch block (either right or left) is commonly chronic and permanent, but it may occur intermittently. An intermittent bundle branch block may occur depending on the heart rate (rate-dependent), or it may be unrelated to the heart rate (rate-independent).

The term *bifascicular block* (BFB) is used when two fascicles are blocked simultaneously. BFB is a form of incomplete bilateral bundle branch block (BBBB) (Table 4-2). The most common BFB is a combination of RBBB and LAHB. BFB consisting of RBBB and LPHB is a rather uncommon occurrence.

In broad terms, trifascicular block can be defined as a simultaneous block (complete or incomplete) in any three of the five ventricular conducting fascicles: the His bundle, the right bundle branch, the left bundle branch, and the anterior and posterior divisions of the left bundle branch. However, the term *TFB* is used specifically when a block involves simultaneously the three peripheral fascicles—namely the right bundle branch and the anterior and posterior divisions of the left bundle branch. Thus, TFB is an expression of BBBB (see Table 4-2).

When all three peripheral fascicles are completely blocked, needless to say, *complete atrioventricular (AV) block* (complete TFB) is the end result. In this case, ventricular escape (idioventricular) rhythm with a very slow ventricular rate is produced (see Chapter 11). The diagnosis of TFB is certain when the same patient exhibits a combination of RBBB and LPHB on one occasion and RBBB with LAHB on another occasion. However, various ECG manifestations are produced when one or more of the three fas-

Table 4-2. Diagnostic criteria of bilateral bundle branch block (bifascicular block and trifascicular block)

Right bundle branch block with left anterior hemiblock

Right bundle branch block with left posterior hemiblock

Alternating left and right bundle branch block

Left or right bundle branch block with first- or second-degree AV block (not every case)

Left or right bundle branch block with prolonged H-V interval >55 msec

Left bundle branch block on one occasion and right bundle branch block on another occasion

Mobitz type II AV block

Any combination of the above findings

Complete AV block with ventricular escape (idioventricular) rhythm

AV = atrioventricular.

cicles are incompletely blocked, intermittently blocked, or both. Extremely complicated ECG findings can result when the degree of incomplete block is different in the three fascicles. AV block of varying degree associated with RBBB or LBBB and/or anterior or posterior hemiblock is usually a typical example of incomplete TFB.

Mobitz type II AV block is an expression of incomplete TFB in which the QRS complexes nearly always disclose RBBB or LBBB, hemiblocks, or BFB. When 2:1 AV block is associated with RBBB, LBBB, or BFB, the block represents Mobitz type II AV block in nearly all cases (see Chapter 11).

Various ECG manifestations of bilateral bundle branch block are summarized in Table 4-2.

RIGHT BUNDLE BRANCH BLOCK

Definition

RBBB is characterized by delayed activation of the right ventricle as a result of a block in the right bundle branch system.

Diagnostic Criteria (Fig. 4-4)

- A QRS interval of 0.12 second or more
- rSR' or an M pattern of QRS complex in leads V_{1-3}
- Deep and slurred S waves in leads I, aVL, and V_{4-6}
- Secondary S-T and T wave change in leads V_{1-3}

Diagnostic Pearls

In RBBB, the initial ventricular septal activation is normal because the conduction disturbance involves only the terminal ventricular activation force. All of the above findings are needed for the diagnosis.

Figure 4-4
Right bundle branch block.

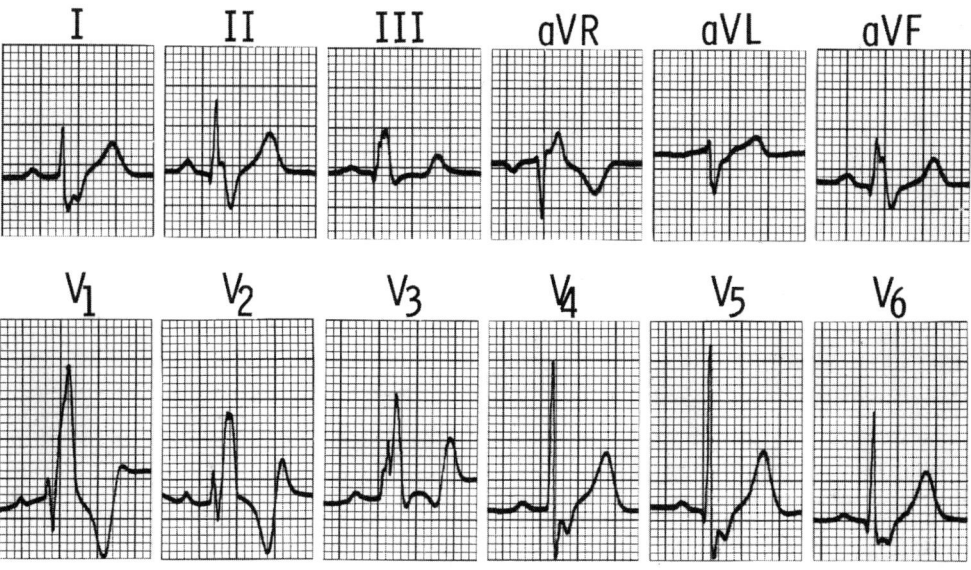

LEFT BUNDLE BRANCH BLOCK

Definition

LBBB is characterized by delayed activation of the left ventricle as a result of a block in the left bundle branch system (above the bifurcation of the fascicles).

Diagnostic Criteria (Fig. 4-5)

- QRS interval of 0.12 second or more
- Absence of septal q waves in leads I, aVL, and V_{4-6}
- rSR', an M pattern, or broad R waves in leads I, aVL, and V_{4-6}
- Broad Q-S or rS waves in leads V_{1-3}
- Secondary, S-T, and T wave change in leads I, aVL, and V_{4-6}

Diagnostic Pearls

The most important ECG finding in LBBB is an alteration of the initial vector during ventricular septal activation, wherein the initial septal activation begins from right to left (see Fig. 4-2) instead of the normal direction of left to right. This reversed ventricular septal vector is responsible for the absence of a physiologic (septal) q wave in leads V_{4-6}. In approximately two-thirds of the cases of LBBB, the initial vector is directed from right to left and anteriorly. In the remaining one-third of the cases of LBBB, the initial vector is directed from right to left and posteriorly. Depending on the direction of the initial vector, the amplitude of the R waves in leads V_{1-3} may be almost or even completely absent, or they may be relatively tall. All of the above findings are needed for the diagnosis.

Figure 4-5
Left bundle branch block.

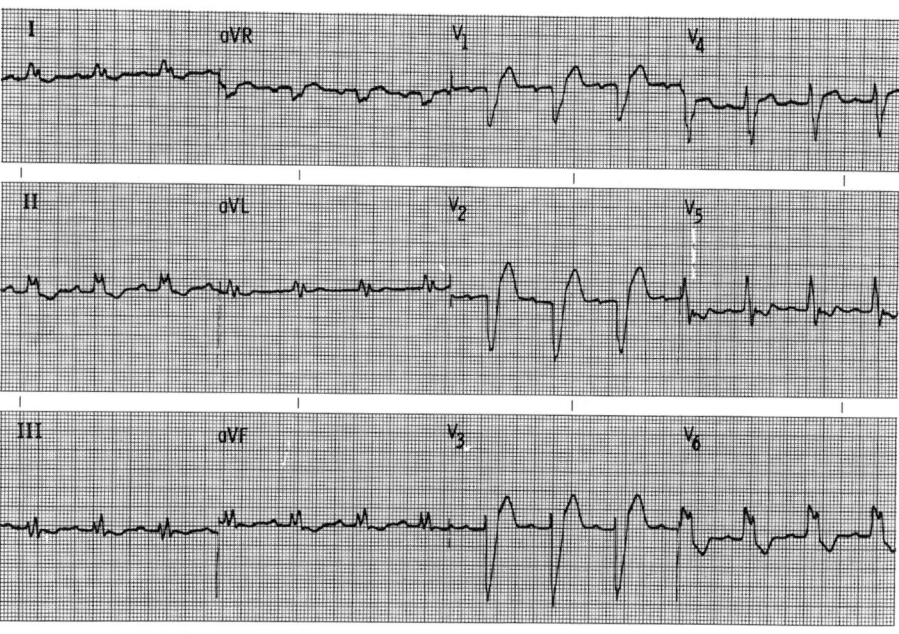

INTERMITTENT BUNDLE BRANCH BLOCK

Definition

Intermittent bundle branch block is characterized by the intermittent occurrence of LBBB or RBBB that may be related to the heart rate (rate-dependent) or unrelated to the heart rate (rate-independent).

Diagnostic Criteria

The diagnostic criteria of RBBB and LBBB are described previously. Rate-dependent bundle branch block (Fig. 4-6) is much more common than rate-independent bundle branch block.

Diagnostic Pearls

When LBBB or RBBB occurs alternately with a normal QRS complex, the ECG finding superficially mimics ventricular premature contractions, causing ventricular bigeminy. Ventricular tachycardia may be closely simulated when LBBB or RBBB occurs periodically. A full understanding of LBBB or RBBB will clarify the differential diagnosis under these circumstances.

Figure 4-6
*Intermittent left bundle
branch block (rate-depen-
dent) and a ventricular
premature contraction (the
seventh beat).*

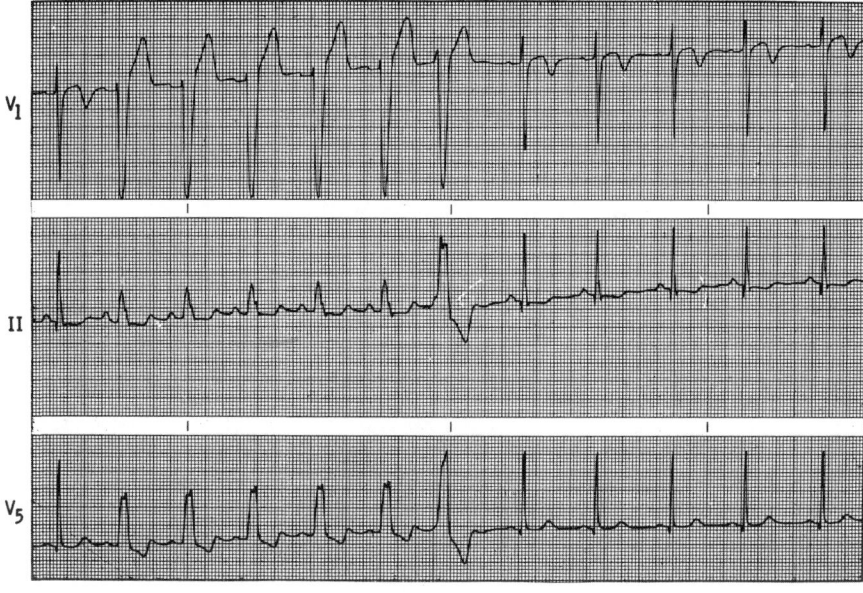

LEFT ANTERIOR HEMIBLOCK

Definition

LAHB is characterized by marked LAD of the QRS complexes as a result of a block in the anterior (superior) division (fascicle) of the left bundle branch system.

Diagnostic Criteria (Fig. 4-7)

- Marked LAD (−45 to −90 degrees) of QRS complexes
- A small q wave in lead I and a small r wave in lead III
- Little or no prolongation of the QRS interval
- No evidence of other factors responsible for LAD (true or pseudo)

Diagnostic Pearls

There are various other causes of LAD of the QRS complexes (e.g., diaphragmatic myocardial infarction). This aspect should be carefully considered before making the diagnosis of LAHB. LAHB often coexists with RBBB, leading to BFB (see Table 4-2). All of the above findings are needed for the diagnosis.

Figure 4-7
*Left anterior hemi-
block.*

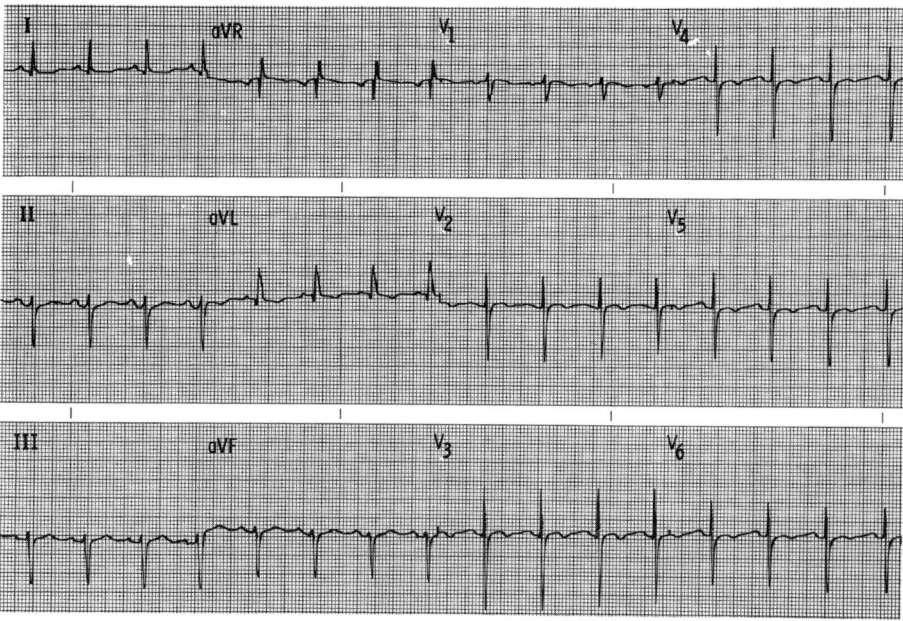

LEFT POSTERIOR HEMIBLOCK

Definition

LPHB is characterized by marked RAD of the QRS complexes as a result of a block in the posterior (inferior) division (fascicle) of the left bundle branch system.

Diagnostic Criteria (Fig. 4-8)

- Marked RAD (+105 to +180 degrees) of the QRS complexes
- A small r wave in lead I and a small q wave in lead III
- Little or no prolongation of the QRS interval
- No evidence of other factors responsible for RAD (true or pseudo).

Diagnostic Pearls

Before making the diagnosis of LPHB, it should be certain that there are no other factors producing RAD of the QRS complexes (e.g., right ventricular hypertrophy, high lateral myocardial infarction). LPHB often coexists with RBBB, leading to BFB (see Table 4-2). All of the above findings are needed for the diagnosis.

Figure 4-8
Left posterior hemiblock associated with anterior myocardial infarction. Note a ventricular premature contraction (VPC) (lead V₁).

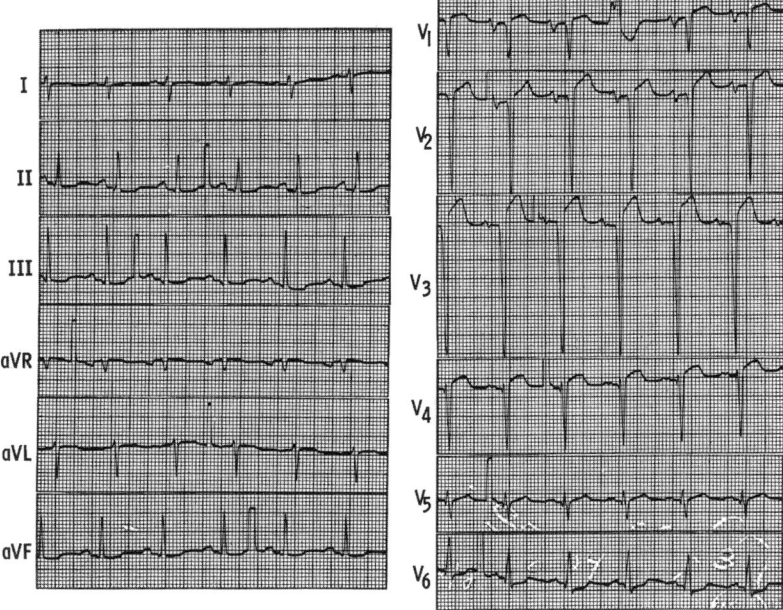

BIFASCICULAR BLOCK (RIGHT BUNDLE BRANCH BLOCK ASSOCIATED WITH LEFT ANTERIOR HEMIBLOCK)

Definition

BFB (RBBB associated with LAHB) is the most common form of incomplete bilateral bundle branch block (BBBB).

Diagnostic Criteria (Fig. 4-9)

To make the diagnosis of BFB (RBBB associated with LAHB), the following must be present:

- RBBB in the precordial leads, and
- LAHB in the limb leads.

Diagnostic Pearls

LAD of the QRS complexes should be at least –45 degrees, and the characteristic features of RBBB (described earlier in this chapter) should be present. This is the most common form of BBBB (see Table 4-2).

Figure 4-9
Bifascicular block consisting of right bundle branch block and left anterior hemiblock.

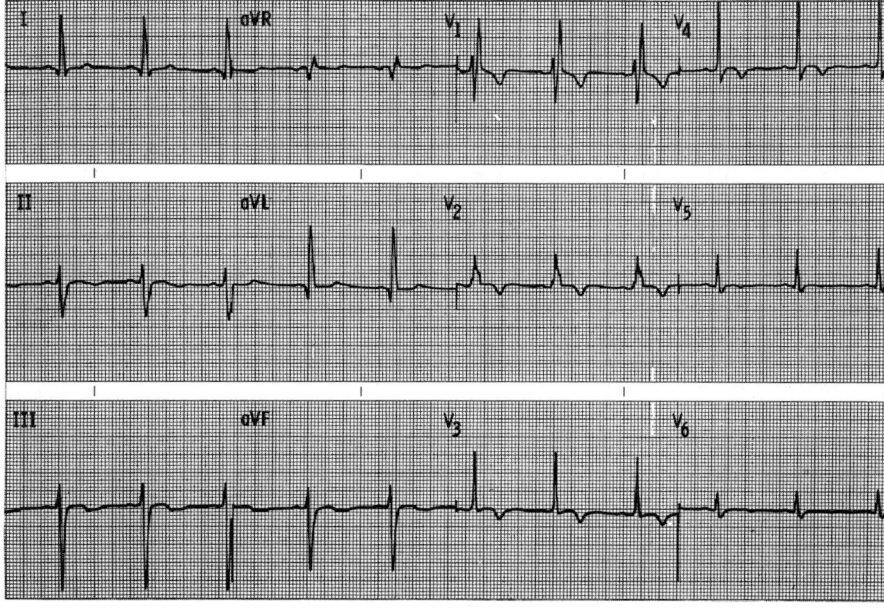

BIFASCICULAR BLOCK (RBBB ASSOCIATED WITH LEFT POSTERIOR HEMIBLOCK)

Definition

BFB (RBBB associated with LPHB) is the less common form of incomplete BBBB.

Diagnostic Criteria (Fig. 4-10)

To make the diagnosis of BFB (RBBB associated with LPHB), the following must be present:

- RBBB in the precordial leads, and
- LPHB in the limb leads.

Diagnostic Pearls

It should be certain that there are the characteristic features of RBBB in the chest leads and that the QRS complexes in the limb leads show marked RAD (≥+105 degrees).

Figure 4-10
*Bifascicular block consisting of
right bundle branch block and left
posterior hemiblock associated
with anteroseptal myocardial
infarction.*

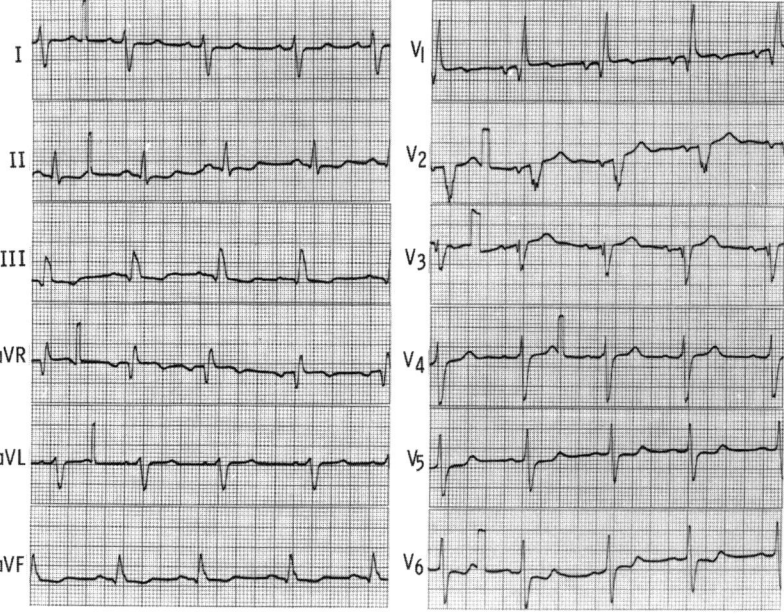

ADVANCED BILATERAL BUNDLE BRANCH BLOCK

Definition

Advanced BBBB is advanced AV block (see Chapter 11) associated with intermittent LBBB, RBBB, or both.

Diagnostic Criteria

To make the diagnosis of advanced BBBB, a combination of the following must be present (Fig. 4-11):

• Advanced AV block;
• Intermittent RBBB, LBBB, or both; and
• Intermittent LAHB, LPHB and/or BFB
• Intermittent ventricular escape rhythm.

Diagnostic Pearls

It should be certain that two or more of the above-mentioned diagnostic criteria are present in the same ECG tracing. Other ECG tracings obtained from the same patient often reveal other forms of BBBB (see Table 4-2).

Figure 4-11
Sinus rhythm (indicated by arrows) with advanced atrioventricular block, producing intermittent ventricular escape rhythm (marked X) and a right bundle branch block. These ECG findings represent advanced incomplete trifascicular block (incomplete bilateral bundle branch block). Note the frequent ventricular fusion beats (FB).

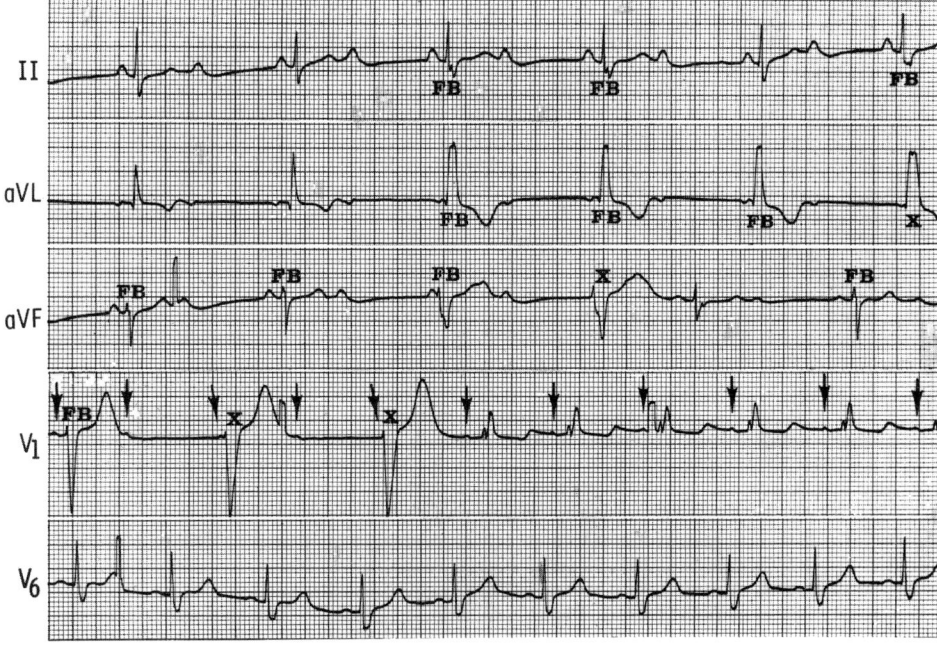

DIFFUSE (NONSPECIFIC) INTRAVENTRICULAR BLOCK

Definition

Diffuse (nonspecific) intraventricular block is characterized by broad QRS complexes as a result of conduction delay within the ventricles diffusely (not due to a localized block in the bundle branch system).

Diagnostic Criteria (Fig. 4-12)

In order to make a diagnosis of diffuse (nonspecific) intraventricular block, the following must be present:

- A broad QRS complex of 0.12 second or more
- No evidence of RBBB or LBBB

Diagnostic Pearls

It should be certain that the broad QRS complex is not due to RBBB or LBBB. Various factors causing diffuse intraventricular block are listed in the Table 4-1. Extremely marked diffuse intraventricular block is produced by two main underlying problems: severe hyperkalemia and toxicity from quinidine or other similar antiarrhythmic agents.

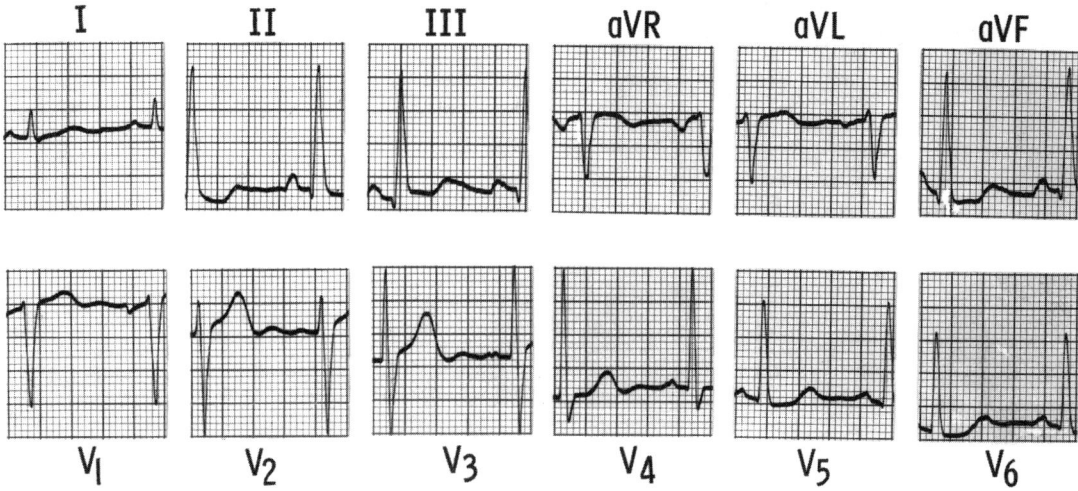

Figure 4-12
Diffuse intraventricular block.

BUNDLE BRANCH BLOCK ASSOCIATED WITH MYOCARDIAL INFARCTION

Bundle branch block associated with myocardial infarction is discussed in Chapter 5.

5

Myocardial Ischemia, Injury, and Infarction

There has been a drastic change in the terminology, classification, and diagnostic criteria of myocardial infarction (MI). The recognition of abnormal (pathologic) Q waves is no longer necessary in every case to diagnose MI because approximately 25–40% of the patients admitted to cardiac care units suffer from non–Q wave MI.

At present, MI is classified into two major categories—namely, *Q wave MI* and *non–Q wave MI*. As their names designate, Q wave MI produces the characteristic abnormal (pathologic) Q waves, whereas non–Q wave MI fails to produce abnormal Q waves. Q wave MI represents transmural MI, whereas non–Q wave MI is considered to be nontransmural MI, or subendocardial MI. In general,

non–Q wave MI is diagnosed by recognizing persisting S-T segment depression (horizontal or down-sloping), T wave inversion, or both, providing that the diagnosis of acute MI is supported by the serum enzyme elevation and clinical findings.

Electrocardiographically, three stages of abnormalities can be produced in experimental animal studies by occlusion of the coronary artery. These electrocardiographic (ECG) abnormalities correlate reasonably well with those found in coronary artery disease (CAD) in humans. The three stages—namely myocardial ischemia, injury, and infarction (necrosis)—may be observed depending on the degree of the impairment of the blood supply to the myocardium. Myocardial ischemia and injury are reversible changes, whereas MI often produces irreversible change. Myocardial ischemia is the earliest finding and is manifested by alteration of the T waves, whereas MI is the most advanced stage, which is manifested by alteration of the QRS complex when dealing with Q wave MI. Myocardial injury, which is manifested by alteration of the S-T segment, is the intermediate stage between myocardial ischemia and Q wave MI. An early phase of acute Q wave MI produces characteristically all three stages of ischemia (outer layer of the heart), injury (middle layer of the heart), and necrosis (center of the heart) as shown in Figure 5-1. It should be noted, however, that subendocardial (non–Q wave) MI produces no QRS change.

The majority of cases of myocardial ischemia, injury, and infarction are due to CAD, but on rare occasions they may be due to other causes such as cardiac trauma or acute anemia.

The location of myocardial ischemia, injury, and infarction is expressed according to the abnormality shown in specific ECG leads. For example, abnormalities shown in leads II, III, and aVF indicate diaphragmatic (inferior) wall involvement. Involvement of the anterior wall is best shown in leads V_{1-6}. In posterior wall involvement, only indirect evidence (reciprocal change) is shown in leads V_{1-3} because there is no ECG lead facing the posterior wall. Atrial MI and right ventricular MI are difficult to diagnose by the ordinary 12-lead ECG, but more reliable diagnostic criteria of right ventricular MI have been established.

Clinically, ECG findings recorded while patients with angina pectoris are resting are often normal. It is common to observe myocardial ischemia or injury on the ECG only during chest pain, and then the ECG returns to normal when the pain subsides. This is particularly so when dealing with coronary artery spasm. The exercise ECG test, Holter monitor ECG, myocardial imaging, or coronary arteriography in patients with angina pectoris often show a significant abnormality.

Characteristic ECG findings (see Fig. 5-1) are observed in approximately 80–85% of patients with acute Q wave MI. However, the ECG may only show S-T segment or T wave abnormalities even in proven cases of acute MI, particularly in non–Q wave MI (subendocardial infarction), right ventricular MI, diaphragmatic (inferior) MI, and posterior MI. In addition, when MI becomes old, the ECG may become completely normal, especially in cases of diaphrag-

Figure 5-1
*Myocardial ischemia, injury, and infarction
compared with a normal myocardium.
During acute myocardial infarction, the electrocardiogram discloses all three stages,
including ischemia (outer layer of heart),
injury (middle layer of heart), and necrosis
(center of heart), as shown in diagram D.
(A = normal myocardium; B = myocardial
ischemia; C = myocardial injury and ischemia;
D = myocardial ischemia, injury, and necrosis
(acute myocardial infarction); E = subacute
myocardial infarction; F = old myocardial
infarction.)*

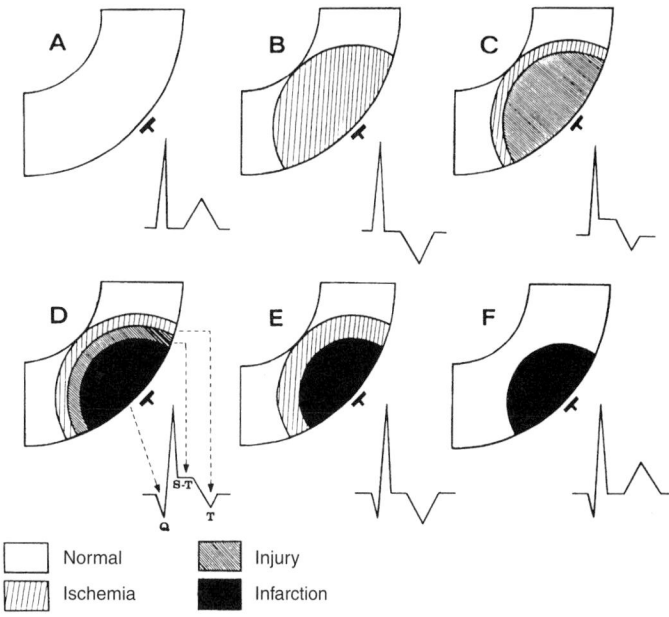

matic MI or posterior MI. Therefore, a normal ECG, particularly when the patient is at rest, by no means excludes CAD. Conversely, an abnormal ECG does not necessarily mean a diseased heart.

Various ECG findings that may resemble CAD (*pseudo-MI*) are discussed later in this chapter. The diagnosis of MI is often difficult in the presence of bundle branch block, especially left bundle branch block (LBBB). This aspect is also discussed later in this chapter. It should be noted that LBBB or right bundle branch block (RBBB) and bifascicular block themselves may actually be due to acute MI (Table 5-1).

As described in Chapters 1 and 2, the repolarization process moves from epicardium to endocardium in a normal heart (see Fig 1-4). In subendocardial ischemia, a delayed recovery in the subendocardial layers does not reverse the direction of the repolarization process because the repolarization is primarily influenced by the intact subepicardial recovery process. As a result, subendocardial ischemia produces prolongation of the Q-T interval. In addition, the magnitude of the T wave is usually increased because the subendocardial ischemic layers continue to repolarize for a time after opposing repolarization potentials from intact subepicardial layers have begun to subside. Thus, a characteristic finding of subendocardial ischemia is the presence of tall and upright T waves with prolonged Q-T intervals. It should be noted that subendocardial ischemia may resemble ECG findings due to hyperkalemia, quinidine effects, or central nervous system (CNS) disorders (see Chapters 16 and 17).

When ischemic change takes place in the subepicardial layers, the onset of the repolarization process is markedly delayed in the subepicardium as compared to the repolarization process in the subendocardium. Thus, intact subendocardial layers start the repolarization process before the ischemic subepicardial layers. Namely, the direction of the repolarization process is reversed (from endocardium to epicardium) in subepicardial ischemia. Thus, subepicardial ischemia is manifested by inverted T waves that are primary T wave changes. When both subendocardial and subepicardial layers develop ischemia, the end result is the same as subepicardial ischemia. Characteristically, subepicardial ischemia is manifested by a deeply and symmetrically inverted T wave.

Subepicardial ischemia can be recognized in the presence of an artificial pacemaker-induced ventricular rhythm, LBBB, or RBBB because the primary T wave change replaces the secondary T wave change.

Table 5-1. Pseudomyocardial infarction patterns

Wolff-Parkinson-White syndrome
    Diaphragmatic MI
    Anteroseptal MI
    Posterior MI
Idiopathic hypertrophic subaortic stenosis
    Diaphragmatic MI
    Posterior MI
    Diaphragmatic posterolateral MI
Left bundle branch block and left ventricular hypertrophy
    Anteroseptal MI
    Anterior MI
    Diaphragmatic MI
Left anterior hemiblock and left axis deviation
    Diaphragmatic MI
    Anterior MI
Chronic pulmonary obstructive disease and right
    ventricular hypertrophy due to other causes
    Diaphragmatic MI
    Posterior MI
    Anteroseptal MI
    Anterior MI

Cardiomyopathy
    Any MI pattern
Chest deformity
    Anteroseptal MI
    Anterior MI
    Anterolateral MI
    Diaphragmatic MI
Normal variant
    Anteroseptal MI
    Anterior MI
    Posterior MI
Ectopic beats and rhythm
    Any MI pattern
Miscellaneous (many different patterns)
    Pericarditis
    Mitral valve prolapse syndrome
    Pulmonary embolism
    Central nervous system disorders
    Hyperkalemia

MI = myocardial infarction.

It should be emphasized that persisting T wave inversion may indicate non–Q wave MI (subendocardial infarction), provided that the diagnosis of acute MI is established by serum enzyme elevation and clinical findings (discussed later in this chapter).

Various conditions may produce alteration of the S-T segment on the ECG. However, a horizontal to down-sloping depression or elevation of the S-T segment usually indicates myocardial injury. More specifically, subendocardial injury produces S-T segment depression, whereas subepicardial injury produces S-T segment elevation. When both subendocardial and subepicardial layers are injured, the end result is the same finding as a pure subepicardial injury. This is observed because the electrical potential is much greater in the subepicardial injury. During the early phase (the first 24–72 hours) of acute Q wave MI, there is always evidence of subepicardial injury. When there is marked subendocardial or subepicardial injury, the lead facing opposite to the injured area may produce significant reciprocal S-T segment changes.

As far as the fundamental mechanism responsible for the production of the S-T segment depression in subendocardial injury is concerned, the concept of the blocking of depolarization is generally accepted. It is postulated that the depolarization process is blocked at the boundaries of the injured zone. As a result, the injured zone retains fewer positive charges at a time when the uninjured zone elsewhere has been completely depolarized. Because of the fewer positive charges, just prior to repolarization, the systolic current of injury moves toward the injured zone. Namely, the systolic current of injury moving away from the electrode produces S-T segment depression in subendocardial injury.

Transient subepicardial injury is rather uncommon as compared with subendocardial injury. Angina pectoris, which produces S-T segment elevation (subepicardial injury) rather than depression (subendocardial injury), is considered to be due to coronary artery spasm in many cases. Coronary artery spasm may occur spontaneously, but it may easily be produced by various provocative tests, including ergonovine injection and the cold pressor test. Coronary artery spasm may or may not coexist with fixed coronary artery stenosis. Coronary artery spasm may cause acute MI or even sudden death.

Persisting subepicardial injury almost always progresses to acute Q wave MI. It is also common to observe marked subepicardial injury without significant Q waves during the very early phase of acute Q wave MI.

Subepicardial injury is usually associated with significant reciprocal S-T segment depression in leads facing the area opposite to the injured zone. For example, diaphragmatic subepicardial injury produces a reciprocal S-T segment depression in leads I and aVL. Posterior subepicardial injury, on the other hand, is diagnosed by recognizing only reciprocal S-T segment depression in leads V_{1-3} as indirect evidence because no lead is available to record posterior injury directly.

The fundamental mechanism responsible for the production of the S-T segment elevation in subepicardial injury can be explained in the same manner as described for the subendocardial injury. That is, the systolic current injury, just prior to repolarization, moves toward the injured zone in the subepicardium. The S-T segment elevation is produced because the systolic current in subepicardial injury is moving toward the electrode.

It is important to remember that Q wave MI can be diagnosed only when the abnormality involves two or more ECG leads facing the same damaged area. An abnormal Q wave in only one lead is *not* diagnostic of MI. This is especially true in lead III. It is generally observed that a Q wave in lead III not due to MI usually disappears or becomes very small during deep inspiration. Thus, lead III may be taken during inspiration whenever a Q wave is present in this lead.

The ECG diagnostic criteria of abnormal Q waves are summarized as follows:

- A Q wave width of 0.04 second or more
- A Q wave depth of 25% or more of the R wave depth

The ECG diagnostic criteria of MI from the viewpoint of involved location are summarized as follows:

- In anteroseptal MI, Q or Q-S waves in leads V_{1-3}
- In anterior (localized) MI, Q or Q-S waves in leads V_{2-4}
- In anterolateral MI, Q or Q-S waves in leads V_{4-6}
- In high lateral MI, Q or Q-S waves in leads I and aVL
- In extensive anterior MI, Q or Q-S waves in leads I, aVL, and V_{1-6}
- In diaphragmatic (inferior) MI, Q or Q-S waves in leads II, III, and aVF

- In posterior MI, tall (or relatively tall) R waves in leads V_{1-3}

MI can involve more than one location simultaneously or on separate occasions. It is common to observe MI involving the diaphragmatic and lateral walls simultaneously (diaphragmatic and lateral MI). In addition, MI involving the posterior, diaphragmatic, and lateral walls together (diaphragmatic posterolateral MI [DPLMI]) is not uncommon. At times, the anterior and diaphragmatic walls are infarcted.

Isolated right ventricular MI is a rare occurrence, observed in no more than 2% of autopsy data. In most cases, right ventricular MI is associated with diaphragmatic MI of the left ventricle. It has been shown that 20–40% of cases of diaphragmatic MI reveal coexisting right ventricular MI.

The diagnosis of right ventricular MI is rather difficult because the characteristic ECG findings are often not registered in the conventional 12-lead ECG. One of the main reasons for this is that any change in the right ventricle may not be recorded on the routine ECG because the electrical potential generated by right ventricular activation is negligible in comparison with that of left ventricular activation. Therefore, the additional right precordial leads (leads V_{3R-6R}) are often necessary to diagnose right ventricular MI.

In recent years, the diagnosis of right ventricular MI has been made more frequently because the entity is readily recognizable by physicians with up-to-date knowledge. On the conventional 12-lead ECG, the most reliable finding to establish the diagnosis of right ventricular MI is marked S-T segment elevation (of ≥1 mm) in leads V_{1-3}. The S-T segment elevation is most pronounced in lead V1 and the magnitude of S-T segment elevation progressively reduced toward leads V_5 and V_6. This ECG finding resembles acute anteroseptal MI.

Atrial MI usually occurs in conjunction with massive ventricular MI. Therefore, the diagnosis of atrial infarction should not be made when no evidence of ventricular infarction is present. Although the **diagnosis of atrial infarction** is never certain, the following findings may indicate atrial MI:

- Elevation or depression of the P-R segment
- Sudden appearance of atrial arrhythmias
- Bizarre configuration of P waves

When MI is complicated by bundle branch block, the diagnosis of MI is often difficult or even impossible. The recognition of MI in the presence of RBBB is relatively easy. The reason for this is that the MI usually alters the initial portion of the QRS complex, whereas the RBBB produces marked alteration of the terminal 0.04-second vectors during ventricular activation. The recognition of MI is extremely difficult or at times impossible in the presence of LBBB because the alteration of the QRS complex is primarily influenced by the latter. Old MI is more difficult to recognize than acute MI under this circumstance.

When acute MI develops in the presence of bundle branch block, alteration of the S-T segment and T wave is observed because of ischemia and injury. For example, instead of the secondary T wave change in bundle branch block, the primary T wave change occurs and replaces the secondary T wave change. In addition, the S-T segment elevation is observed when the S-T segment depression is expected to be present in uncomplicated bundle branch block (leads V_{4-6} in LBBB and leads V_{1-3} in RBBB). These S-T segment and T wave changes will not be observed when MI becomes old.

SUBENDOCARDIAL ISCHEMIA

Definition

Subendorcardial ischemia is myocardial ischemia involving primarily the subendocardial zone of the left ventricle.

Diagnostic Criteria (Fig. 5-2)

- Increased amplitude of T waves in two or more ECG leads facing the ischemic zone
- Often associated with broad T waves
- Often associated with a prolonged Q-T interval

Diagnostic Pearls

Subendocardial ischemia is usually a transient ECG phenomenon, but a persisting subendocardial ischemia may lead to acute MI. Subendocardial ischemia should be differentiated from hyperkalemia and CNS disorders (see Chapters 16 and 17).

Figure 5-2
Diffuse subendocardial ischemia.

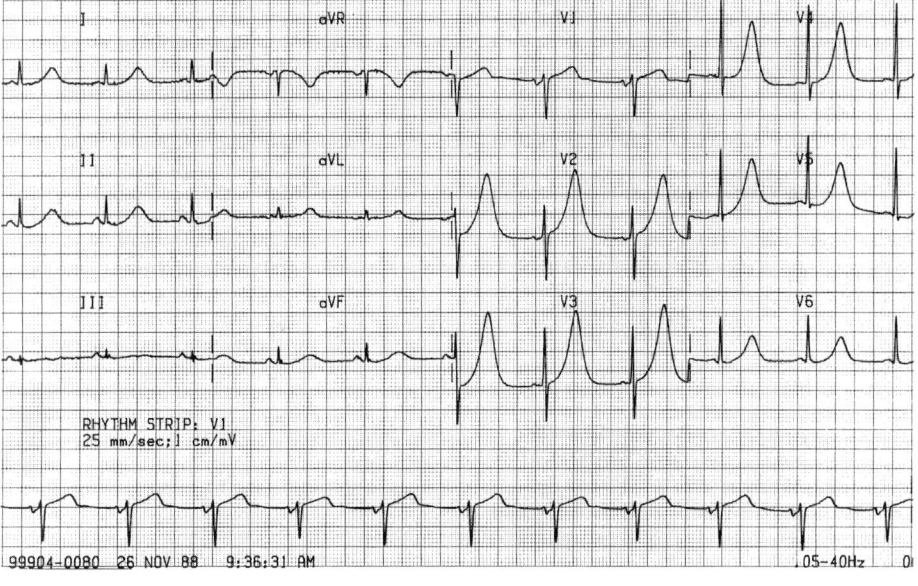

SUBEPICARDIAL ISCHEMIA

Definition

Subepicardial ischemia is myocardial ischemia involving primarily the subepicardial zone of the left ventricle.

Diagnostic Criteria (Fig. 5-3)

- Deeply and symmetrically inverted T waves in two or more ECG leads facing the ischemic zone
- Little or no prolongation of T wave width or Q-T interval

Diagnostic Pearls

Inverted T waves should involve two or more leads facing subepicardial ischemia. When subendocardial and subepicardial ischemia occur simultaneously, the end result is the same as a pure subepicardial ischemia. Subepicardial ischemia may mimic myocarditis, pericarditis, or even CNS disorders (see Chapter 17).

Figure 5-3
Diffuse subepicardial ischemia.

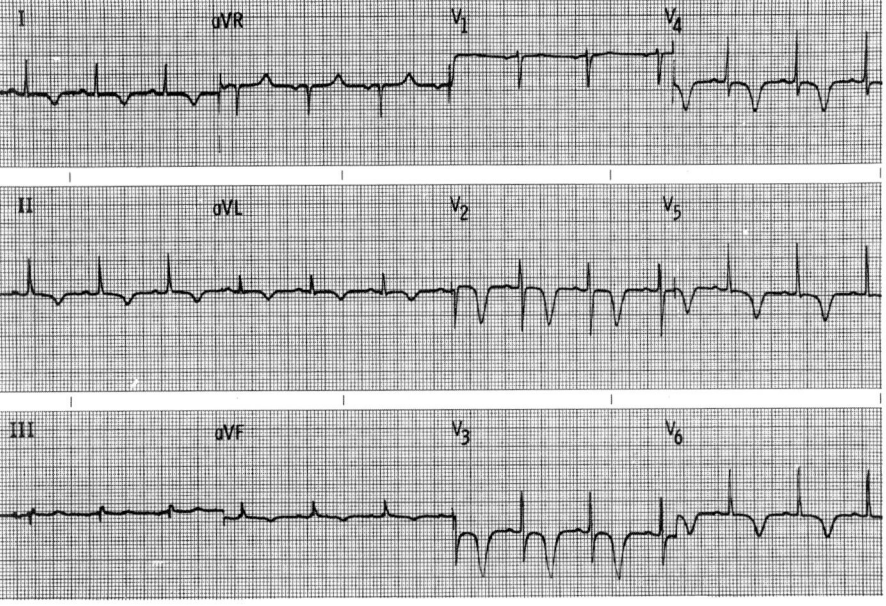

SUBENDOCARDIAL INJURY

Definition

Subendocardial injury is myocardial injury primarily involving the subendocardial zone of the left ventricle.

Diagnostic Criteria (Fig. 5-4)

- Horizontal to down-sloping S-T segment depression (usually ≥1 mm) in two or more ECG leads facing the injured zone.
- Any factors causing the S-T segment depression (e.g., digitalis effect, LVH, LBBB, etc.) should be absent.
- S-T segment depression may be associated with biphasic to slightly inverted (not symmetric) T waves.

Diagnostic Pearls

Subendocardial injury is often a transient phenomenon, but persisting subendocardial injury may lead to non–Q wave MI. It is important to remember that there are many factors that may cause ECG findings closely mimicking subendocardial injury. Typically, digitalis effects in some cases superficially resemble subendocardial injury. Subendocardial injury is frequently provoked by physical exercise in patients with CAD.

Figure 5-4
Subendocardial injury. The rhythm strips A, B, and C are not continuous (lead II).

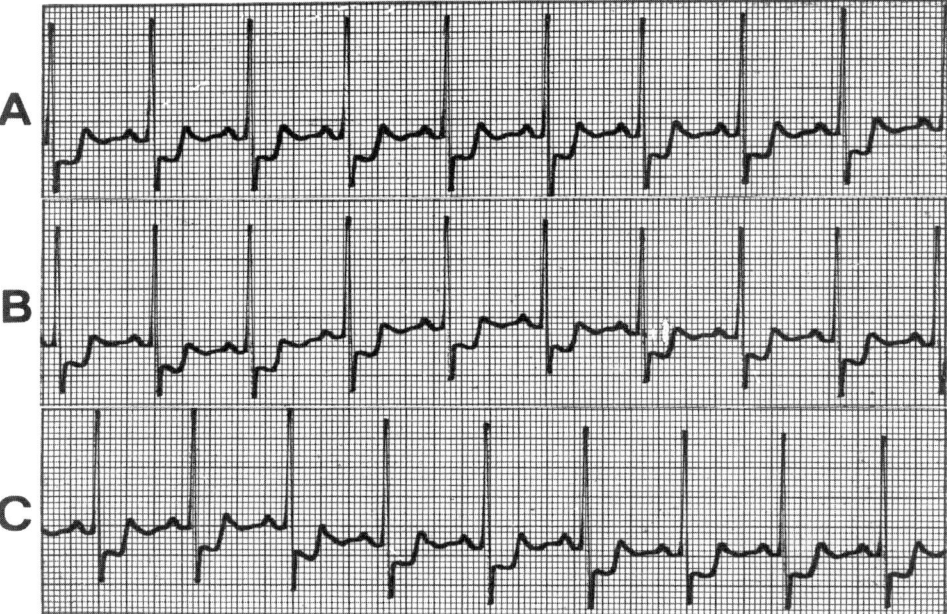

SUBEPICARDIAL INJURY

Definition

Subepicardial injury is myocardial injury primarily involving the subepicardial zone of the left ventricle.

Diagnostic Criteria (Fig. 5-5)

- S-T segment elevation (≥1 mm up-sloping or horizontal) in two or more ECG leads facing injured zone
- Reciprocal S-T segment depression in other ECG leads in the opposite area from the injured zone

Diagnostic Pearls

Subepicardial injury is often a transient phenomenon, but persisting S-T segment elevation frequently leads to acute MI. When S-T segment elevation involves practically every ECG lead diffusely, acute pericarditis is most likely the diagnosis (see Chapter 17). Subepicardial injury should be distinguished from the early repolarization pattern (normal variant), in which "J-point elevation" is the main ECG finding (see Chapter 2).

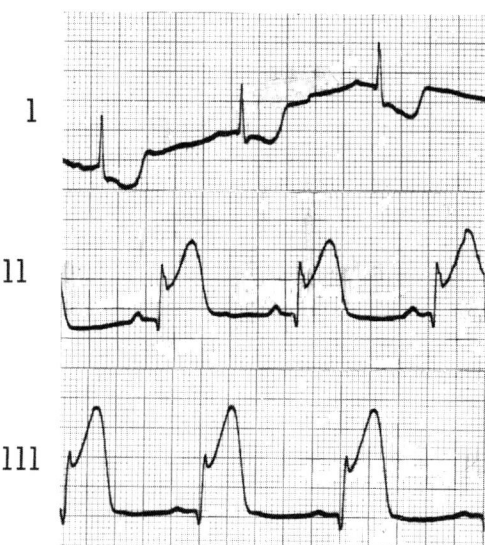

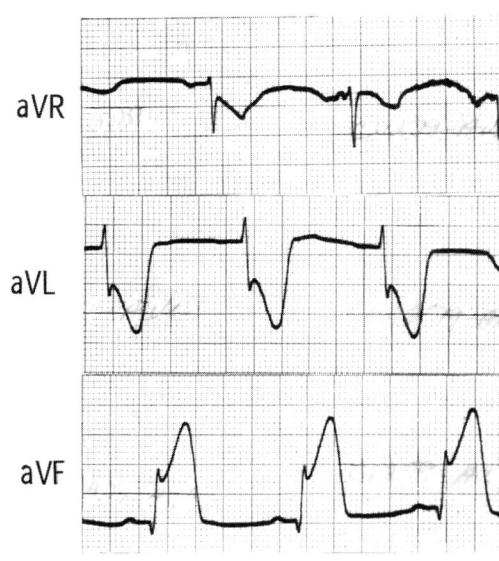

Figure 5-5
Diaphragmatic (inferior) subepicardial injury.

CORONARY ARTERY SPASM

Definition

Coronary artery spasm involves one or more coronary arteries and is associated with chest pain. Coronary artery spasm may or may not be associated with underlying fixed coronary artery lesion(s).

Diagnostic Criteria

The following are present in coronary artery spasm (Fig. 5-6):

- S-T segment elevation in two or more ECG leads facing the involved artery associated with chest pain.
- Coronary artery spasm may occur spontaneously, but it may be provoked by various maneuvers, including the ergonovine test, cold pressor test, and so forth.
- Coronary artery spasm may involve only one artery, but multiple arteries may be involved.
- ECG findings may return to normal when coronary artery spasm subsides.

Diagnostic Pearls

Coronary artery spasm should be differentiated from acute pericarditis, subepicardial injury not due to spasm, and early ECG findings of acute MI and an early repolarization pattern (see Chapters 2 and 17). It should be pointed out that coronary artery spasm may lead to acute MI and sudden death in severe cases.

Figure 5-6

A 41-year-old man was admitted to the hospital because of recurrent chest pain even at rest. Tracing A was obtained on admission while he was complaining of chest pain. Tracing B was taken several hours later when the pain had subsided. In A, there is a marked elevation of the S-T segment in leads II, III, aVF, V_5, and V_6, accompanied by reciprocal S-T segment depression in leads aVR, aVL, and V_{1-3}. These findings indicate diaphragmatic posterolateral subepicardial injury. In B, however, taken several hours after A—when he was free of chest pain—the electrocardiogram is normal. This transient S-T segment elevation is considered to be due to coronary artery spasm.

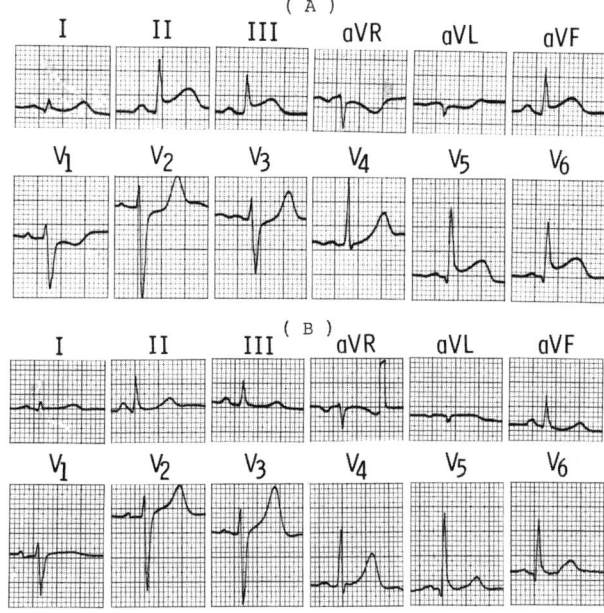

NON–Q WAVE MYOCARDIAL INFARCTION

Definition

Non–Q wave MI involves the subendocardial zone of the left ventricle. Non–Q wave MI has other ECG terms, including subendocardial MI and nontransmural MI.

Diagnostic Criteria (Fig. 5-7)

• No abnormal Q wave
• Persisting S-T segment depression (horizontal to down-sloping) of 1 mm or more
• Persisting symmetric T wave inversion
• Elevation of creatine phosphokinase (CPK) with MB isoenzyme

Diagnostic Pearls

When the ECG changes are transient (<30 minutes) without serum CPK elevation, the diagnosis of angina pectoris has to be made (*not* non–Q wave MI). The findings of persisting S-T segment depression and/or T wave inversion without serum CPK elevation are difficult to label clinically. All other underlying disorders or drugs that produce S-T segment depression and/or T wave inversion should be considered for the differential diagnosis.

Figure 5-7
Anterior non–Q wave myocardial infarction. Note marked S-T segment depression in all precordial leads. Other electrocardiographic abnormalities include low voltage (see Chapter 17) and a remote possibility of diaphragmatic myocardial infarction.

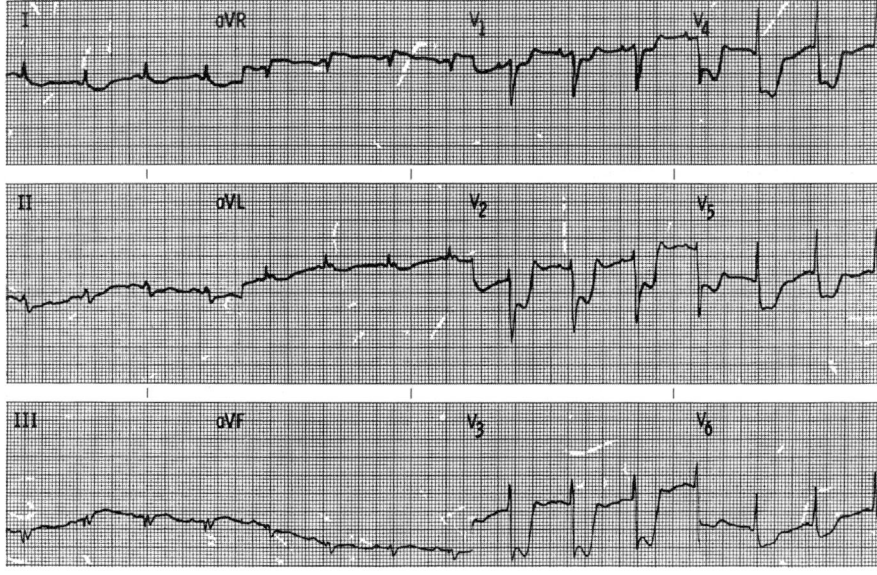

ANTEROSEPTAL MYOCARDIAL INFARCTION

Definition

Anteroseptal myocardial infarction (ASMI) involves the ventricular septum of the left ventricle.

Diagnostic Criteria (Fig. 5-8)

- Abnormal Q waves in leads V_{1-3} (up to lead V_4 in some cases)
- The S-T segment elevation and T wave inversion during the first 72 hours in the same ECG leads

Diagnostic Pearls

In the very early stage of acute ASMI, the S-T segment elevation in leads V_{1-3} may resemble acute right ventricular MI; however, no Q wave is observed in right ventricular MI. The T wave inversion in leads V_{1-3} may last for many weeks, months, or even years after acute ASMI.

Figure 5-8
Recent anteroseptal myocardial infarction with diffuse anterior ischemia.

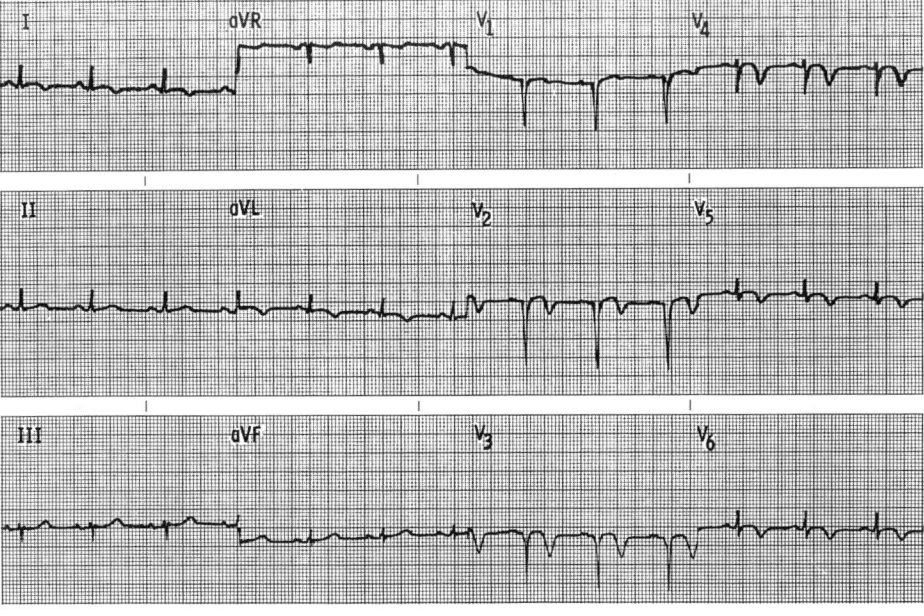

ANTERIOR (LOCALIZED) MYOCARDIAL INFARCTION

Definition

Anterior (localized) myocardial infarction (AMI) involves the anterior wall (localized) of the left ventricle.

Diagnostic Criteria (Fig. 5-9)

- Abnormal Q waves in leads V_{2-4} (only in leads V_{3-4} in some cases)
- The S-T segment elevation with T wave inversion in these ECG leads during the first 72 hours

Diagnostic Pearls

In AMI, the ventricular septal activation is normal. Thus, lead V_1 shows the expected small R wave in AMI. The T wave inversion may last for many weeks, months, or even years in leads V_{2-4} after acute AMI.

Figure 5-9
Localized anterior myocardial infarction. Note a ventricular premature contraction in lead V_6 (marked V).

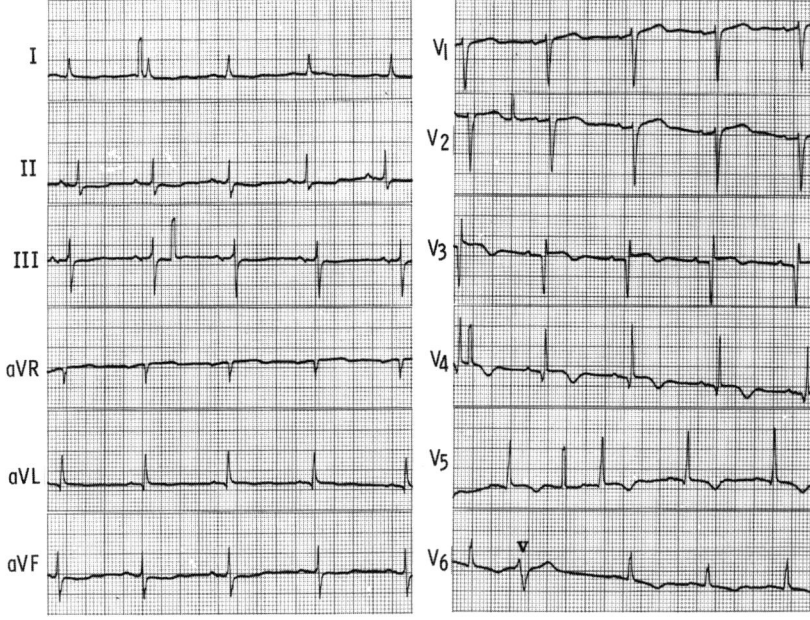

ANTEROLATERAL MYOCARDIAL INFARCTION

Definition

Anterolateral myocardial infarction (ALMI) involves the lateral wall of the left ventricle.

Diagnostic Criteria (Fig. 5-10)

- Abnormal Q waves in leads V_{4-6} (only in leads V_{5-6} in some cases)
- S-T segment elevation with T wave inversion in these ECG leads during the first 72 hours

Diagnostic Pearls

ALMI is often called lateral MI (same meaning). ALMI often coexists with high lateral MI, diaphragmatic (inferior) MI, and posterior MI.

Figure 5-10
Anterolateral myocardial infarction associated with acute diaphragmatic (inferior) myocardial infarction.

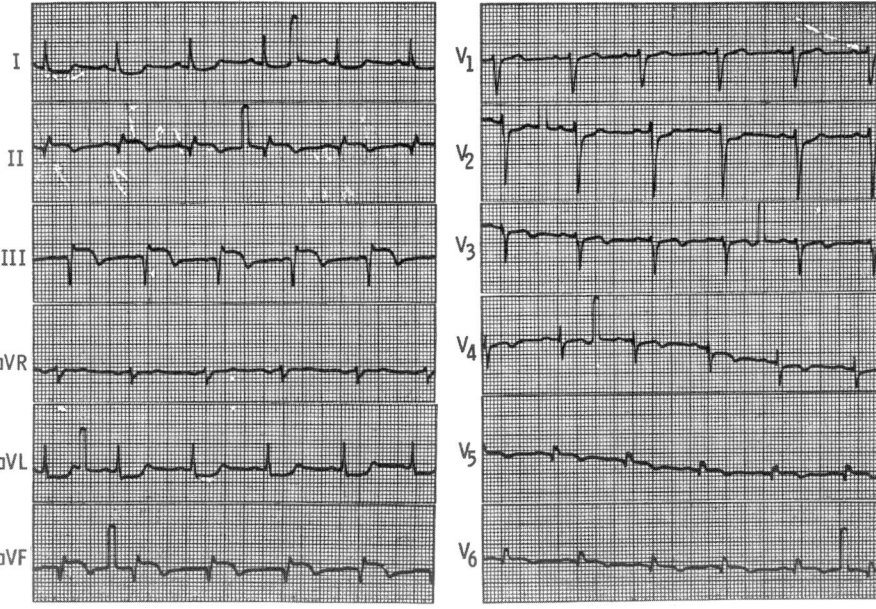

HIGH LATERAL MYOCARDIAL INFARCTION

Definition

High lateral myocardial infarction (HLMI) involves the higher portion of the left ventricular lateral wall.

Diagnostic Criteria (Fig. 5-11)

- Abnormal Q waves in leads I and aVL
- S-T segment elevation with T wave inversion in these ECG leads during the first 72 hours

Diagnostic Pearls

HLMI often coexists with posterior MI, diaphragmatic MI, and ALMI. HLMI is frequently missed by inexperienced readers.

Figure 5-11
High lateral myocardial infarction. Note Q wave or Q-S wave in leads I and aVL associated with T wave inversion. In addition, a possibility of posterior myocardial infarction is considered (see Fig. 5-14).

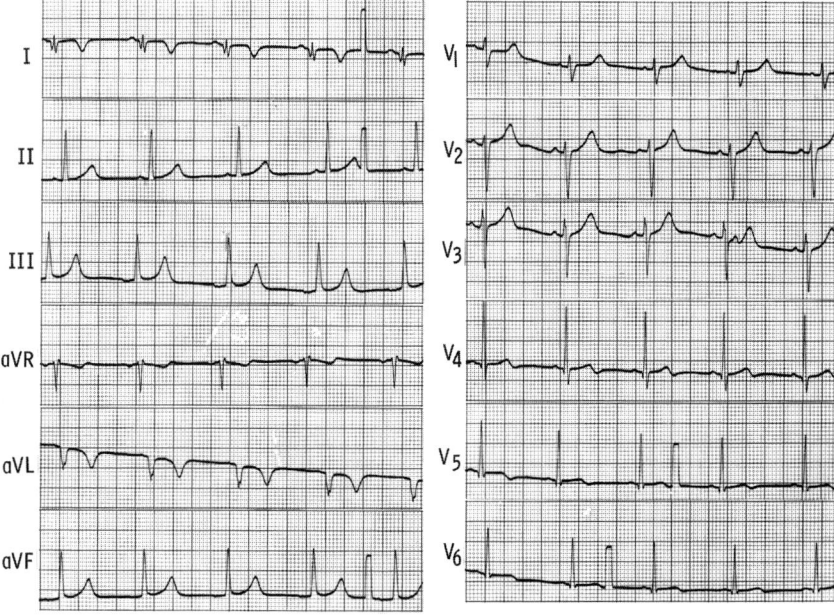

EXTENSIVE ANTERIOR MYOCARDIAL INFARCTION

Definition

Extensive anterior MI involves the entire anterior wall of the left ventricle.

Diagnostic Criteria

The following are present in extensive anterior MI (Fig. 5-12):

- Abnormal Q waves in leads V_{1-6}
- Abnormal Q waves in leads I and aVL (not an essential finding)
- S-T segment elevation with T wave inversion in these ECG leads during the first 72 hours

Diagnostic Pearls

Extensive anterior MI is frequently called massive anterior MI. Extensive anterior MI is actually a combination of ASMI, AMI, ALMI, and HLMI. The presence of HLMI is not essential for the diagnosis of extensive anterior MI.

Figure 5-12
Acute extensive anterior myocardial infarction.

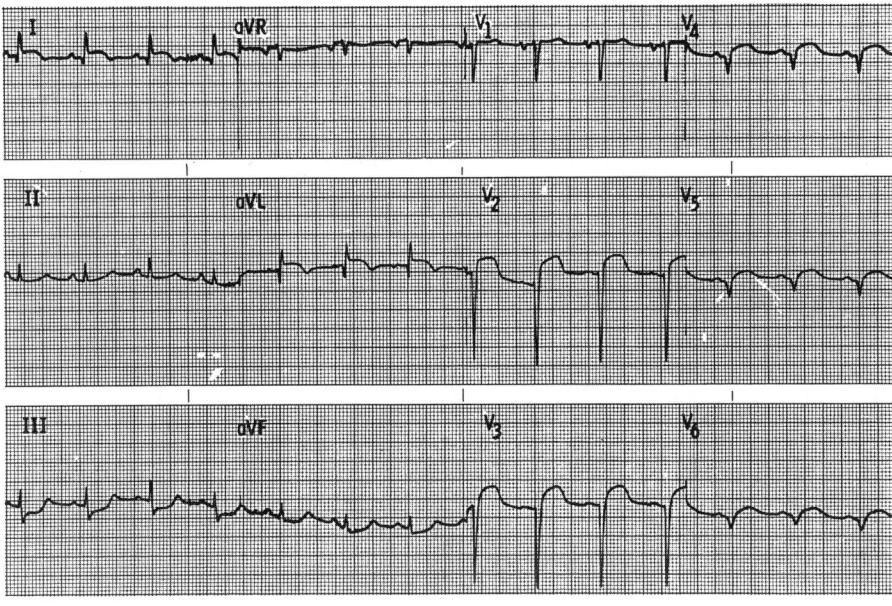

DIAPHRAGMATIC (INFERIOR) MYOCARDIAL INFARCTION

Definition

Diaphragmatic (inferior) myocardial infarction (DMI) involves the inferior wall of the left ventricle.

Diagnostic Criteria (Fig. 5-13)

- Abnormal Q waves in leads II, III, and aVF (in at least two of these leads)
- The S-T segment elevation with T wave inversion in these ECG leads during the first 72 hours

Diagnostic Pearls

DMI often coexists with posterior MI and lateral MI, leading to DPLMI. The Q-S waves are *not* reliable findings to diagnose DMI.

Figure 5-13
Recent diaphragmatic (inferior) myocardial infarction.

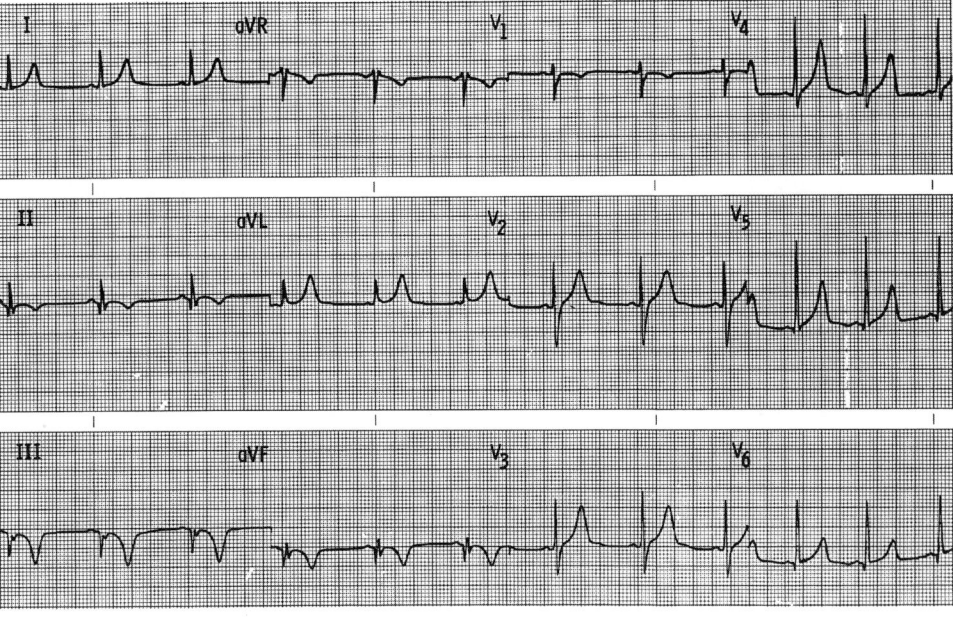

POSTERIOR MYOCARDIAL INFARCTION

Definition

Posterior myocardial infarction (PMI) involves the posterior wall of the left ventricle.

Diagnostic Criteria (Fig. 5-14)

- Tall (or relatively) tall R waves in leads V_{1-3} (only in V_{1-2} in some cases)
- The S-T segment (horizontal) depression with upright T waves in these ECG leads during the first 72 hours

Diagnostic Pearls

PMI fails to produce abnormal Q waves because there are no ECG leads facing the posterior wall. Thus, the above-mentioned diagnostic ECG findings of PMI are reciprocal ECG changes. PMI often coexists with diaphragmatic and lateral MI, leading to DPLMI (Fig. 5-15). PMI is frequently missed by inexperienced readers.

Figure 5-14
Posterior myocardial infarction. Note a tall R wave in lead V_1 with an upright and tall T wave. In addition, lateral ischemia is considered (inverted/biphasic T wave in lead V_6).

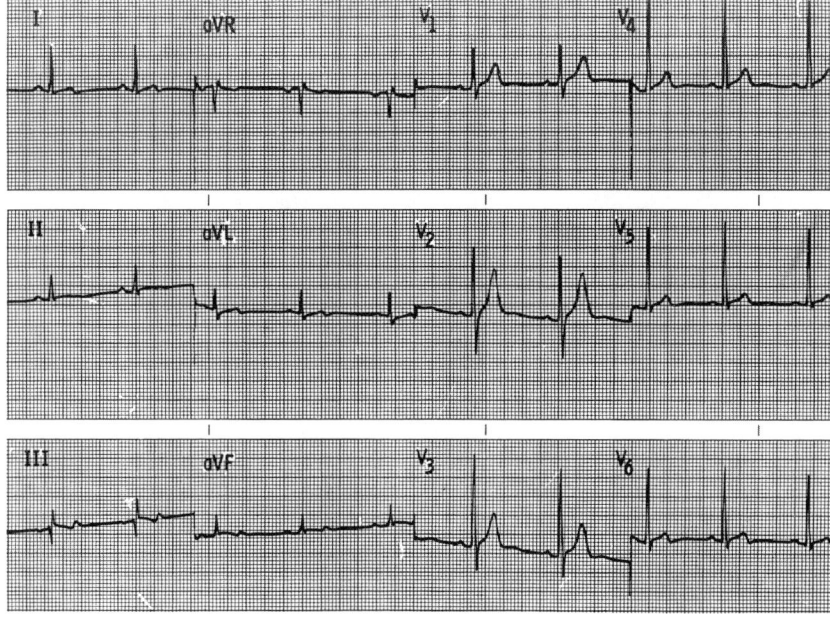

DIAPHRAGMATIC POSTEROLATERAL MYOCARDIAL INFARCTION

Definition

DPLMI involves the inferior, posterior, and lateral walls of the left ventricle diffusely.

Diagnostic Criteria (Fig. 5-15)

- Abnormal Q waves in leads II, III, aVF, and V_{4-6}
- Tall (or relatively tall) R waves in leads V_{1-3}
- S-T segment elevation with T wave inversion in leads II, III, aVF, and V_{4-6} during the first 72 hours
- Reciprocal S-T segment depression in leads V_{1-3} with upright (often tall) T waves in these leads during the first 72 hours
- Abnormal Q waves in leads I and aVL with S-T segment elevation and T wave inversion during the first 72 hours in some cases

Diagnostic Pearls

DPLMI is actually a combination of DMI, PMI, and ALMI. Often, the high lateral wall of the left ventricle is involved together (HLMI). DPLMI is frequently misdiagnosed by inexperienced readers.

Figure 5-15
Diaphragmatic posterolateral myocardial infarction. Note Q waves in leads I, II, III, aVF, and V$_{4-6}$ associated with tall R waves in leads V$_1$ and V$_2$ with tall T waves.

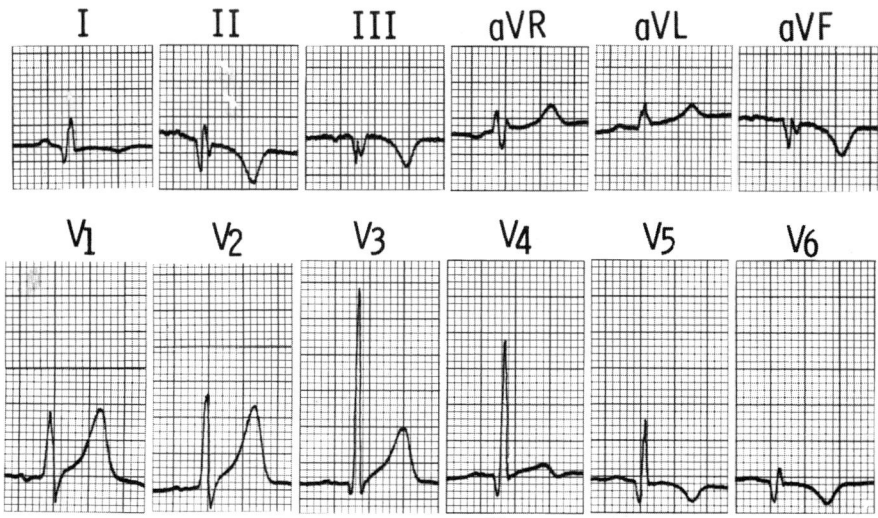

RIGHT VENTRICULAR MYOCARDIAL INFARCTION

Definition

Myocardial infarction involving the right ventricle.

Diagnostic Criteria (Fig. 5-16)

- S-T segment elevation (of ≥1 mm) in leads V_{1-3}
- S-T segment elevation (of ≥1 mm) in leads V_1 and V_{3R-6R}
- S-T segment elevation in leads V_{1-6} (marked in lead V_1 and least in lead V_6)
- Often associated with acute DMI of the left ventricle
- Reduction of R' wave amplitude in leads V_{1-2} with reduction of depth of S waves in leads V_{4-6} in the presence of RBBB

Diagnostic Pearls

In right ventricular MI, abnormal Q waves are *not* produced. An early stage of ECG finding in acute ASMI of the left ventricle superficially resembles right ventricular MI, but ASMI eventually produces the characteristic abnormal Q waves (or Q-S waves; see Fig. 5-8). Taking additional right precordial leads (leads V_{3R-6R}) is often beneficial in the diagnosis of right ventricular MI.

Figure 5-16
Acute right ventricular MI. Note marked S-T segment elevation in leads V$_{1-3}$ (most pronounced in lead V$_1$).

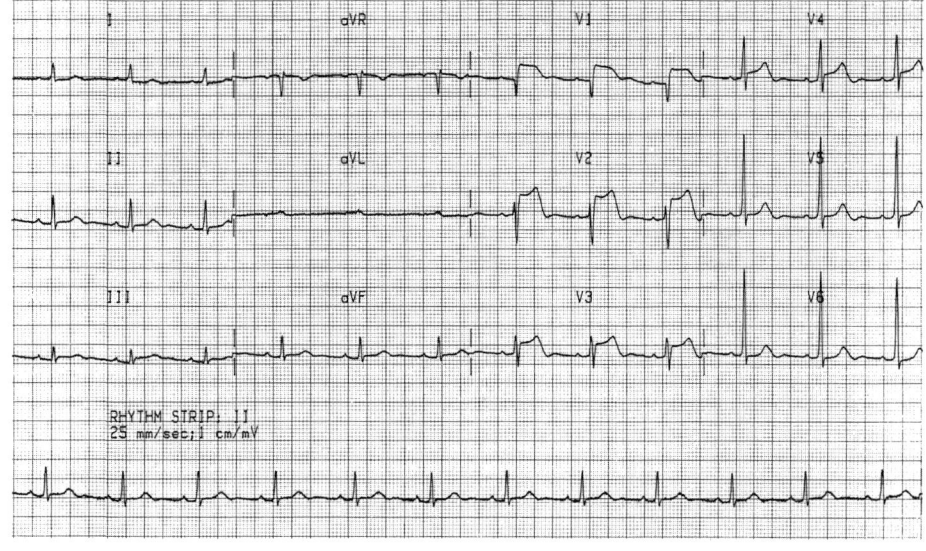

RIGHT BUNDLE BRANCH BLOCK ASSOCIATED WITH ANTEROSEPTAL MYOCARDIAL INFARCTION

Definition

RBBB associated with ASMI is ASMI with preexisting RBBB or RBBB due to ASMI.

Diagnostic Criteria (Fig. 5-17)

- Abnormal Q waves in leads V_{1-3}
- S-T segment elevation with T wave inversion in these ECG leads during the first 72 hours
- Diagnostic criteria of RBBB (discussed previously)

Diagnostic Pearls

The ECG finding is actually a combination of ASMI and RBBB. The diagnosis is relatively easy because the first half of the QRS complex is abnormal in leads V_{1-3} due to ASMI, whereas the last half of the QRS complex is abnormal as a result of RBBB. Nevertheless, inexperienced readers often fail to recognize ASMI in the presence of RBBB.

Figure 5-17
Acute anteroseptal myocardial infarction associated with right bundle branch block (see Fig. 4-4). Other electrocardiographic abnormalities include low voltage (see Chapter 17) and a remote possibility of diaphragmatic myocardial infarction.

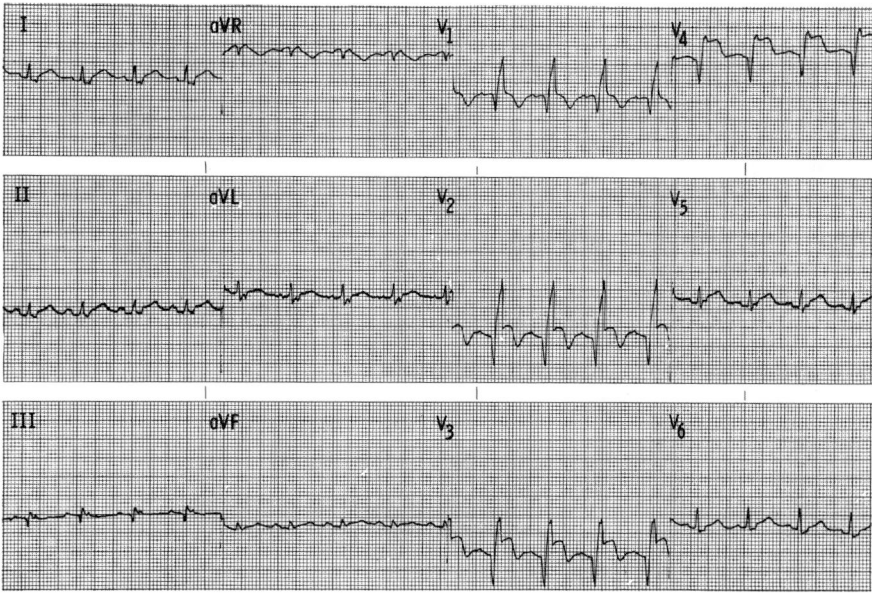

RIGHT BUNDLE BRANCH BLOCK ASSOCIATED WITH DIAPHRAGMATIC MYOCARDIAL INFARCTION

Definition

DMI occurs in the presence of preexisting or new RBBB.

Diagnostic Criteria (Fig. 5-18)

- Abnormal Q waves in leads II, III, and aVF
- S-T segment elevation with T wave inversion in these ECG leads during the first 72 hours
- Diagnostic criteria of RBBB (discussed previously)

Diagnostic Pearls

The characteristic ECG finding of RBBB is shown in the precordial leads, but there are diagnostic Q waves in leads II, III, and aVF.

Figure 5-18
Diaphragmatic (inferior) myocardial infarction associated with right bundle branch block (see Fig. 4-4). Other ECG finding is diffuse anterior ischemia (inverted T waves in all precordial leads).

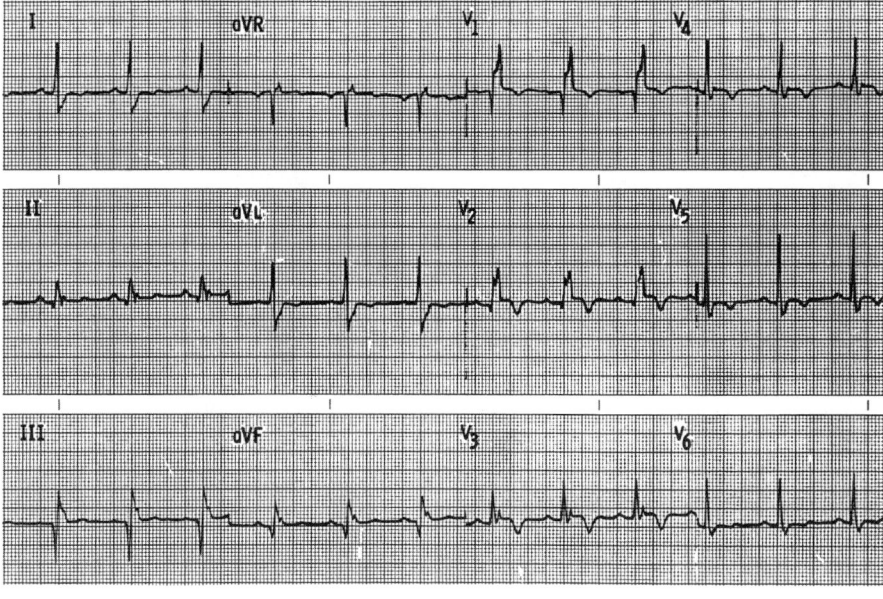

RIGHT BUNDLE BRANCH BLOCK ASSOCIATED WITH DIAPHRAGMATIC POSTEROLATERAL MYOCARDIAL INFARCTION

Definition

DPLMI occurs in the presence of preexisting or new RBBB.

Diagnostic Criteria (Fig. 5-19)

- Abnormal Q waves in leads II, III, aVF, and V_{4-6}
- S-T segment elevation with T wave inversion in these ECG leads during the first 72 hours
- Tall (or relatively tall) R waves in leads V_{1-3}
- Reciprocal S-T segment depression with upright (often tall) T waves in leads V_{1-3} during the first 72 hours
- Abnormal Q waves in leads I and aVL in some cases
- Diagnostic criteria of RBBB (described previously)

Diagnostic Pearls

The diagnosis of DMI and ALMI is relatively easy in the presence of RBBB. However, recognizing PMI is somewhat difficult in the presence of RBBB. Under this circumstance, PMI is diagnosed because the amplitude of the initial R waves in leads V_{1-3} is taller than expected in the presence of RBBB.

Figure 5-19
Diaphragmatic posterolateral myocardial infarction (see Fig. 5-15) associated with right bundle branch block (see Fig. 4-4).

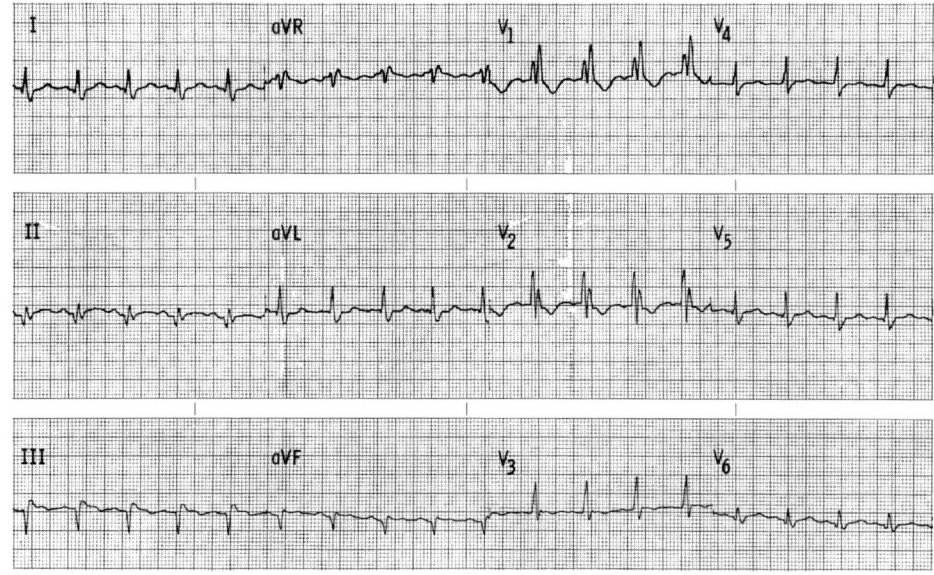

LEFT BUNDLE BRANCH BLOCK ASSOCIATED WITH ACUTE MYOCARDIAL INFARCTION

Definition

Acute MI occurs in the presence of preexisting LBBB or LBBB as a result of acute MI.

Diagnostic Criteria (Fig. 5-20)

- Primary T wave change replacing the secondary T wave change (symmetrically and deeply inverted T waves replacing biphasic or slightly inverted T waves in leads I, aVL, and V_{4-6})
- Upright or tall T waves replacing the biphasic or slightly inverted T waves in the above-mentioned ECG leads
- S-T segment elevation replacing the S-T segment depression in any ECG leads (particularly leads V_{4-6})
- Reappearance of Q waves in leads I and V_{4-6} in the presence of LBBB
- The diagnostic criteria of LBBB (described previously)

Diagnostic Pearls

The diagnostic clue of acute MI in the presence of LBBB is recognizing the primary T wave change replacing the secondary T wave change, especially in leads V_{4-6}. Old MI is often difficult or even impossible to recognize in the presence of LBBB.

Figure 5-20
Left bundle branch block (see Fig. 4-5) associated with acute anterior myocardial infarction. Note symmetric and deeply inverted T waves in all precordial leads.

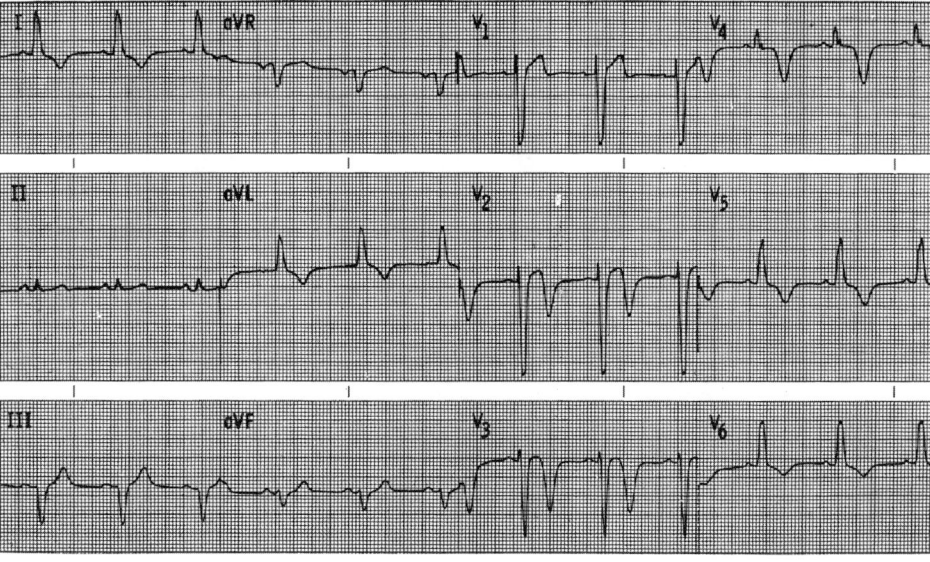

6

Diagnostic Approach to Cardiac Arrhythmias

For a detailed analysis of cardiac arrhythmias, it is preferable to have a long rhythm strip of lead II, or sometimes leads III or aVF, because these leads show the P wave most clearly. Occasionally, lead V_1 shows the P wave more clearly than the above-mentioned leads. Ideally, long rhythm strips of leads II and V_1 should be used for detailed analysis.

In selected cases, electrophysiologic studies (EPSs) may be necessary to diagnose various cardiac arrhythmias more accurately, especially when dealing with tachyarrhythmias with broad QRS complexes. By and large, the diagnostic approach to cardiac arrhythmias is summarized as follows:

1. Evaluation of the atrial activity
2. Evaluation of the QRS configuration
3. Evaluation of Ashman's phenomenon
4. Evaluation of the R-R cycles
5. Evaluation of the postectopic pause
6. Evaluation of the coupling intervals
7. Evaluation of the heart rate
8. Evaluation of the response to carotid sinus stimulation (CSS)
9. Evaluation of findings from exercise electrocardiographic testing, Holter monitor electrocardiogram (ECG), and EPS in selected cases

When the suspected cardiac arrhythmias are not recorded by repeated 12-lead ECGs, the ambulatory ECG (Holter monitor ECG) should be taken for 24–72 hours. In addition, exercise (stress) electrocardiographic testing may be indicated in selected cases when any cardiac arrhythmia is considered to be related to physical exercise. Furthermore, exercise electrocardiographic testing often provides a clinical guideline to determine the nature of a given arrhythmia in conjunction with the proper therapeutic approach.

The various cardiac arrhythmias are classified as follows:

1. Disturbances of impulse formation
2. Conduction disturbances
3. Combination of no. 1 and no. 2
4. Artificial pacemaker-induced rhythm

Various conduction disturbances may be expressed as heart blocks, but there are many types, depending on the site of the heart blocks. Not uncommonly, two or more sites may show conduction disturbances simultaneously. For instance, sinoatrial (SA) block and atrioventricular (AV) block often coexist in a patient with acute diaphragmatic myocardial infarction. Various conduction disturbances are summarized as follows:

1. SA block
2. Intra-atrial block
3. AV block
4. Intra-His block
5. Intraventricular block, including left bundle branch block (LBBB), right bundle branch block (RBBB), hemiblock, bifascicular block, trifascicular block, and nonspecific (diffuse) intraventricular block
6. Exit block
7. Combined conduction disturbances

To interpret a cardiac arrhythmia accurately, clinical significance of a given arrhythmia should always be considered. In particular, the presence or absence of significant underlying heart disease is extremely important for the proper diagnostic and therapeutic approaches to various arrhythmias. The general underlying causes of various cardiac arrhythmias are summarized as follows:

1. Cardiac diseases (e.g., coronary artery disease, rheumatic heart disease)
2. Noncardiac diseases (e.g., hyperthyroidism)
3. Electrolyte imbalances (e.g., hypokalemia, hyperkalemia)
4. Drug-induced conditions (e.g., digitalis toxicity)
5. Cocaine, coffee, alcohol, smoking, anxiety, etc.

One of the most important points to remember is to identify various artifacts that may cause electrocardiographic findings very similar to true cardiac arrhythmias. The best example is muscle tremors due to Parkinson's disease, which commonly produce artifacts superficially mimicking various cardiac arrhythmias (Figs. 6-1 and 6-2).

As described earlier (see Chapter 1), rapid heart action may originate from any portion of the heart. Thus, rapid heart action may be sinus or ectopic in origin. In addition, tachyarrhythmias may occur in paroxysmal and nonparoxysmal forms. The nonparoxysmal form may originate from a primary or ectopic pacemaker, whereas paroxysmal tachyarrhythmias are always ectopic in origin. Since sinus tachycardia can be diagnosed without any difficulty in most instances, primarily ectopic tachyarrhythmias are discussed.

Furthermore, the main discussion is focused on the differential diagnosis between various supraventricular tachyarrhythmias with wide QRS complexes and ventricular tachyarrhythmias because of their practical importance.

It should be pointed out that any supraventricular tachyarrhythmias may coexist with any ventricular tachyarrhythmias, leading to double or even triple ectopic tachyarrhythmias. On the other hand, multifocal supraventricular tachyarrhythmias, such as a combination of atrial fibrillation (AF) or atrial flutter with independent AV junctional tachycardia (JT) or double AV JT, may occur. Needless to say, these multifocal tachyarrhythmias are rare forms of AV dissociation.

Although it has been known for many years that the differential diagnosis between supraventricular tachyarrhythmias and ventricular tachyarrhythmias is extremely important in view of their management and prognosis, it is often difficult to distinguish between them. The reason for this is that supraventricular tachyarrhythmias, regardless of the fundamental mechanism involved, may closely resemble ventricular tachyarrhythmias when the QRS complex is wide in the former.

Although differential diagnosis between supraventricular tachyarrhythmias and ventricular tachyarrhythmias is

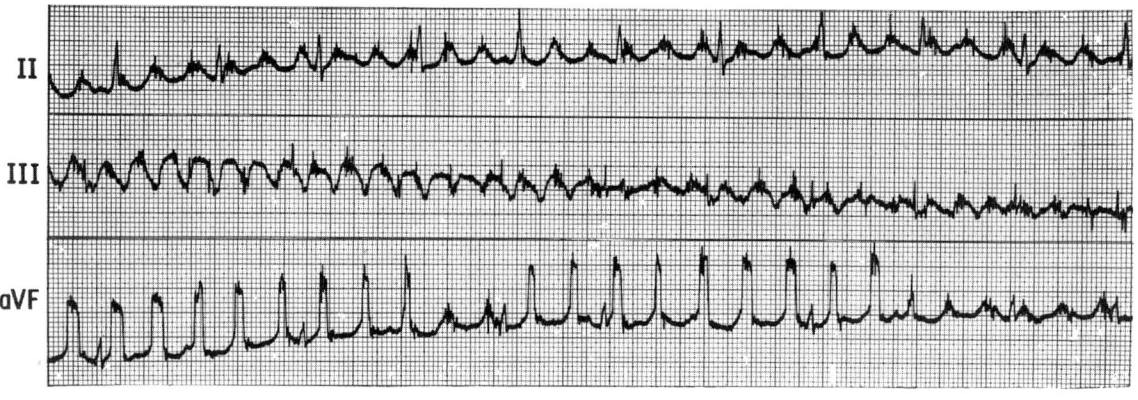

Figure 6-1
This electrocardiogram tracing shows artifacts due to muscle tremors closely resembling atrial flutter or even ventricular tachycardia.

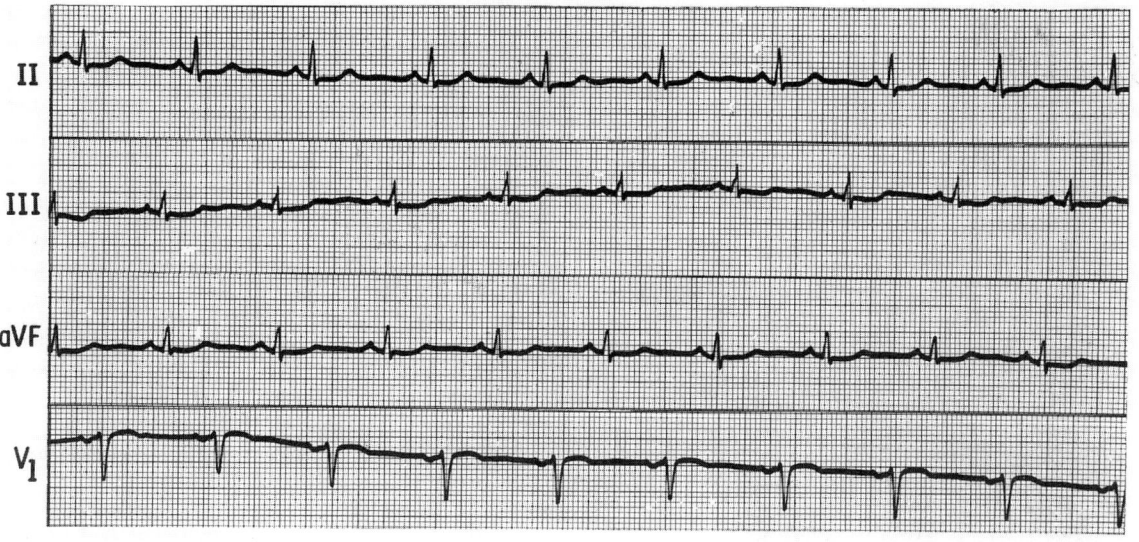

Figure 6-2
This electrocardiogram tracing taken on the same patient (see Fig. 6-1) after eliminating the muscle tremors reveals normal sinus rhythm without any artifact.

not always possible in every instance, the following may be used to distinguish them:

1. Identification of the atrial activity
   a. Determination of the relationship between atrial and ventricular activities
   b. Comparison of atrial and ventricular cycles
2. Evaluation of the configuration of the QRS complexes during the tachyarrhythmia
   a. Comparison of the QRS complexes during the tachyarrhythmia and isolated ectopic beats preceding or following the rapid heart action
   b. Comparison of the QRS complex during the tachyarrhythmia and ventricular captured beats
   c. Determination of preexisting LBBB or RBBB
   d. Determination of preexisting Wolff-Parkinson-White (WPW) syndrome
   e. Determination of aberrant ventricular conduction
3. Evaluation of the response to CSS
4. Determination of the regularity of R-R cycles
5. Evaluation of the coupling intervals and the post-tachyarrhythmias pause
6. Determination of the heart rate
7. Identification of the His bundle potential in relationship to the atrial and ventricular activity

IDENTIFICATION OF ATRIAL ACTIVITY

Identifying atrial activity is the first step in determining the origin of the tachyarrhythmia. When the P wave is definitely present, the relationship between the P wave and the QRS complex must be determined. When the ectopic P waves precede the QRS complexes, regardless of the configuration of the latter, the tachycardia is supraventricular in origin. In this circumstance, the tachycardia is atrial in origin if the axis of the ectopic P wave is similar to that of the sinus P wave. On the other hand, AV JT or reciprocating tachycardia can be diagnosed when the retrograde P wave (inverted P wave in lead II and upright P wave in lead aVR) precedes the QRS complex, regardless of its configuration. When the QRS complex is wide, bizarre, or both, either because of preexisting or rate-dependent bundle branch block or because of aberrant ventricular conduction, it closely mimics VT even if there are P waves preceding the QRS complexes. VT may be closely simulated even in sinus tachycardia when there is bundle branch block.

When the ectopic P waves, which are conducted in a retrograde fashion, follow the QRS complexes, the origin of the ectopic impulses may be either in the AV junction or in the ventricles. In this circumstance, AV JT is probably present when the QRS complex is narrow. However, VT may produce retrograde P waves that may resemble AV JT.

Comparison between atrial and ventricular cycles is important because the atrial-ventricular conduction ratio may be 1:1, but it may be any multiple of each other, or it may show Wenckebach phenomenon.

In the presence of regularly occurring P waves (either sinus or ectopic), the QRS complexes may independently originate from either the AV junction or the ventricles, leading to complete or incomplete AV dissociation. Thus, the presence of AV dissociation does not favor or exclude the diagnosis of AV JT or VT. In addition, AV JT or VT may develop in the presence of atrial tachyarrhythmias, including AF, atrial flutter, and tachycardia, leading to AV dissociation. In these circumstances, the comparison of the configuration of the QRS complex during the tachycardia with a ventricular captured beat is often the only clue to distinguish between them. This aspect of the differential diagnosis is discussed later in this chapter. The differential diagnosis between AV JT with a wide QRS complex and VT is one of the most difficult problems in the interpretation of cardiac arrhythmias because each may closely simulate the other. The most common cause of a wide QRS complex in an AV JT is preexisting bundle branch block (Figs. 6-3 and 6-4).

EVALUATION OF CONFIGURATION OF QRS COMPLEXES DURING TACHYARRHYTHMIAS

Evaluation of the configuration of the QRS complexes during tachycardia and comparison with that of isolated ectopic beats preceding or following the rapid heart action is often the only clue to identifying the exact location of the ectopic impulse formation. This is true because the same ectopic focus is believed to be capable of producing isolated ectopic beats as well as tachycardia. For example, isolated atrial premature contractions (APCs) often lead to atrial group beats, atrial tachycardia, AF, or atrial flutter, and these atrial tachyarrhythmias are often followed by isolated APCs on termination of the rapid heart action. This information is extremely valuable when the QRS complex is wide, bizarre, or both dur-

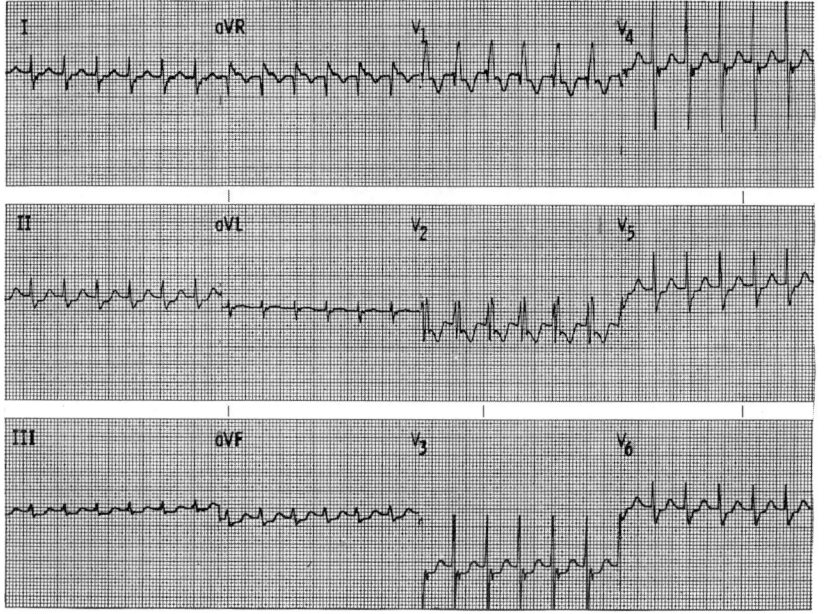

Figure 6-3
This figure and Figure 6-4 were taken on the same patient on different occasions. This figure shows a regular tachycardia (rate: 150 bpm) with wide QRS complexes. This tachycardia could be diagnosed as either supraventricular (probable atrioventricular junctional) tachycardia with a right bundle branch block or as ventricular tachycardia. Ventricular tachycardia is definitely excluded, however, because this patient had right bundle branch block during sinus rhythm on another occasion (see Fig. 6-4).

Figure 6-4
Right bundle branch block during sinus rhythm (rate: 63 bpm).

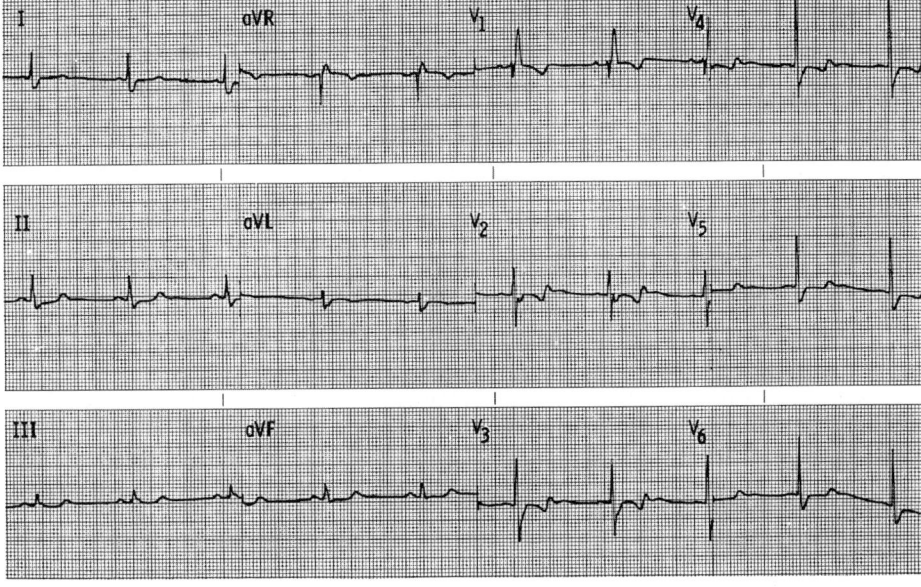

ing the tachyarrhythmias and during isolated APCs resulting either from preexisting or rate-dependent bundle branch block or from aberrant ventricular conduction.

The most practical point in the differential diagnosis is to compare the configuration of the QRS complex during the tachycardia with isolated ventricular premature contractions (VPCs) before and after the tachycardia. When the configurations of the QRS complexes of the isolated VPCs and tachycardia are identical, the diagnosis of VT is certain (Fig. 6-5).

Comparison of QRS configuration during the tachycardia and the ventricular captured beats (or reciprocal beats) is another important aspect of the differential diagnosis in the presence of incomplete AV dissociation. When the QRS complexes of ventricular captured beats or reciprocal beats have the same configuration as that of the tachycardia, regardless of whether the QRS complex is narrow or wide, the tachycardia is AV junctional in origin. Conversely, if the contours of the QRS complexes in the ventricular captured beats or reciprocal beats and the tachycardia are different, the diagnosis of VT can be made.

It should be emphasized that the presence of ventricular fusion beats favors a diagnosis of VT.

Determination of preexisting LBBB or RBBB is, at times, the only clue to distinguish between supraventricular tachycardia and ventricular tachycardia, particularly when the atrial activity is not discernible or is independent of the QRS complex and the QRS complex is wide, bizarre, or both. Thus, when the ECG that was taken preceding or following an episode of rapid heart action shows LBBB or RBBB and when the QRS contour is identical to that seen during the tachyarrhythmia, the diagnosis of ventricular tachycardia is definitely excluded (see Figs. 6-3 and 6-4). Similarly, AF or atrial flutter with preexisting or rate-dependent LBBB or RBBB also closely mimics ventricular tachycardia. In these circumstances, grossly irregular R-R cycles and identification of fibrillation or flutter waves exclude VT.

Knowledge of preexisting WPW syndrome is also very helpful in differentiating various rapid heart actions. This syndrome is known to be associated with various supraventricular tachyarrhythmias with wide QRS complexes due to anomalous AV conduction, thus closely resembling ventricular tachyarrhythmias. A detailed description of the various supraventricular tachyarrhythmias associated with WPW syndrome is found in Chapter 12.

Recognition of aberrant ventricular conduction in supraventricular tachyarrhythmias is extremely important to distinguish them from ventricular tachyarrhythmias.

Figure 6-5
Sinus rhythm with frequent ventricular premature contractions (marked X) and intermittent nonsustained ventricular tachycardia (rate: 200 bpm). All rhythm strips are continuous.

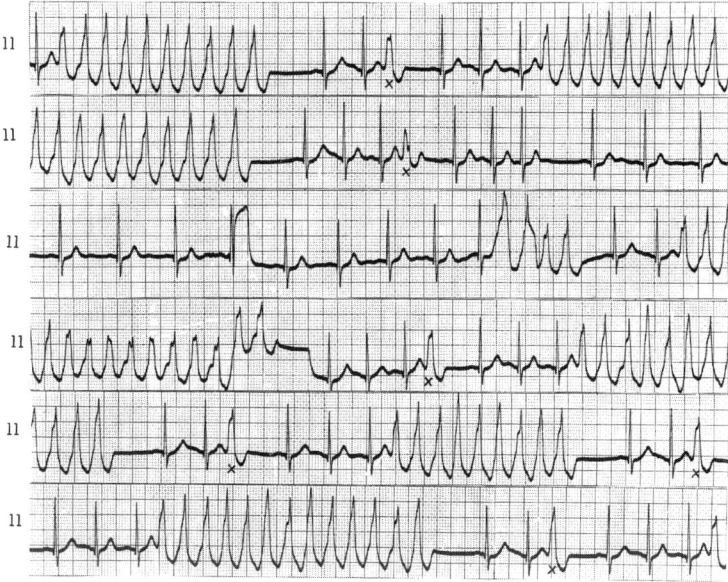

Aberrant ventricular conduction is favored by the following findings: RBBB pattern, absence of the post-tachyarrhythmia pause, varying coupling intervals, a long cycle preceding the coupling interval (Ashman's phenomenon), identical or similar initial vectors between the abnormal beat and the normally conducted beat, etc.

Ashman's Phenomenon

The most important factor for the production of aberrant ventricular conduction is Ashman's phenomenon (Fig. 6-6). In 1945, Ashman described the electrocardiographic finding that aberrant ventricular conduction tends to occur following a long ventricular cycle (R-R interval) preceding the coupling interval (the interval from a bizarre beat to the normal beat of the basic rhythm). It can be said that the longer the ventricular cycle (R-R interval), the longer is the refractory period following it; the shorter the ventricular cycle, the shorter is the refractory period.

Diagnostic criteria of Ashman's phenomenon are as follows:

- Ashman's phenomenon may be recognized in any cardiac rhythm when aberrant ventricular conduction occurs following a long ventricular cycle (R-R interval).

- The aberrant ventricular conduction is more pronounced in a ventricular complex following the longest ventricular cycle as a result of marked Ashman's phenomenon.
- Atrial or AV junctional bigeminy nearly always shows aberrant ventricular conduction in atrial or AV junctional premature beats because of Ashman's phenomenon. This is observed because atrial or AV junctional premature beats must follow a long ventricular cycle (postectopic pause) during atrial or AV junctional bigeminy.
- The P-R interval of atrial or AV junctional premature beats is often long during bigeminy, again as a result of Ashman's phenomenon. For the same reason, blocked APCs are common during atrial bigeminy (blocked atrial bigeminy).
- Ashman's phenomenon is pronounced when the ventricular cycle becomes suddenly shortened following a long ventricular cycle, particularly in AF. As a result, aberrant ventricular conduction occurs (see Fig. 6-6). It is not uncommon to observe consecutively occurring aberrant ventricular conduction once it is initiated by Ashman's phenomenon (see Fig. 6-6). This electrocardiographic finding closely simulates VT.

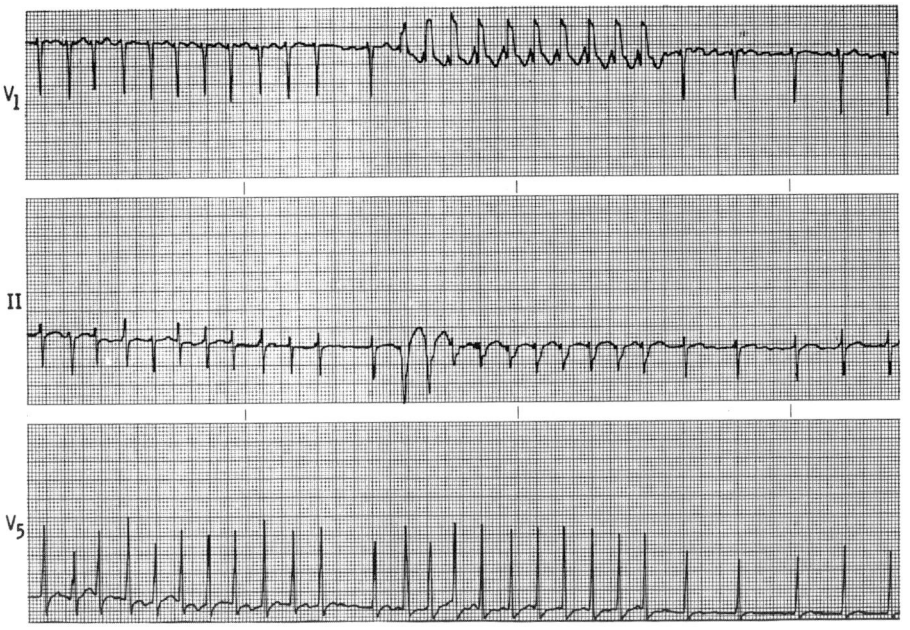

Figure 6-6
Atrial fibrillation with consecutively occurring aberrant ventricular conduction initiated by Ashman's phenomenon. Ventricular tachycardia is closely simulated, but a lack of any pause following many bizarre beats excludes the possibility of ventricular tachycardia.

- Ashman's phenomenon may be encountered in multifocal atrial tachycardia (MAT), which leads to aberrant ventricular conduction.
- Occasionally, a sinus beat (ventricular captured beat) during incomplete AV dissociation may show aberrant ventricular conduction as a result of Ashman's phenomenon.
- The configuration of the QRS complex during aberrant ventricular conduction as a result of Ashman's phenomenon is commonly (about 80–85% of cases) that of a RBBB pattern (see Fig. 6-6), and only 15–20% may show LBBB pattern. Not uncommonly, aberrantly conducted beats may reveal an electrocardiographic finding of a bifascicular block pattern consisting of a RBBB pattern and left anterior or posterior hemiblock pattern. At times, aberrantly conducted beats may show both a LBBB pattern and a RBBB pattern in the same electrocardiographic tracing. The alternation of the QRS contour in aberrant ventricular conduction represents functional (not true) bundle branch block, hemiblock, or both.
- Secondary T wave changes are observed in an aberrantly conducted QRS complex. The T wave alteration in this circumstance is analogous to that of VPCs, LBBB, or RBBB.

Various electrocardiographic findings causing broad (bizarre) QRS complexes are summarized in Table 6-1; various electrocardiographic findings that support (or favor) ventricular ectopy are summarized in Table 6-2. Various electrocardiographic findings that support aberrant ventricular conduction are summarized in Table 6-3. When the ectopic beat reveals an incomplete RBBB pattern, the impulse is considered to be originating from one of the fascicles of the left bundle branch system.

EVALUATION OF RESPONSE TO CAROTID SINUS STIMULATION

The response to CSS is different, depending on the nature and origin of the various tachyarrhythmias (Table 6-4). Sinus tachycardia is only transiently slowed by carotid sinus stimulation, and the original sinus rate returns soon after the procedure is over. At times, however, varying degrees of AV block may be produced by CSS in sinus tachycardia.

When CSS is applied for atrial tachycardia, there may be three different responses: There may be no response at all, sinus rhythm may be restored (Fig. 6-7), or there may

Table 6-1. Electrocardiogram findings causing broad (bizarre) QRS complexes

Ventricular ectopy
  Ventricular premature contractions
  Ventricular parasystole
  Ventricular tachycardia
  Ventricular escape beats or rhythm
  Ventricular fibrillation or flutter
Intraventricular block
  Right bundle branch block
  Left bundle branch block
  Bifascicular or trifascicular block
  Diffuse (nonspecific) intraventricular block
Aberrant ventricular conduction
  Ashman's phenomenon
  Short coupling interval
  Very rapid supraventricular tachyarrhythmias of
    various origins or mechanisms
Wolff-Parkinson-White syndrome
Artificial pacemaker-induced ventricular beats or rhythm

Table 6-2. Electrocardiogram findings that support (or favor) ventricular ectopy

Full compensatory pause during sinus rhythm (occasionally interpolated)—no disturbance on the sinus P-P cycle
Significant pause after a bizarre QRS complex in atrial fibrillation or atrial flutter
No premature P wave preceding a bizarre QRS complex
Extremely broad and bizarre QRS complex
No evidence of Ashman's phenomenon
Left bundle branch block pattern or multiformed
Bizarre QRS complex in elderly or cardiac patients and/or toxicity

be a slowing of the ventricular rate resulting from increased AV block, especially when the underlying cause is digitalis intoxication. The response of AV JT to carotid sinus stimulation is similar to that of atrial tachycardia. That is, AV JT (usually paroxysmal) may convert to sinus rhythm, or it may not be influenced by the procedure. In reciprocating

Table 6-3. Electrocardiographic findings that support aberrant ventricular conduction

Ashman's phenomenon

Bizarre QRS complex preceded by ectopic P wave during sinus rhythm

No long pause following bizarre beat(s)

Irregular R-R cycles during consecutive aberrant ventricular conduction in atrial fibrillation, atrial flutter, or multifocal atrial tachycardia

Very short coupling interval

Extremely rapid ventricular rate in supraventricular tachyarrhythmias

Right bundle branch block pattern (80–85% of cases)

Identical initial vector

tachycardia, slowing of the ventricular rate may be produced as a result of increased AV block by CSS.

When CSS is applied to AF or atrial flutter, a slowing of the ventricular rate is invariably produced because of the increased AV block. Occasionally, a long ventricular standstill may result when CSS is applied to elderly patients with AF or atrial flutter. In contrast to supraventricular tachyarrhythmia, ventricular tachyarrhythmia, as a rule, does not respond to CSS. Thus, no response to the procedure does not diagnose or exclude supraventricular tachyarrhythmia or ventricular tachyarrhythmia. In other words, VT is excluded if there is any response to CSS.

DETERMINATION OF REGULARITY OF R-R CYCLES

Although it has been said that VT often shows a slight irregularity of the R-R cycles, it is rather uncommon to recognize any appreciable irregularity except when VT transforms to ventricular fibrillation (VF). Conversely, supraventricular (atrial or AV junctional) tachycardia may produce a slight irregularity of the cardiac cycle, particularly in the initial portion of the paroxysm. Thus, slight irregularity of the R-R cycles is not a useful criterion for the differential diagnosis of supraventricular and ventricular tachyarrhythmia.

Table 6-4. Various responses to carotid sinus stimulation during cardiac arrhythmias*

Arrhythmias	Responses
Sinus tachycardia	Transient slowing of sinus (atrial) rate
	Varying degree AV block (less common)
Atrial tachycardia	Termination
	No response
	Slowing of ventricular rate due to increased AV block (less common)
	Increased atrial rate (less common)
Atrial fibrillation or flutter	Slowing of ventricular rate due to increased AV block
AV junctional tachycardia	
Paroxysmal	Termination
	No response
Nonparoxysmal	No response
Ventricular tachycardia	No response (rare exceptions)
Wolff-Parkinson-White syndrome	Vary
Parasystole	Vary

AV = atrioventricular.
*Carotid sinus stimulation is not recommended in digitalis intoxication or in hypersensitive individuals.

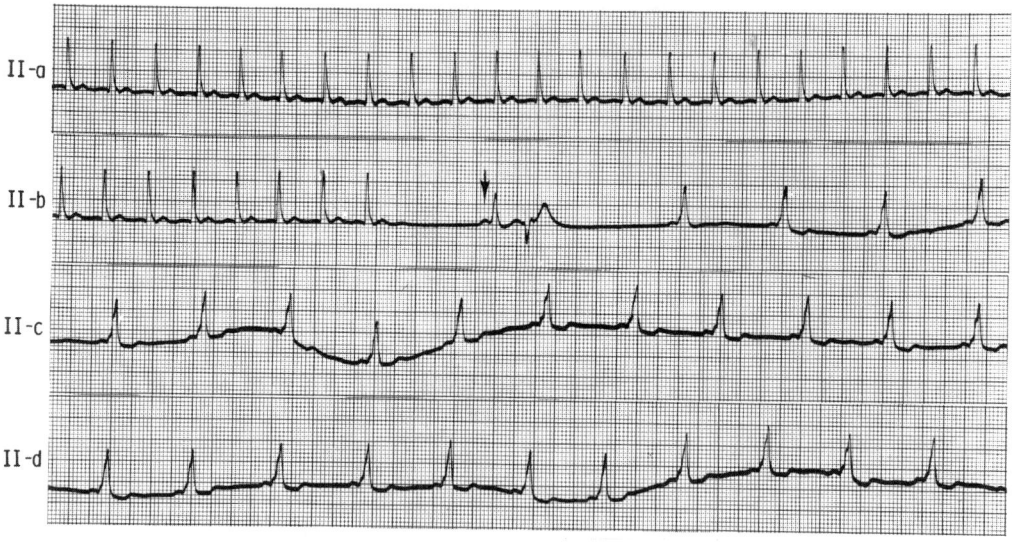

II-a

II-b

II-c

II-d

Figure 6-7 *Supraventricular (reciprocating) tachycardia due to Wolff-Parkinson-White syndrome is terminated by carotid sinus stimulation (indicated by arrow). Note a ventricular premature contraction (the tenth beat in lead II b). Delta wave is present during sinus rhythm. Leads II a–d are continuous.*

Grossly irregular R-R cycles, regardless of the configuration of the QRS complex, are nearly always due to AF and less commonly may be due to atrial flutter or tachycardia with varying AV response or VF. When the QRS complex is wide, bizarre, or both, due to either preexisting or rate-dependent bundle branch block or to aberrant ventricular conduction (see Fig. 6-6) or to anomalous AV conduction in the WPW syndrome, VT is closely simulated. On the other hand, when the R-R cycles show a regular irregularity, the tachycardia often arises from the AV junction, and the irregularity is often due to Wenckebach exit block or the periodic occurrence of reciprocal beats.

EVALUATION OF COUPLING INTERVALS AND POST-TACHYARRHYTHMIA PAUSE

In general, the coupling intervals are constant in VT or VPCs. Conversely, wide and/or bizarre QRS complexes due to aberrant ventricular conduction in AF always have varying coupling intervals (see Fig. 6-6). In addition, VT is always followed by a post-tachycardia pause, whereas aberrantly conducted beats in AF are *not* followed by a long pause (see Fig. 6-6).

DETERMINATION OF HEART RATE

Although various tachyarrhythmias produce different rate ranges (see Chapter 1), the heart rate is *not* a reliable index to use for the differential diagnosis of supraventricular and ventricular tachyarrhythmias because of the overlap of the heart rates. Nevertheless, a ventricular rate beyond 200 beats per minute (bpm) usually favors supraventricular tachyarrhythmias, and a ventricular rate faster than 250 bpm nearly always indicates AF or atrial flutter, regardless of the width of the QRS complex.

IDENTIFICATION OF HIS BUNDLE POTENTIAL IN RELATION TO VENTRICULAR ACTIVITY

Study of the His bundle potential has been used to locate the precise origin of the ectopic focus or conduction defect. When the ventricular activity is preceded by a His bundle potential, the rapid heart action is due to a supraventricular tachycardia. Conversely, in ventricular tachycardia, the QRS complex is *not* preceded by the His bundle potential.

CONCLUSION

The differential diagnosis between supraventricular tachy-arrhythmias and ventricular tachyarrhythmias is often diffi-cult and at times impossible because many features mimic each other. Yet, it is extremely important to distinguish the two because their management and prognosis differ.

When the QRS complexes of supraventricular tachy-arrhythmias are wide, bizarre, or both, the following may be used to distinguish them from VT:

1. Determination of the relationship between atrial and ventricular activities
2. Comparison of the QRS complexes during tachy-arrhythmias with those of ventricular captured beats
3. Comparison of the QRS complexes during tachy-arrhythmias with those of isolated ectopic beats before or after the episode of rapid heart action
4. Recognition of a preexisting or rate-dependent LBBB or RBBB
5. Recognition of a preexisting WPW syndrome
6. Recognition of aberrant ventricular conduction and Ashman's phenomenon
7. Evaluation of the response to CSS
8. Determination of the regularity of the R-R cycles
9. Identification of the His bundle potential in relation-ship to ventricular activity

7

Disturbances of Sinus Impulse Formation and Conduction

When any of the five criteria necessary for the diagnosis of normal sinus rhythm (normal axis of the P wave, constant and normal P-R interval, constant P wave configuration in a given lead, rate between 60 and 100 beats per minute [bpm], and constant P-P or R-R cycle) are lacking, a cardiac arrhythmia of sinus origin is considered to be present. Such arrhythmias include sinus premature contraction (extrasystole), sinus bradycardia, sinus tachycardia, sinus arrhythmia, wandering pacemaker in the sinus node, sinus arrest (pause or standstill), and sinoatrial (SA) block.

SICK SINUS SYNDROME

There has been an increasing awareness of the clinical entity known as sick sinus syndrome (SSS) in recent years because the syndrome is found to be relatively common in daily practice, particularly among the elderly, and it can be successfully treated with artificial cardiac pacing in most cases. The term has been used to describe a broad spectrum of clinical manifestations (e.g., syncope or near syncope, dizziness, increased congestive heart failure and/or angina, and palpitations) that result from a dysfunctioning sinus node. Electrocardiographic manifestations in SSS are summarized as follows:

1. Marked and persisting sinus bradycardia
2. Sinus arrest, SA block, or both
3. Drug-resistant (e.g., resistant to atropine or isoproterenol [Isuprel]) sinus bradyarrhythmias
4. Long pause following an atrial premature contraction (APC)
5. Prolonged sinus node recovery time determined by atrial pacing
6. Chronic atrial fibrillation (AF) or repetitive occurrence of AF (less commonly atrial flutter) (a) with slow ventricular rate and (b) preceded or followed by sinus bradycardia, sinus arrest, or SA block
7. Atrioventricular (AV) junctional escape rhythm (JER) (with or without slow and unstable sinus activity)
8. Carotid sinus syncope (Fig. 7-1)
9. Failure of restoration of sinus rhythm following cardioversion
10. Brady-tachyarrhythmia syndrome (Fig. 7-2)
11. Common coexisting AV block, intraventricular block, or both
12. Any combination of the above

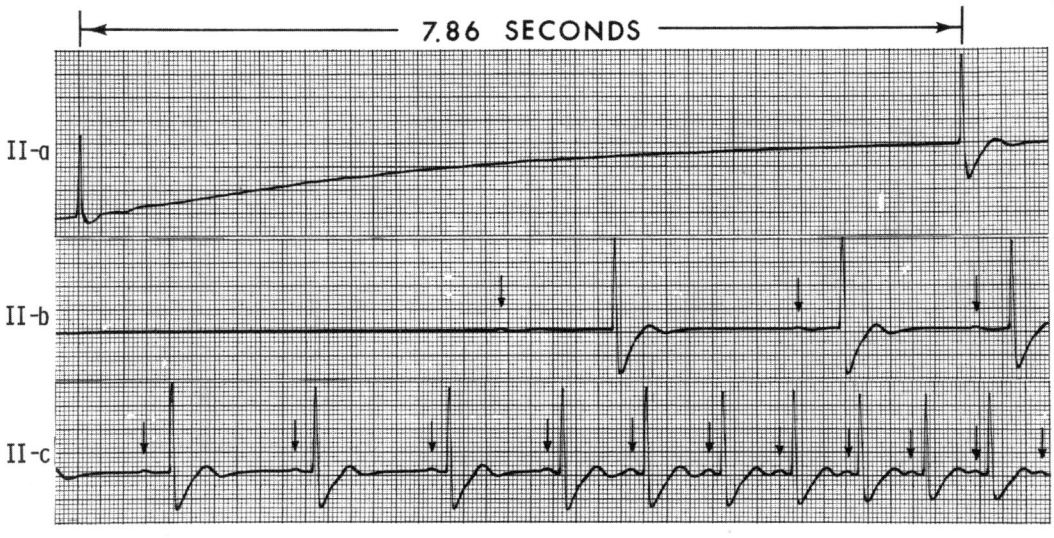

Figure 7-1

Carotid sinus syncope manifested by sinus arrest (7.86 seconds) and occasional atrioventricular junctional escape beats. The arrows indicate sinus P waves. Leads II a, b, and c are continuous. These electrocardiographic findings strongly suggest sick sinus syndrome.

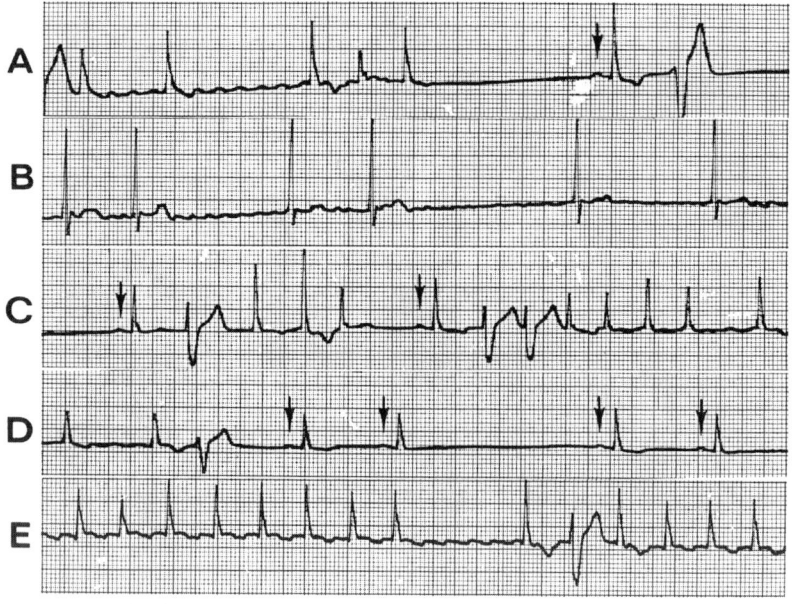

Figure 7-2
Brady-tachyarrhythmia syndrome manifested by unstable sinus bradycardia (marked with arrows), intermittent atrial flutter with rapid ventricular response, ventricular premature contractions, and occasional aberrant ventricular conduction. These electrocardiographic findings indicate advanced sick sinus syndrome. The Holter monitor rhythm strips A to E are not continuous.

SINUS BRADYCARDIA

Definition

Sinus bradycardia is a cardiac rhythm originating from the sinus node with a rate slower than 60 bpm.

Diagnostic Criteria (Fig. 7-3)

- P wave of sinus origin (normal mean axis of the P wave)
- Constant and normal P-R interval (0.12–0.20 second)
- Constant P wave configuration in each given lead
- Rate of 45–59 bpm (cyclic length >1 second)
- Regular or slightly irregular P-P (or R-R) cycle

Diagnostic Pearls

Sinus bradycardia should be distinguished from various slow heart rhythms due to many other mechanisms, including AV JER, second-degree or advanced AV block, frequent blocked APCs, SA block, and sinus arrest. In sinus bradycardia, the P waves are always upright in lead II and inverted in aVR. One or more AV junctional escape beats may occur in the presence of marked sinus bradycardia, leading to incomplete AV dissociation (see Chapter 9). In addition, sinus bradycardia often coexists with sinus arrhythmia.

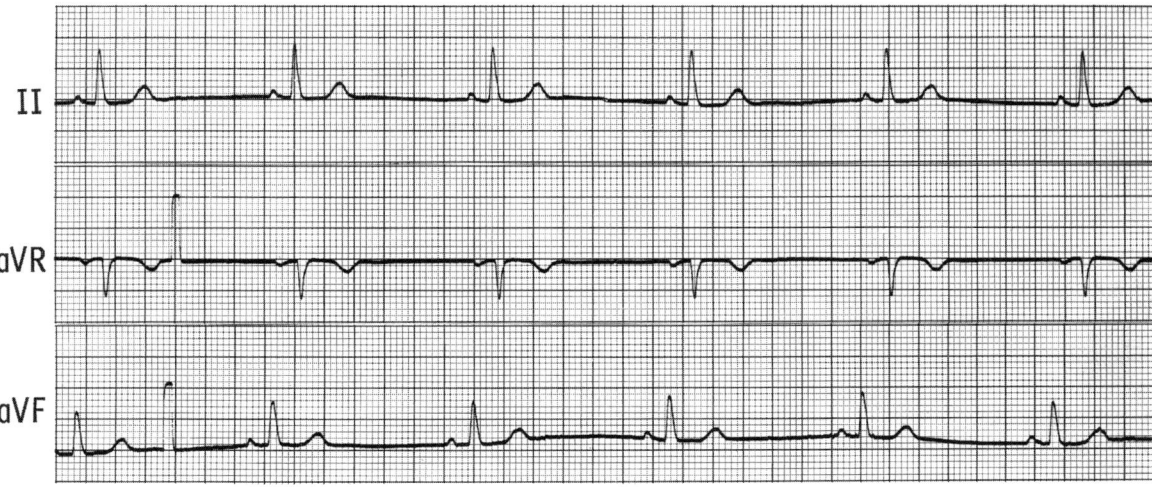

Figure 7-3
Sinus bradycardia with a rate of 45 bpm.

SINUS TACHYCARDIA

Definition

The cardiac rhythm originating from the sinus node with a rate of more than 100 bpm.

Diagnostic Criteria (Fig. 7-4)

- P wave of sinus origin (normal mean axis of P waves)
- Constant and normal P-R interval (0.12–0.20 second)
- Constant P wave configuration in each given lead
- Rate of 101–160 bpm (up to 200 bpm in some cases) (cycle length <0.60 second)
- Regular or slight irregular P-P cycle

Diagnostic Pearls

Sinus tachycardia should be distinguished from various tachyarrhythmias originating from ectopic foci, including atrial tachycardia, AV JT, AF, atrial flutter, and multifocal atrial tachycardia (MAT). In sinus tachycardia, the P waves are always upright in lead II and inverted in lead aVR. It is important to emphasize that sinus tachycardia does not start or stop abruptly. In other words, sinus tachycardia is *not* paroxysmal in nature. Conversely, various ectopic tachyarrhythmias (e.g., paroxysmal atrial tachycardia) possess paroxysmal in nature.

Figure 7-4
Sinus tachycardia with a rate of 147 bpm.

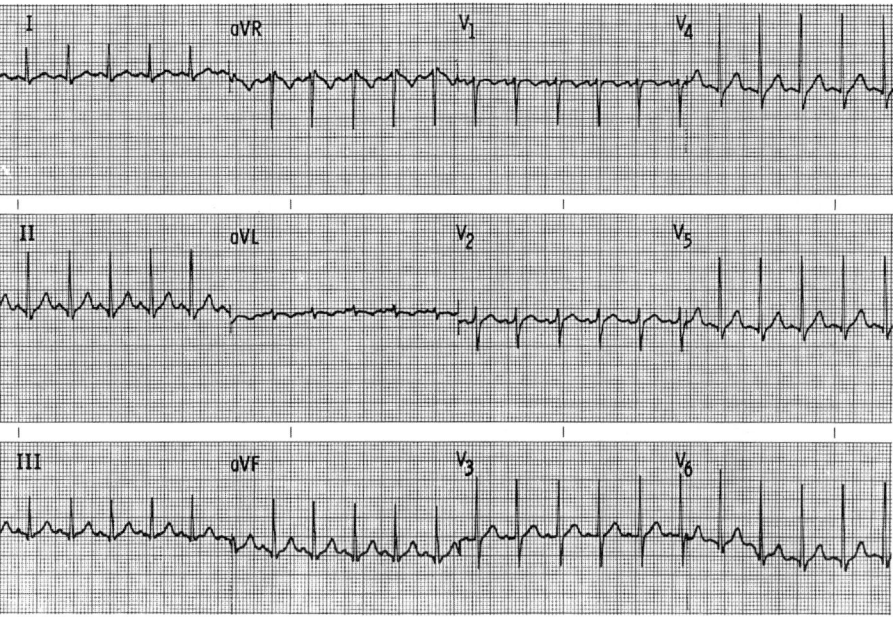

SINUS ARRHYTHMIA

Definition

Sinus arrhythmia is an irregular cardiac rhythm originating from the sinus node. There are two major types of sinus arrhythmia: respiratory and nonrespiratory. In the respiratory form, the sinus rate increases with inspiration and slows with expiration. The nonrespiratory form has no relationship to respiration. The respiratory form is extremely common in children and young adults—a benign normal variant. The nonrespiratory form is common in elderly individuals—often called idiopathic. The rare form is ventriculophasic sinus arrhythmia (see Chapter 11).

Diagnostic Criteria (Fig. 7-5)

- P wave of sinus origin (normal mean axis of the P wave)
- Constant and normal P-R interval (0.12–0.20 second)
- Constant P wave configuration in each given lead
- Rate of 45–100 bpm (occasionally <45 bpm or >100 bpm)
- Irregular P-P (or R-R) cycle (variation of P-P interval ≥0.16 second)

Diagnostic Pearls

Sinus arrhythmia often coexists with sinus bradycardia and is occasionally associated with a wandering pacemaker or sinus tachycardia. Sinus arrhythmia should be distinguished from various irregular cardiac rhythms due to other mechanisms, such as frequent APCs, AF with advanced AV block, sinus rhythm with Wenckebach AV block, SA block, and sinus arrest. In sinus arrhythmia, the P waves are always upright in lead II and inverted in lead aVR.

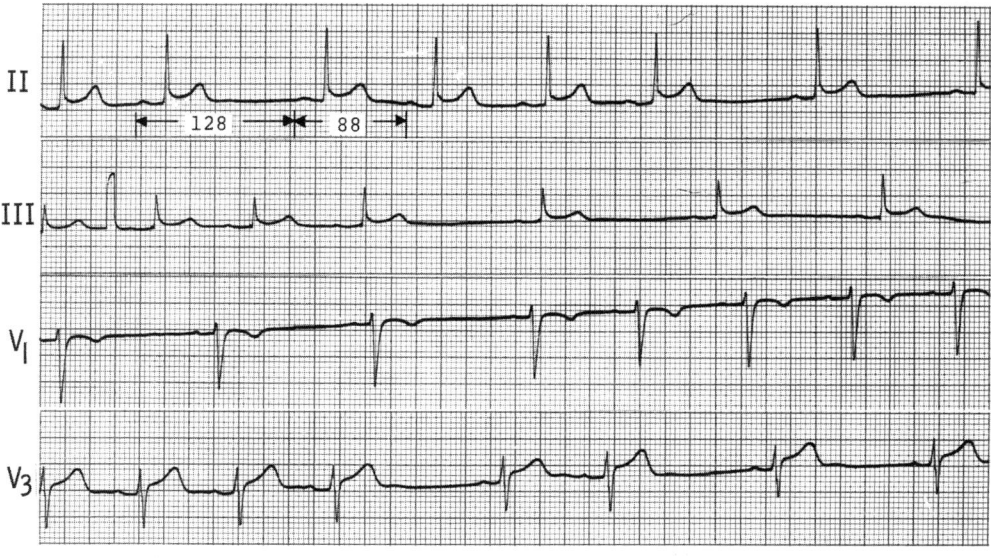

Figure 7-5
Sinus arrhythmia. The numbers represent hundredths of a second.

WANDERING PACEMAKER IN THE SINUS NODE

Definition

In wandering pacemaker in the sinus node, the pacemaker shifts from one part of the sinus node to another so that the P wave configuration changes from beat to beat.

Diagnostic Criteria (Fig. 7-6)

- P wave of sinus origin (normal mean axis of the P wave)
- Varying P wave configuration in each given lead
- Relatively constant P-R interval (may vary between 0.12 and 0.20 second)
- Slightly irregular or regular P-P cycles
- Rate of 45–100 beats/minute (rarely <45 bpm or >100 bpm)

Diagnostic Pearls

Wandering pacemaker in the sinus node is considered to be a variant of sinus arrhythmia or an exaggerated form of sinus arrhythmia. Thus, sinus arrhythmia is commonly associated with wandering pacemaker. It should be emphasized that wandering pacemaker may be closely simulated by artifacts of various origins.

Figure 7-6
Sinus arrhythmia with wandering atrial pacemaker.

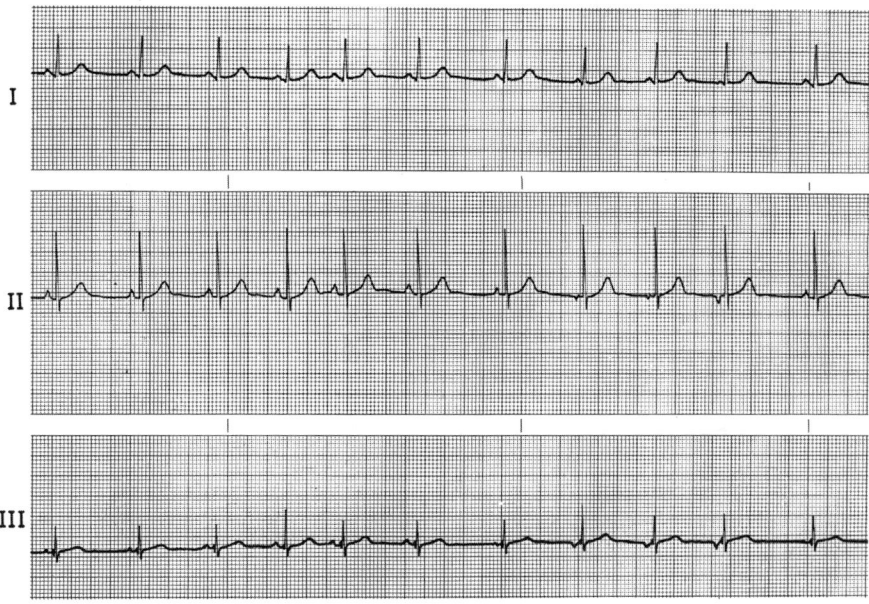

I

II

III

SINUS ARREST (PAUSE OR STANDSTILL)

Definition

Sinus arrest is defined as a failure of impulse formation in the sinus node leading to an absence of P waves.

Diagnostic Criteria (Fig. 7-7)

- Absence of P waves of sinus origin
- No relationship between the duration of sinus arrest and the basic P-P cycle
- Common occurrence of AV junctional or ventricular escape beats
- Chronic sinus arrest often leading to chronic AF

Diagnostic Pearls

Sinus arrest should be distinguished from SA block because both conditions produce an absence of P waves. The P-P interval in sinus arrest has no relationship to the basic P-P cycle, whereas the P-P interval in SA block shows either multiples of the basic P-P cycle (Fig. 7-8) or a regular irregularity (Fig. 7-9).

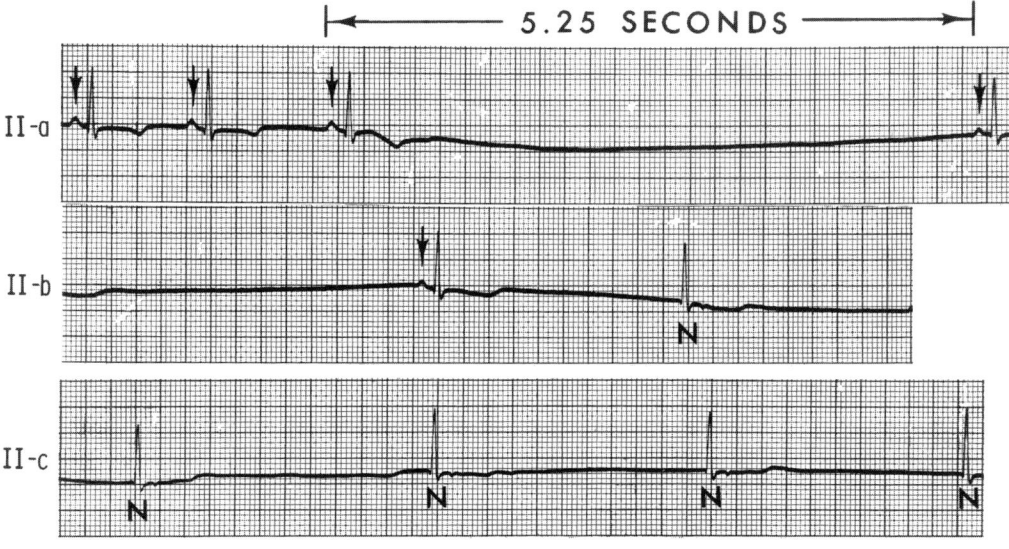

Figure 7-7
Sinus rhythm (marked with arrows) with intermittent sinus arrest (5.25 seconds) leading to slow atrioventricular junctional escape rhythm (marked N). These electrocardiographic findings indicate advanced sick sinus syndrome.

MOBITZ TYPE II SINOATRIAL BLOCK

Definition

Mobitz type II SA block is a block of the sinus impulse transmission at the SA junction leading to an occasional absence of the P waves of the sinus origin.

Diagnostic Criteria (Fig. 7-8)

- Occasional absence of one or more P waves of the sinus origin.
- The long P-P interval due to SA block is exactly (or almost exactly) a multiple of the basic P-P cycle.
- Type II SA block may occur periodically at regular or irregular intervals.
- One or more AV junctional or ventricular escape beats may occur in SA block.

Diagnostic Pearls

Type II SA block should be distinguished from sinus arrest (see Fig. 7-7), marked sinus arrhythmia, and sinus brady-cardia (see Figs. 7-3 and 7-5).

Figure 7-8
*Sinus rhythm (marked
with arrows) with inter-
mittent type II sinoatrial
block. Note that the
long P-P interval is
twice the short P-P
cycle. The numbers rep-
resent hundredths of a
second. The Holter
monitor rhythm strips
A–D are not continuous.*

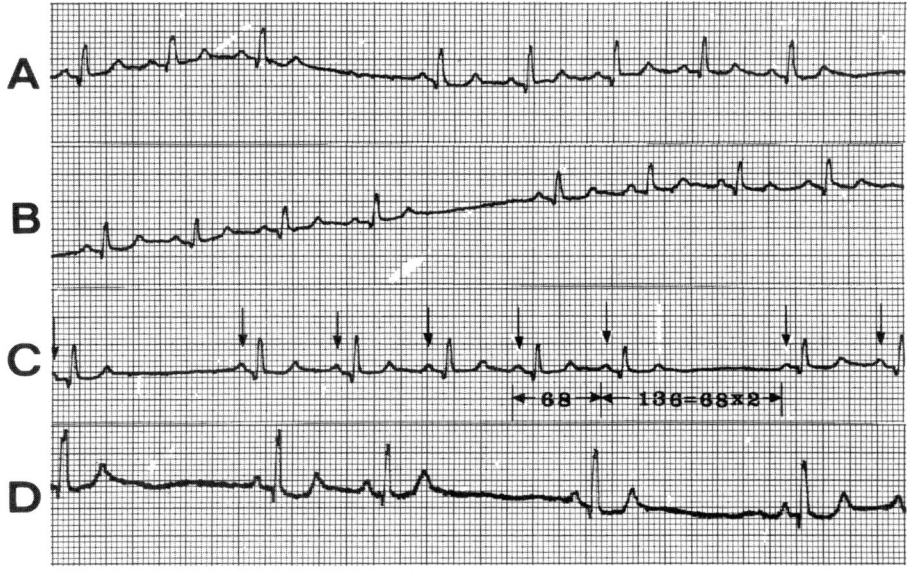

WENCKEBACH (MOBITZ TYPE I) SINOATRIAL BLOCK

Definition

Wenckebach (Mobitz type I) SA block is characterized by progressive increments of the refractoriness at the SA junction followed by no conduction of the sinus impulse leading to an occasional absence of the P waves of the sinus origin (Wenckebach conduction of the sinus impulses at the SA junction).

Diagnostic Criteria (Fig. 7-9)

- Progressive shortening of the sinus P-P intervals followed by a long pause (long P-P interval).
- Long P-P interval is less than two basic P-P cycles.
- Wenckebach SA block may occur periodically at regular or irregular intervals.
- One or more AV functional or ventricular escape beats may occur.

Diagnostic Pearls

Wenckebach SA block is one of the most difficult cardiac arrhythmias to diagnose because the long P-P interval due to SA block is *not* a multiple of the basic P-P cycles. Wenckebach SA block superficially resembles marked sinus arrhythmia, blocked APC, sinus arrest, or sinus bradycardia. Progressive shortening of the P-P cycles is the clue to diagnose Wenckebach SA block.

Figure 7-9
Patient with acute diaphragmatic myocardial infarction in a coronary care unit. Leads II a, b, and c are continuous. Arrows indicate sinus P waves. Long and short P-P cycles alternate throughout the tracing. The long cycle is shorter than two P-P cycles. This regular irregularity of the P-P cycles represents a 3:2 Wenckebach sinoatrial block. In addition, there is a Wenckebach atrioventricular conduction without actual blocked P waves throughout the tracing except for an early portion of lead II a. A blocked P wave in lead II a is indicated by P.

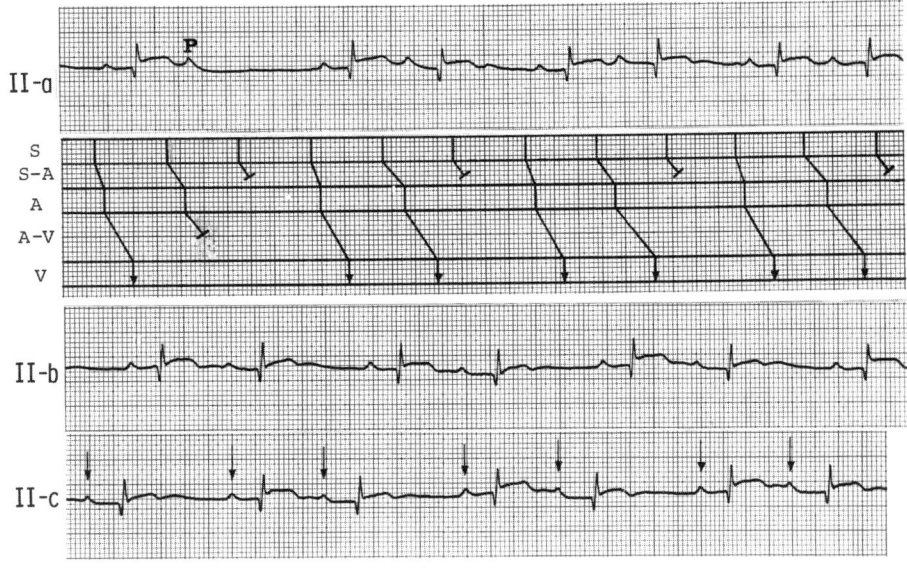

8

Atrial Arrhythmias

Atrial arrhythmias may originate from anywhere in the atria other than the sinus node. Atrial arrhythmias are almost always generated by active impulse formation. Thus, some form of rapid atrial arrhythmia will result. Common atrial arrhythmias include atrial premature contractions (APCs), atrial tachycardia (AT), atrial flutter, and atrial fibrillation (AF). These arrhythmias are closely interrelated with each other in terms of mechanism and clinical significance. It has been suggested that an ectopic focus in the atria that produces an isolated APC may be capable of producing AT, atrial flutter, and AF. The relationship between atrial flutter and AF is very close. Thus, it is common to observe one changing to the other, even on the same electrocardiographic tracing. Although atrial tachyarrhythmias are classified into AT, atrial flutter, and AF primarily on the basis of atrial rate, it is not uncommon to observe a transitional (or intermediate) rhythm between these atrial tachyarrhythmias. This is particularly true when the atrial rate is faster than 350 beats/minute (bpm) (up to 400 bpm), but the flutter cycle is still regular. This rhythm is termed *atrial impure flutter*. On the other hand, the term *atrial flutter-fibrillation* is used when the rhythm is a mixture of atrial flutter and AF. The atrial rates in AT, atrial flutter, and AF are 160–250 bpm, 250–350 bpm, and 400–650 bpm, respectively, but these rates are arbitrarily divided. Atrial rates are often altered by various drugs, particularly quinidine and digitalis. The ventricular rates in untreated atrial tachyarrhythmias are generally 160–200 bpm simply because the atrioventricular (AV) junctional tissue is unable to conduct extremely rapid atrial impulses. This is due to the longer refractory period in the AV junction than in the atria. When the ventricular rate is around 80 bpm or slower in AF, the rhythm is called AF with advanced AV block.

Atrial tachyarrhythmias may occur in a paroxysmal or chronic form. AF often persists for a long period of time when the underlying disorder is rheumatic heart disease, particularly mitral stenosis and sick sinus syndrome. Atrial tachyarrhythmias may occur in healthy subjects as well as in diseased hearts. However, AF or atrial flutter is more commonly encountered in diseased hearts. In addition, thyrotoxicosis is frequently associated with paroxysmal AF. The common occurrence of various tachyarrhythmias associated with Wolff-Parkinson-White (WPW) syndrome is well-known. AT with varying AV block (usually Wenckebach AV block) that occurs during digitalization almost always indicates digitalis intoxication (often termed *paroxysmal atrial tachycardia with block*). By and large, the

incidence of various atrial arrhythmias increases progressively with age.

Less common atrial arrhythmias include atrial parasystole, left atrial rhythm, slow atrial tachycardia (rate of 120–140 bpm), and atrial dissociation (see Chapter 13). Multifocal atrial tachycardia (MAT) is not uncommon, and atrial escape rhythm is only occasionally observed. Atrial standstill is rarely encountered; if it occurs, it is almost always found in terminal cardiac patients and in severe digitalis intoxication.

APCs may originate anywhere in the atria outside the sinus node. In most instances, the impulse from the atrial premature focus activates the entire atria, including the sinus node. The sinus node is prematurely discharged, and its inherent sinus impulse discharge is suppressed momentarily. Thus, the sinus node automaticity is reset following an APC. The propagation of the impulse in the atria from an atrial ectopic focus is usually different from that of the sinus impulse, but conduction below the AV node is identical to that in normal sinus rhythm.

It should be noted that an APC is *not* followed by a full compensatory pause in most cases, whereas a ventricular premature contraction (VPC) is almost always followed by a full compensatory pause (see Chapter 10). APCs may occur every other beat (atrial bigeminy), every third beat (atrial trigeminy) or every fourth beat (atrial quadrigeminy). When APCs reveal broad QRS complexes as a result of aberrant ventricular conduction or bundle branch block, the electro-cardiographic finding closely simulates VPCs. The term *blocked*, or *nonconducted*, APC is used when the premature P waves are not followed by QRS complexes.

Various atrial arrhythmias are summarized as follows:

1. Common atrial arrhythmias
   a. APCs
   b. AT
   c. AF
   d. Atrial flutter
   e. Atrial flutter-fibrillation
2. Less common atrial arrhythmias
   a. Slow atrial tachycardia
   b. MAT
   c. Atrial escape rhythm
   d. Left atrial rhythm
   e. Right atrial rhythm
3. Rare atrial arrhythmias
   a. Atrial parasystole
   b. Atrial dissociation
   c. Atrial standstill

ATRIAL PREMATURE CONTRACTION

Definition

APC is the premature occurrence of ectopic P waves originating from any portion of the atria.

Diagnostic Criteria (Fig. 8-1)

• Premature occurrence of ectopic P wave in the presence of sinus rhythm.
• Constant coupling interval (interval from the ectopic beat to the preceding beat of the basic rhythm).
• The premature ectopic P wave is usually upright in lead II and inverted in lead aVR.
• The QRS complex of an APC is usually normal (narrow).
• The QRS complex of an APC may be broad and bizarre because of aberrant ventricular conduction (AVC), right bundle branch block (RBBB), left bundle branch (LBBB), or WPW syndrome.
• APC may *not* be followed by a QRS complex, in which case it is called a blocked, or nonconducted, APC.

• APCs may occur consecutively (up to five beats in a row) and are then called grouped APCs.
• On rare occasions, an APC may show inverted P waves in leads II, III, and aVF (often up to leads I and V_{4-6}) and upright P waves in leads aVR and V_1 when the ectopic impulse originates from the left atrium (called left APC).

Diagnostic Pearls

When APCs reveal broad and bizarre QRS complexes, VPCs are closely simulated (see Chapter 6). In most cases, an APC is *not* followed by a full compensatory pause, whereas a VPC is almost always followed by a full compensatory pause. When an APC is *not* followed by a QRS complex (blocked APC), the electrocardiographic finding may easily be misdiagnosed as many other cardiac arrhythmias, including sinus arrhythmia, sinus arrest, sinoatrial block, and advanced AV block (see Chapters 6 and 7). It should be noted that the premature P wave is often superimposed on the T wave of the preceding beat, leading to a false absence of the ectopic P wave. Careful observation is essential to identify the premature P wave.

Figure 8-1
Sinus rhythm with frequent atrial premature contractions (indicated by arrows) producing atrial bigeminy.

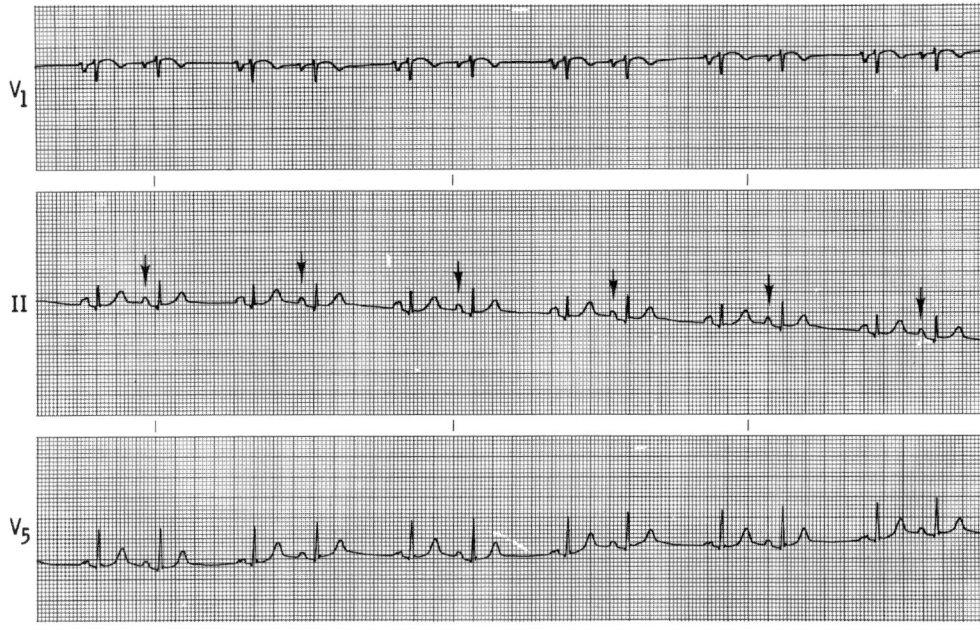

ATRIAL PREMATURE CONTRACTION WITH ABERRANT VENTRICULAR CONDUCTION

Definition

APC with AVC is the premature occurrence of ectopic P waves associated with bizarre QRS complex as a result of AVC.

Diagnostic Criteria (Fig. 8-2)

- APC with a bizarre QRS complex because the atrial impulse is conducted to the ventricles during their partial refractory period.
- AVC occurs as a result of a short coupling interval, Ashman's phenomenon, or both (see Chapter 6).

Diagnostic Pearls

APC with AVC closely mimics a VPC (see Chapter 10), especially when the premature P wave is not easily visible. Remember that an APC is *not* followed by a full compensatory pause, whereas a VPC is almost always followed by a full compensatory pause (see Chapter 10).

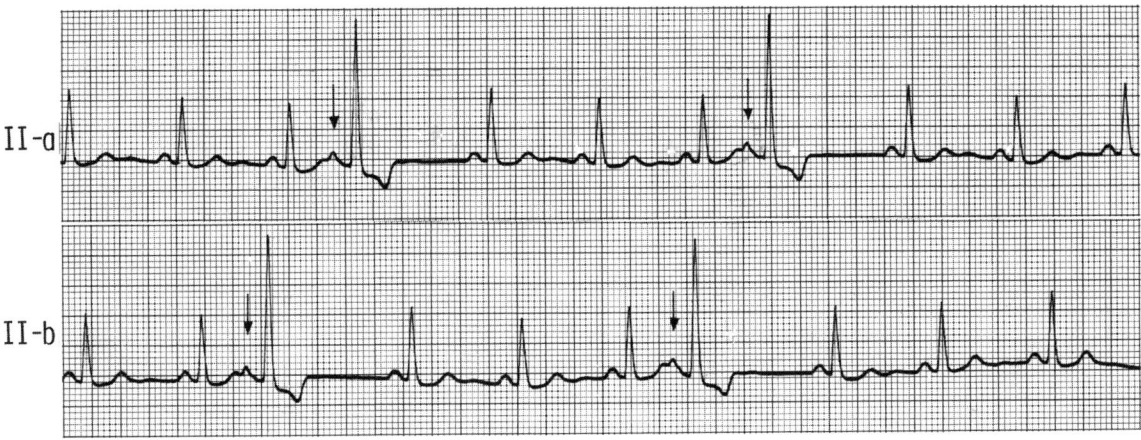

Figure 8-2
Sinus rhythm and atrial premature contractions (indicated by arrows) with aberrant ventricular conduction due to a short coupling interval. Leads II a and b are not continuous.

BLOCKED (NONCONDUCTED) ATRIAL PREMATURE CONTRACTION

Definition

Blocked (nonconducted) APC is the premature occurrence of an ectopic P wave *not* followed by a QRS complex.

Diagnostic Criteria (Fig. 8-3)

- APC *not* followed by a QRS complex because the premature atrial impulse is conducted to the AV junction during its absolute refractory period.
- Blocked APC occurs as a result of a short coupling interval, Ashman's phenomenon, or preexisting AV block.

Diagnostic Pearls

Blocked APC is the most common cause of a ventricular pause. It is extremely important to recognize a premature P wave without a QRS complex to make the correct diagnosis of blocked (nonconducted) APC. Blocked APC superficially resembles marked sinus arrhythmia, second-degree or advanced AV block, sinus arrest, and sinoatrial block. Blocked atrial bigeminy closely mimics marked sinus bradycardia.

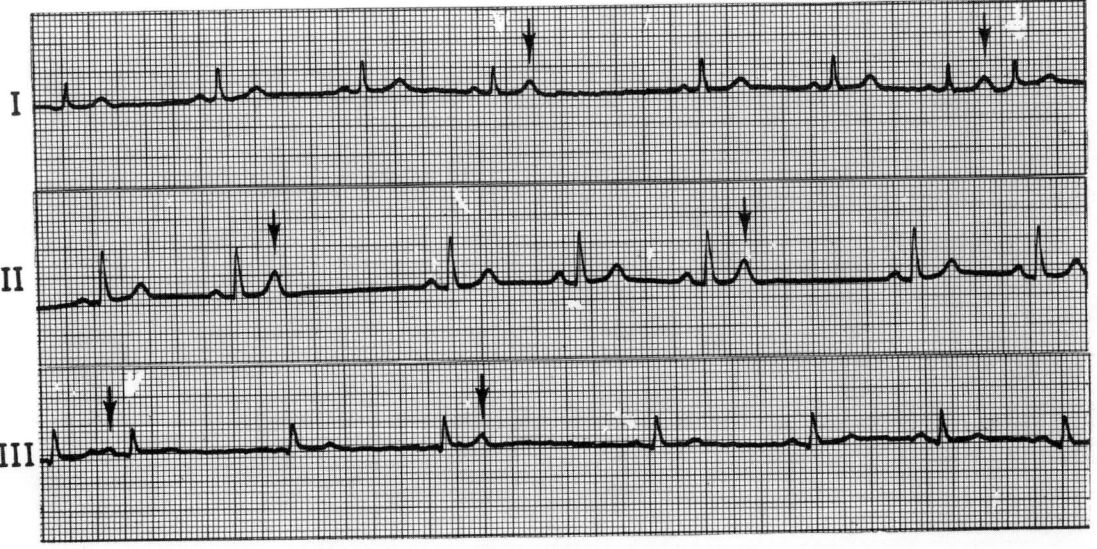

Figure 8-3
Sinus rhythm with frequent atrial premature contractions (marked with arrows) and many atrial premature contractions are not followed by QRS complexes (blocked atrial premature contractions).

ATRIAL TACHYCARDIA

Definition

AT is the regular and rapid cardiac rhythm originating from any position of the atria.

Diagnostic Criteria (Fig. 8-4)

- Regular atrial rhythm with rate of 160–250 bpm (<160 bpm in some cases).
- The ectopic P waves are usually upright in leads II, III, and aVF and inverted in lead aVR.
- AV conduction ratio is usually 1:1, but it may show a 2:1 or Wenckebach AV conduction.
- The QRS complexes are normal in most cases.
- The QRS complexes may be broad and bizarre because of LBBB, RBBB, or AVC.

Diagnostic Pearls

In AT, the ectopic P waves are often superimposed on the T waves of the preceding beats, leading to a false impression of absent P waves. Careful observation is necessary to identify the rapidly occurring P waves. AT is often termed *paroxysmal atrial tachycardia* (PAT) because the tachycardia usually is paroxysmal in nature. In rare cases, the ectopic P waves are inverted in leads II, III, and aVF (often up to leads I and V$_{4-6}$) and upright in leads aVR and V$_1$ in left atrial tachycardia (see Chapter 13). AT is frequently initiated by APCs.

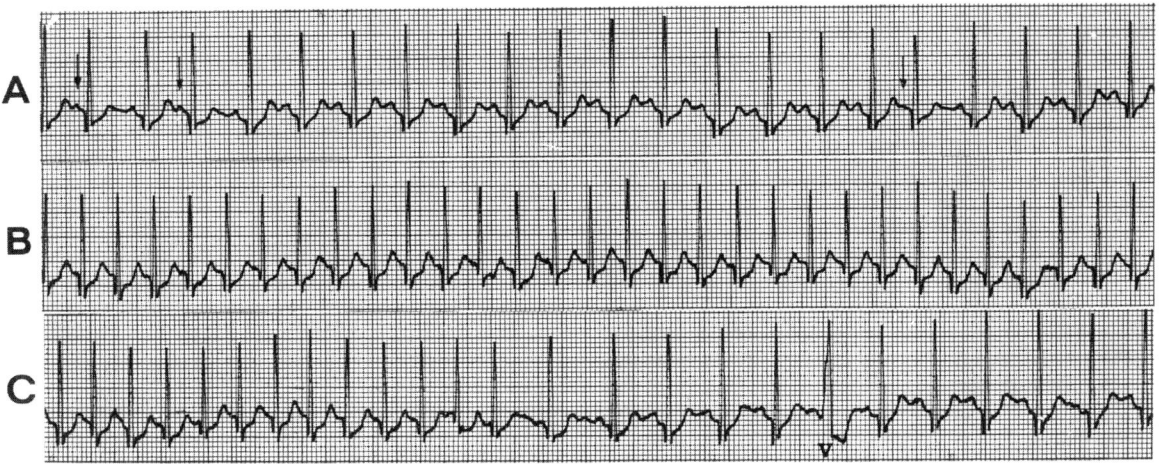

Figure 8-4
Atrial tachycardia (rate of 187 bpm) initiated by frequent atrial premature contractions (marked with arrows). Note a ventricular premature contraction (marked V). The Holter monitor ECG rhythm strips A–C are continuous.

ATRIAL TACHYCARDIA WITH ABERRANT VENTRICULAR CONDUCTION

Definition

AT with AVC is a regular and rapid atrial rhythm originating from any portion of the atria associated with bizarre QRS complexes as a result of AVC.

Diagnostic Criteria (Fig. 8-5)

- Diagnostic criteria described in Figure 8-4.
- AT with AVC because of rapid rate when the rapidly occurring atrial impulses are conducted to the ventricles during their partial refractory period.
- AVC in AT is often initiated by Ashman's phenomenon (see Chapter 6).

Diagnostic Pearls

AT with AVC closely mimics ventricular tachycardia. Proper identification of the rapidly occurring P waves is essential to diagnose AT with AVC. Remember that the ectopic P waves are often superimposed on the T waves of the preceding beats. In-depth understanding of AVC and Ashman's phenomenon is extremely important to make the correct diagnosis of AT with AVC. AT is often initiated by frequent APCs.

Figure 8-5
Sinus rhythm and paroxysmal atrial tachycardia (rate of 210 bpm) with aberrant ventricular conduction of varying degrees. The Holter monitor ECG rhythm strips A–C are not continuous.

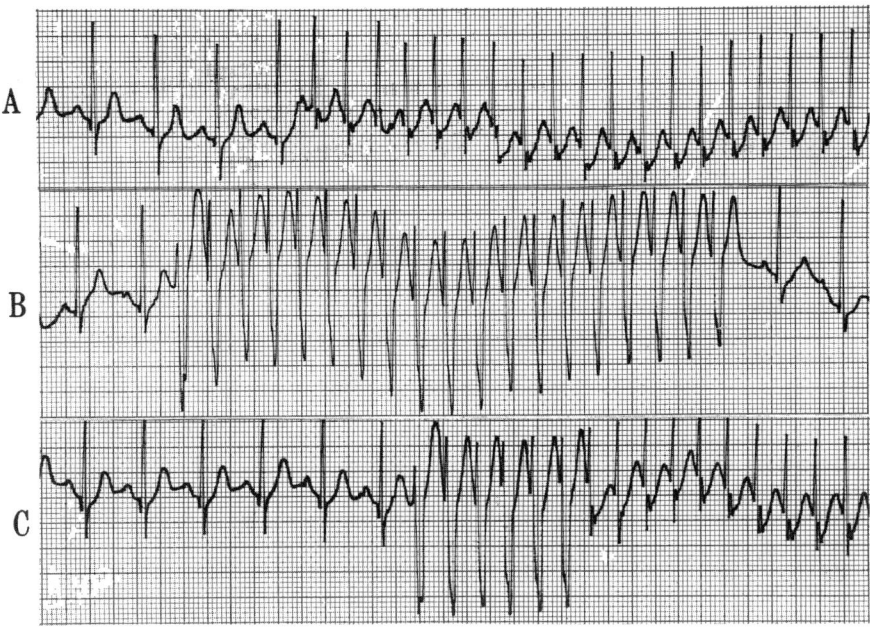

ATRIAL TACHYCARDIA ASSOCIATED WITH ATRIOVENTRICULAR BLOCK

Definition

AT associated with AV block is a rapid and regular atrial rhythm originating from any position of atria associated with AV block.

Diagnostic Criteria (Fig. 8-6)

- Diagnostic criteria described in Figure 8-4
- AT associated with AV block of varying degrees and any types
- AT most commonly associated with Wenckebach AV block
- The AT next most commonly associated with 2:1 AV block

Diagnostic Pearls

PAT is often associated with Wenckebach AV block. Thus, the term *PAT with block* is frequently used to describe this electrocardiographic finding. Clinically, PAT with block is most commonly found in patients with digitalis intoxication.

Since AT with Wenckebach AV block produces irregular ventricular cycles, AF is superficially simulated. Regularly occurring P waves confirm the diagnosis of AT. All readers should read Chapter 11 (Atrioventricular Block) to understand Wenckebach Atrioventricular block during sinus rhythm.

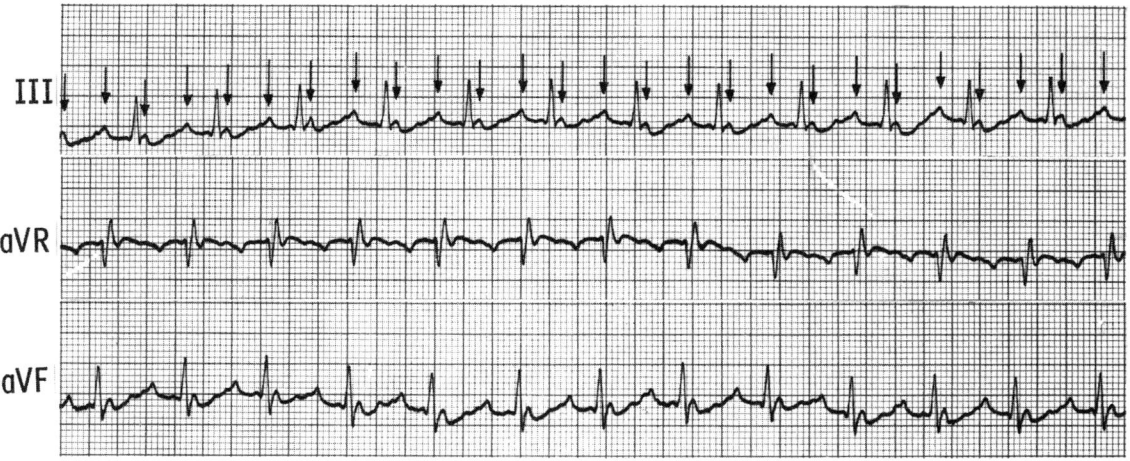

Figure 8-6
Atrial tachycardia (indicated by arrows, rate of 187 bpm) with a 2:1 atrioventricular block.

ATRIAL FLUTTER WITH A 2:1 ATRIOVENTRICULAR CONDUCTION

Definition

Atrial flutter with a 2:1 AV conduction is characterized by regular and rapid atrial waves with a saw-tooth appearance that originate from any portion of the atria, with a 2:1 AV conduction ratio.

Diagnostic Criteria (Fig. 8-7)

- Regular and rapid saw-tooth appearance atrial waves with atrial rate ranging from 250 to 350 bpm.
- Constant 2:1 AV conduction ratio (ventricular rate of 125–175 bpm).
- Atrial rate may be slightly slower than 250 bpm in some cases.

Diagnostic Pearls

Atrial flutter with 2:1 AV conduction is the most common uncomplicated form of atrial flutter. Whenever dealing with any regular tachycardia and normal QRS complexes with a ventricular rate of 125–175 bpm, atrial flutter with 2:1 AV conduction should be considered, especially when the ordinary P waves are *not* discernible. Under this circumstance, the term *2:1 AV conduction (response)* is used instead of 2:1 AV block because the 2:1 ratio is a physiologic phenomenon. Atrial flutter rate is often reduced by quinidine or other similar antiarrhythmic agents. Conversely, atrial flutter rate is accelerated by digitalis. Atrial flutter is one of the most common arrhythmias in humans. Atrial flutter with 2:1 AV conduction is frequently misdiagnosed by inexperienced readers.

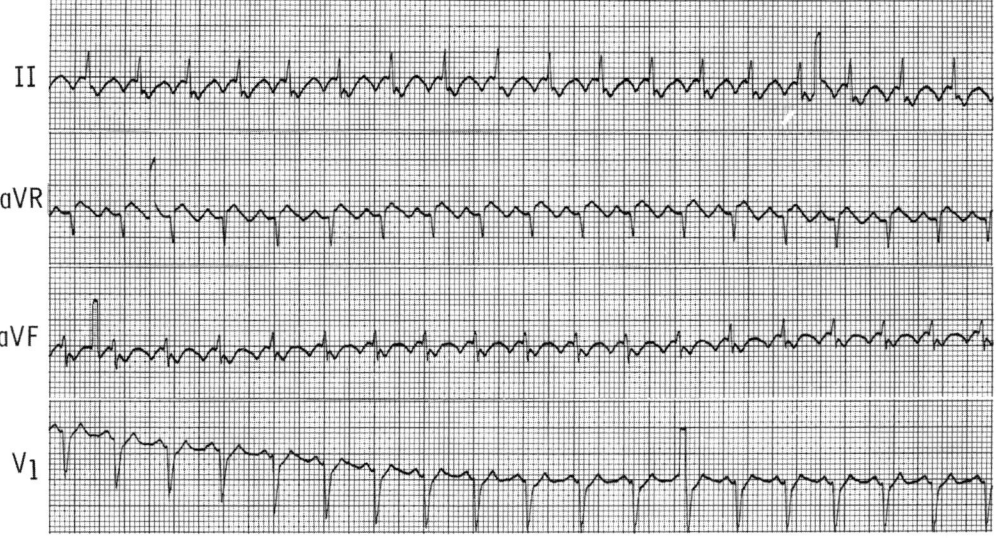

Figure 8-7
Atrial flutter with a 2:1 atrioventricular conduction (ventricular rate of 150 bpm).

ATRIAL FLUTTER WITH A 4:1 ATRIOVENTRICULAR BLOCK

Definition

Atrial flutter with a 4:1 AV block is characterized by regular and rapid atrial waves with a saw-tooth appearance and a 4:1 AV conduction ratio.

Diagnostic Criteria (Fig. 8-8)

- Regular and rapid atrial waves with a saw-tooth appearance
- Atrial rate of 250–350 bpm (slightly <250 bpm in some cases)
- Constant 4:1 AV conduction ratio

Diagnostic Pearls

The 4:1 AV conduction ratio is a pathologic phenomenon (abnormally delayed conduction in the AV junction because of prolonged refractory period). Thus, this arrhythmia is called *atrial flutter with 4:1 AV block*. Recognizing atrial flutter waves is relatively easy because the ventricular rate is relatively slow (around 65–80 bpm).

Figure 8-8
*Atrial flutter with a
4:1 atrioventricular
block (ventricular
rate of 60 bpm).*

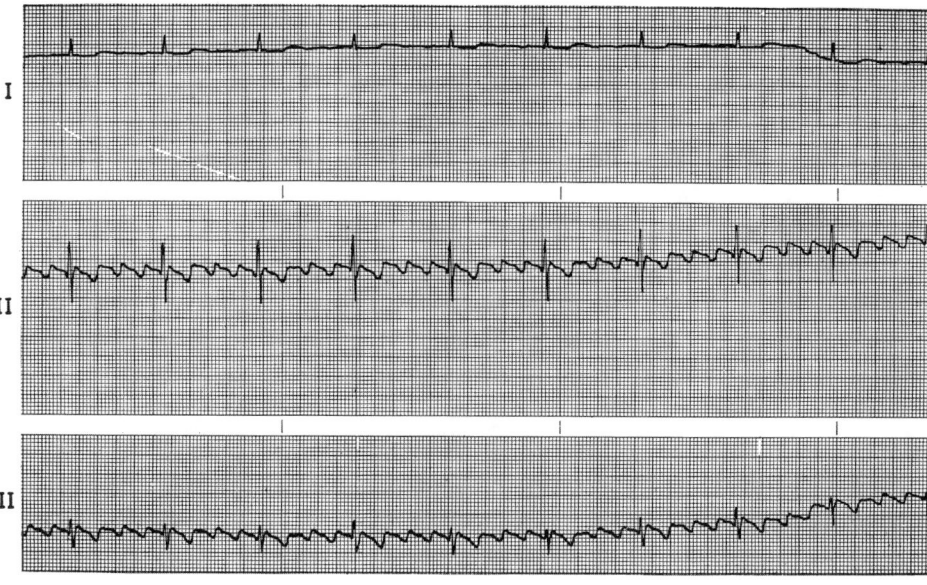

ATRIAL FIBRILLATION

Definition

AF is a very rapid and chaotic atrial rhythm originating from any portion of the atria and having a rapid and irregular ventricular response.

Diagnostic Criteria (Fig. 8-9)

- Grossly irregular and rapid ventricular cycles with no discernible P waves (ventricular rate of 120–180 bpm).
- Very rapid and chaotic AF waves replacing P waves.
- AF waves may be fine or coarse.

Diagnostic Pearls

AF is the most common ectopic rhythm in humans. AF should be considered first whenever dealing with grossly irregular and rapid ventricular cycles with no discernible P waves. Uncomplicated (pure) AF always exhibits a rapid ventricular rate of 120–180 bpm (much faster in some cases). The atrial rate in AF is 400–650 bpm. In a practical sense, however, the atrial rate in AF is rather difficult or even impossible to determine.

Figure 8-9
Atrial fibrillation with very rapid ventricular response (ventricular rate of 190–220 bpm).

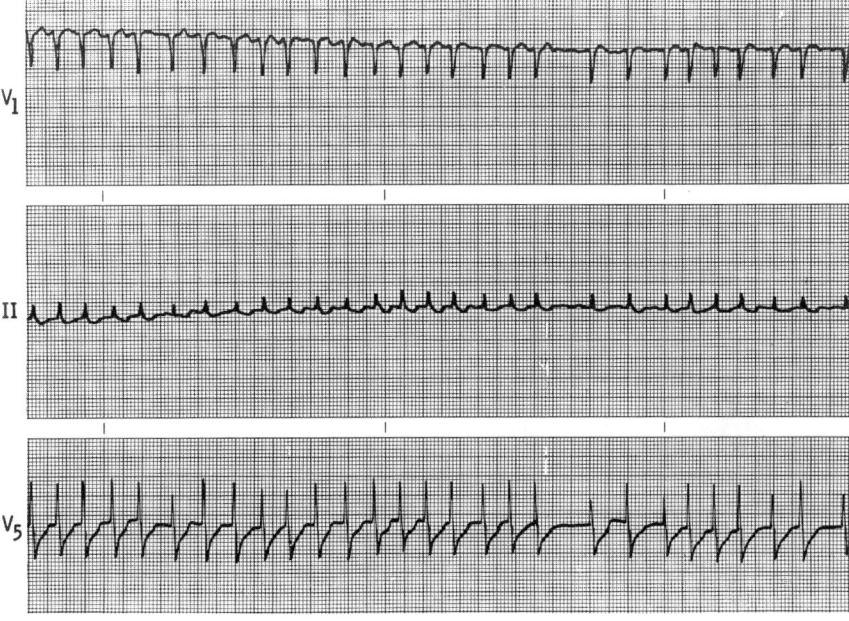

ATRIAL FIBRILLATION WITH BUNDLE BRANCH BLOCK

Definition

AF with bundle branch block is a very rapid and chaotic atrial rhythm originating from any portion of the atria and having grossly irregular ventricular cycles that are associated with LBBB or RBBB.

Diagnostic Criteria (Fig. 8-10)

- Grossly irregular and rapid ventricular cycles with no discernible P waves (ventricular rate of 120–180 bpm)
- LBBB or RBBB (see Chapter 4) in the presence of underlying AF

Diagnostic Pearls

When LBBB or RBBB is associated with underlying AF, ventricular tachycardia is closely simulated. However, grossly irregular ventricular cycles exclude the diagnosis of ventricular tachycardia (see Chapter 10). It is important to differentiate these cardiac arrhythmias because their clinical significance and their therapeutic approaches differ considerably.

Figure 8-10
Atrial fibrillation with rapid ventricular response (rate of 160–185 bpm) and left bundle branch block.

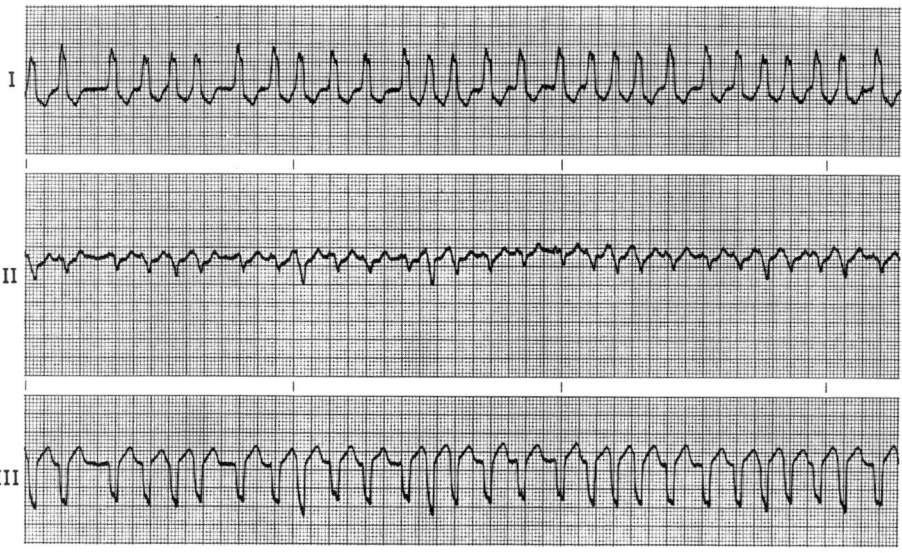

ATRIAL FIBRILLATION WITH ABERRANT VENTRICULAR CONDUCTION

Definition

AF with AVC is a very rapid and chaotic atrial rhythm originating from any portion of the atria having grossly irregular ventricular cycles and occasional bizarre QRS complexes because the atrial impulses are conducted to the ventricles during their partial refractory period.

Diagnostic Criteria (Fig. 8-11)

- Grossly irregular and rapid ventricular cycles (ventricular rate of 120–180 bpm) with no discernible P waves
- Occasional or intermittent bizarre QRS complexes (AVC) as a result of one of three reasons: a short coupling interval, Ashman's phenomenon, or an extremely rapid ventricular rate (see Chapter 6)

Diagnostic Pearls

Occasional occurrence of AVC closely mimics VPCs. Under this circumstance, VPCs are excluded on the basis of a lack of ventricular pause following a bizarre beat and the above-mentioned three reasons responsible for the production of AVC. Consecutively occurring AVC closely resembles ventricular tachycardia (see Fig. 6-6). Again, the above-mentioned differential points confirm the diagnosis. In AF, a lack of ventricular pause following bizarre beats is the most important clue to exclude the diagnosis of VPCs or ventricular tachycardia.

Figure 8-11
Atrial flutter-fibrillation with occasional aberrant ventricular conduction (the eighth and fourteenth beats) due to Ashman's phenomenon.

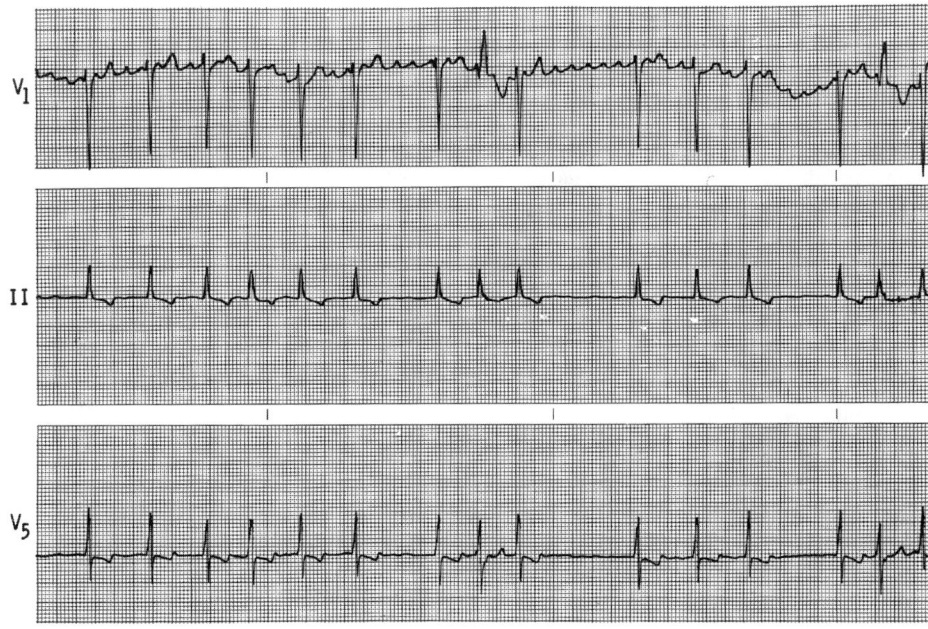

ATRIAL FIBRILLATION WITH ADVANCED ATRIOVENTRICULAR BLOCK

Definition

AF with advanced AV block is AF with a slow ventricular rate as a result of an abnormally prolonged refractory period in the AV junction.

Diagnostic Criteria (Fig. 8-12)

- Grossly irregular ventricular cycles with no discernible P waves
- Ventricular rate slower than 80 bpm as a result of an abnormally prolonged refractory period in the AV junction (advanced AV block)
- Occasional AV junctional (less commonly ventricular) escape beats because of advanced AV block

Diagnostic Pearls

Because of the relatively slow ventricular rate in AF, the rhythm may superficially resemble other bradyarrhythmias, especially when the ventricular rate is slower than 50 bpm. The underlying disorder of AF with advanced AV block is often sick sinus syndrome.

Figure 8-12
Atrial fibrillation with advanced atrioventricular block (rate of 38–45 bpm) producing intermittent atrioventricular junctional escape beats (the third, fifth, and sixth beats) and a ventricular escape beat (the second beat). These electrocardiographic findings represent advanced sick sinus syndrome.

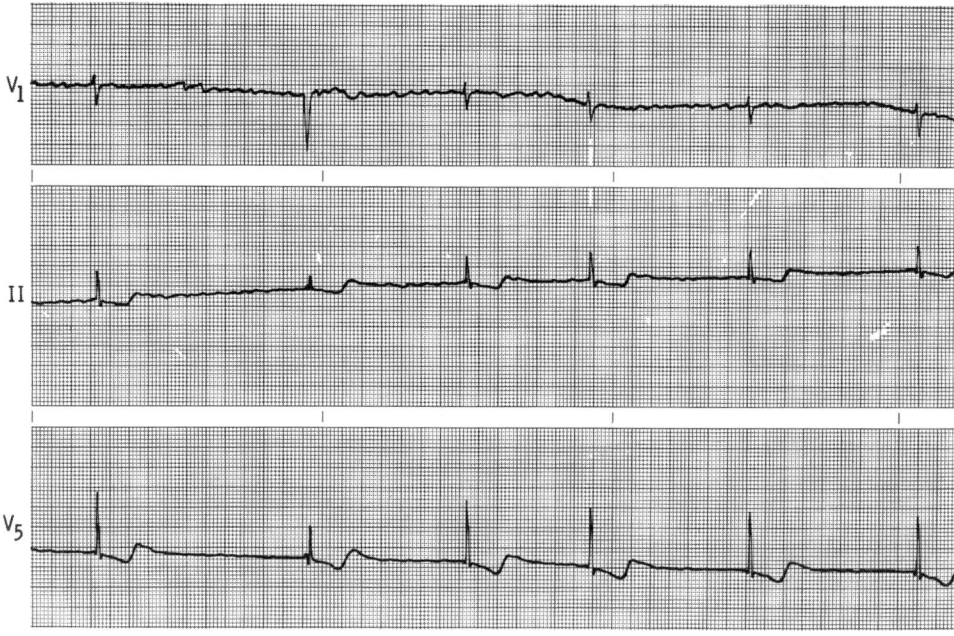

MULTIFOCAL ATRIAL TACHYCARDIA

Definition

MAT is a rapid and irregular cardiac rhythm originating from two or more different portions of the atria.

Diagnostic Criteria (Fig. 8-13)

- Two or more ectopic P waves with different configurations and two or more different ectopic P-P cycles
- Atrial rate of 100–250 bpm (occasionally <100 bpm)
- Isoelectrical line present between P-P intervals
- Frequent occurrence of varying P-R intervals and AV blocks of varying degree (nonconducted ectopic P waves)

Diagnostic Pearls

Because of the irregular ventricular cycles in MAT, AF is superficially simulated. The presence of P waves with various configurations excludes the possibility of AF. MAT is most commonly encountered in patients with chronic obstructive pulmonary disease.

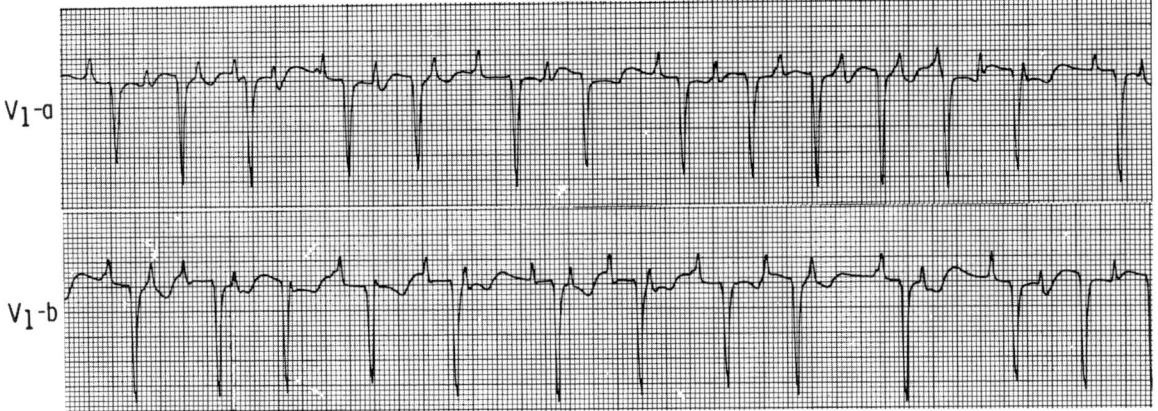

Figure 8-13
Multifocal atrial tachycardia with varying Wenckebach atrioventricular blocks. Leads V₁ a and b are continuous.

9

Atrioventricular Junctional Arrhythmias

Atrioventricular (AV) junctional arrhythmias may originate from any location in the AV junctional tissue. Generally, there are two major fundamental mechanisms responsible for the production of various AV junctional arrhythmias: *active* impulse formation and *passive* impulse formation. Active impulse formation in the AV junction may produce AV junctional premature contractions (JPCs) and AV junctional tachycardia (JT), whereas passive impulse formation results in AV junctional escape beats (JEBs) or rhythm (JER). Active impulse formation occurs because of an abnormal acceleration of impulse formation in the AV junction, regardless of the atrial mechanism. It is common to observe that AV JT is initiated by an isolated AV JPC. There are two types of AV JT: paroxysmal and nonparoxysmal. The former may be observed in apparently healthy individuals, while the latter almost always occurs in organic heart diseases and is particularly associated with digitalis intoxication. AV JEBs or JER, on the other hand, appear only as a physiologic mechanism to control the ventricles when atrial impulses (either sinus or ectopic) are unable to reach the AV junction. This may occur due to various causes, including marked sinus bradycardia, sinus arrest, sinoatrial block, and second- or third-degree AV block.

The electrocardiographic features of each AV junctional beat, regardless of whether it is a response to active or passive impulse formation, are essentially the same, except for the effect on the cardiac rhythm and the time of onset in the cardiac cycle. In other words, the configurations of the P, QRS, and T complexes of isolated AV junctional beats are identical, regardless of the fundamental mechanism involved.

The relationship between atrial and ventricular depolarization will vary, however, depending on the location of the ectopic pacemaker in the AV junction and the status of the antegrade and retrograde conduction systems. In general, the P waves tend to precede the QRS complexes when the ectopic focus is located in the upper portion of the AV junction, when antegrade AV conduction is impaired, or both. Conversely, the QRS complexes tend to precede the P waves when the ectopic focus is located in the lower portion of the AV junction, when retrograde ventriculoatrial conduction is impaired, or both. The P wave may not be discernible if it is superimposed on the QRS complex, in which the atria and the ventricles are activated simultaneously. This may occur when the ectopic focus is located in the middle portion of the AV junction provided that antegrade and retrograde conduction times are identical. P waves may be absent even when the ectopic focus is located in the upper or lower portions of the AV junction if there is a significant impairment of retrograde conduction in the upper portion of the AV junction and of antegrade conduction in the lower portion of the AV junction, however. Furthermore, P waves will be absent when there is a complete block of retrograde conduction, regardless of the location of the ectopic focus in the AV junction. Similarly, only the P wave may appear, without the QRS complex, in an AV junctional beat when there is a complete block of antegrade conduction. This can occur regardless of the location of the ectopic focus in the AV junction. If there is a block in both antegrade and retrograde conduction, needless to say, the P and QRS complexes will be absent; this is a form of exit block.

When P waves are present in AV junctional beats or rhythm (provided that AV dissociation is not present), the P waves are usually inverted in leads II, III, and aVF and upright in lead aVR. This pattern occurs because the atria are activated in a retrograde fashion. The mean electrical axis of the P waves in the frontal plane is usually between −60 and −90 degrees in AV junctional beats or rhythm. The P wave is usually not inverted in lead I. Similarly, the P wave is not inverted in leads V_5 or V_6.

The P-R and the R-P intervals vary depending on the location of the ectopic focus in the AV junction, on the status of antegrade and retrograde conduction, or both. In general, the P-R interval is 0.12 second or less, and the R-P interval is between 0.10 and 0.20 second, provided there is no conduction defect. The reason for the short P-R interval (≤0.12 second) in AV junctional arrhythmias is obvious. Unlike sinus rhythm, the impulse from the ectopic focus in AV junctional arrhythmias does *not* proceed from the atria to the ventricles. The P-R interval in the AV junctional arrhythmias is a difference of the conduction time between antegrade conduction to the ventricles and retrograde conduction to the atria from the ectopic pacemaker in the AV junction, provided that atrial activation occurs earlier than ventricular activation. Therefore, the P-R interval in AV junctional arrhythmias is *not* a true AV conduction time. In general, the P-R interval in AV junctional arrhythmias tends to be shorter when the ectopic pacemaker is located nearer the ventricles, when there is some degree of retrograde conduction defect present, or both. The converse holds true for the R-P interval.

AV dissociation commonly results when AV junctional beats or rhythm develop. AV dissociation is discussed in detail later in this chapter.

The QRS complex in AV junctional beats or rhythm is often normal in appearance, but it may be wide and bizarre, either because of aberrant ventricular conduction (AVC) or preexisting left bundle branch block (LBBB) or right bundle branch block (RBBB).

Reciprocal beats commonly develop when AV junctional beats or rhythm are present. Reciprocal beats and rhythm are discussed in detail in Chapter 13. AV junctional parasystole is a less common AV junctional arrhythmia (see Chapter 13).

Various AV junctional arrhythmias are summarized as follows:

1. Active impulse formation in the AV junction
   a. AV JPCs
   b. AV JT
      (1) Paroxysmal AV JT
      (2) Nonparoxysmal AV JT
2. Passive impulse formation in the AV junction: AV JEBs and JER
3. Uncommon AV junctional arrhythmias
   a. AV junctional parasystole
   b. Reciprocal beats and reciprocating tachycardia

ATRIOVENTRICULAR JUNCTIONAL PREMATURE CONTRACTIONS

AV JPCs may arise from any focus in the AV junctional tissue. In most instances, the impulse from the AV junction activates the entire atria, including the sinus node, unless the underlying rhythm is atrial fibrillation (AF) or atrial flutter. An ectopic impulse originating from the AV junction is conducted in two directions simultaneously. Retrograde conduction activates the atria, whereas antegrade conduction activates the ventricles. Although the onset of retrograde and antegrade conduction is simultaneous, atrial and ventricular activation do not necessarily occur simultaneously. In fact, more often, atrial and ventricular activations are completed at different times.

The sinus node is often prematurely discharged by the ectopic impulse from the AV junction, and the sinus node momentarily loses its inherent pacemaking function (automaticity). Propagation of the impulse in the atria from the ectopic focus in the AV junction is usually in a retrograde conduction, but conduction below the location of the ectopic focus is identical to that of sinus beats.

AV JPCs may occur every other beat (AV junctional bigeminy), every third beat (AV junctional trigeminy), or every fourth beat (AV junctional quadrigeminy). In addition, AV JPCs may occur consecutively (up to five beats in a row); this electrocardiographic finding is called *AV junctional group beats*. When six or more AV JPCs occur consecutively, the finding is termed *AV JT*. AV JPCs may show AVC because of a very short coupling interval or because of Ashman's phenomenon (see Chapter 6). When an AV JPC is not followed by a QRS complex, it is called a *blocked AV JPC*.

ATRIOVENTRICULAR JUNCTIONAL PREMATURE CONTRACTIONS

Definition

AV JPCs are characterized by the premature activation of the atria, ventricles, or both by any focus in the AV junctional tissue.

Diagnostic Criteria (Fig. 9-1)

- Premature retrograde P waves (inverted P waves in leads II, III, and aVF and upright P wave in lead aVR) that may be preceded or followed by QRS complexes in the presence of underlying sinus rhythm.
- The QRS complexes are normal unless there is AVC or bundle branch block (RBBB or LBBB).
- Constant coupling interval (interval from the ectopic beat to the preceding beat of the basic rhythm).
- Premature retrograde P waves not followed by QRS complexes (rare).
- Premature normal (narrow) QRS complexes not preceded or followed by retrograde P waves (not common).

Diagnostic Pearls

The QRS complex of AV JPC is almost always normal unless there is AVC, RBBB, or LBBB. The coupling interval is always constant, and the premature P wave must be conducted in a retrograde fashion (P wave axis ≥ -60 degrees).

Figure 9-1
Sinus rhythm with frequent atrioventricular junctional premature contractions producing atrioventricular junctional bigeminy.

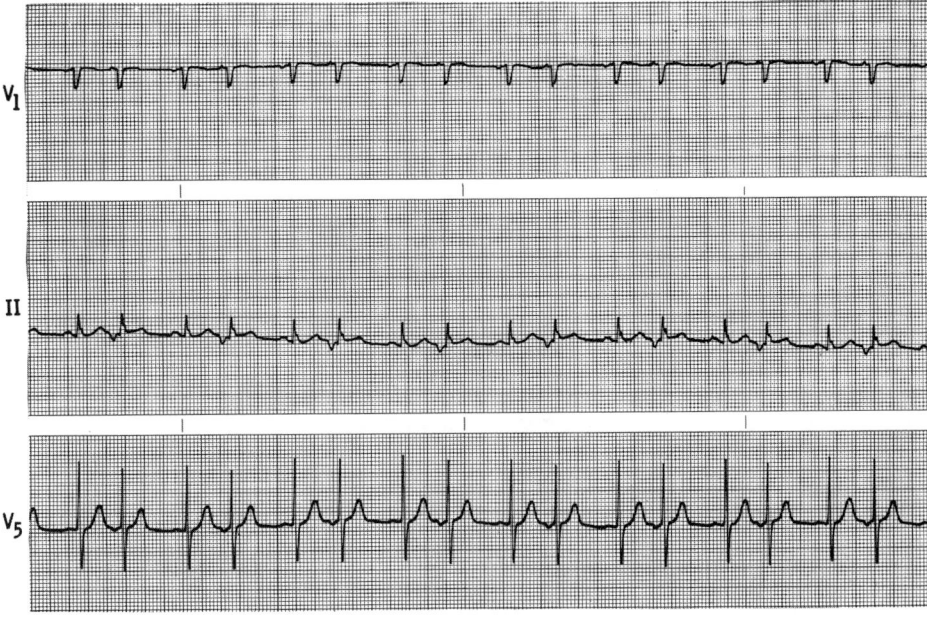

ATRIOVENTRICULAR JUNCTIONAL PREMATURE CONTRACTIONS WITH ABERRANT VENTRICULAR CONDUCTION

Definition

AV JPCs with AVC are characterized by the premature activation of the atria, ventricles, or both by any focus in the AV junctional tissue associated with AVC.

Diagnostic Criteria (Fig. 9-2)

- Criteria described previously (see Fig. 9-1)
- Bizarre QRS complex due to a short coupling interval or Ashman's phenomenon because the AV junctional premature impulse is conducted to the ventricles during their partial refractory period

Diagnostic Pearls

AV JPCs with AVC closely mimic ventricular premature contractions (VPCs) because of bizarre and/or broad QRS complexes. Prematurely occurring retrograde P waves preceding bizarre QRS complexes exclude VPCs.

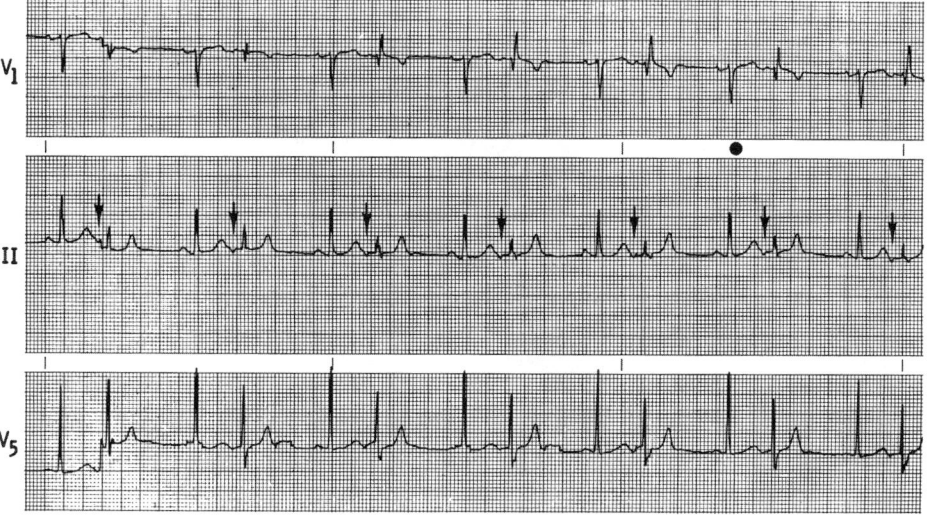

Figure 9-2
Sinus rhythm and frequent atrioventricular junctional premature contractions (marked with arrows) with aberrant ventricular conduction due to Ashman's phenomenon.

ATRIOVENTRICULAR JUNCTIONAL TACHYCARDIA

AV JT may originate from any location in the AV junctional tissue, as seen in AV JPCs. AV JT appears as an active impulse formation, so that the rate of AV junctional impulse discharge is accelerated. As a result, the rate is naturally faster than that of AV JER. In other words, AV JT has a rate faster than the inherent rate (45–60 bpm) of the AV junction.

AV JT is divided into two major categories: *paroxysmal* AV JT and *nonparoxysmal* AV JT. Not only are the nature of the onset and the termination of the two forms of AV JT different, but their usual rates and clinical significance are also different. That is, paroxysmal AV JT produces a rate of 160–250 bpm, which is the same rate range as paroxysmal atrial tachycardia, and may occur in apparently healthy individuals. Conversely, nonparoxysmal AV JT produces a rate of 60–130 bpm, which is the range of normal sinus rhythm and sinus tachycardia, and is practically always found in diseased hearts.

The ectopic focus in the AV junction may activate both the atria and the ventricles. The P-R and R-P intervals vary in this circumstance, depending on the location of the ectopic focus and the status of the antegrade and retrograde conduction systems. In many instances, however, particularly in nonparoxysmal AV JT, there is an independent atrial mechanism, such as AF, leading to AV dissociation. The QRS complex in the AV JT is often normal, but it may be wide and bizarre because of AVC, LBBB, or RBBB.

PAROXYSMAL ATRIOVENTRICULAR JUNCTIONAL TACHYCARDIA

Definition

AV JT is a very rapid and regular tachycardia with normal QRS complexes originating from any portion of the AV junctional tissue. The QRS complexes may be preceded or followed by retrograde P waves.

Diagnostic Criteria (Fig. 9-3)

- Rapid and regular tachycardia (rate of 160–250 bpm) with normal QRS complexes.
- The retrograde P waves (inverted P waves in leads II, III, and aVF and upright P waves in lead aVR) may be preceded or followed by QRS complexes.
- Regular and rapid tachycardia without discernible P waves in some cases.
- Regular and rapid tachycardia with independent sinus P waves or other atrial arrhythmias, causing AV dissociation in some cases.

- The onset and termination of tachycardia is paroxysmal in nature.
- Regular tachycardia may show broad or bizarre QRS complexes because of AVC, LBBB, or RBBB.

Diagnostic Pearls

Paroxysmal AV JT with broad or bizarre QRS complexes due to AVC, RBBB, or LBBB may closely simulate ventricular tachycardia (VT). Under these circumstances, retrograde P waves preceding the QRS complexes support the diagnosis of AV JT. Other differential diagnostic clues are found in Chapters 6 and 10.

Figure 9-3
Paroxysmal atrioventricular junctional tachycardia (rate of 166 bpm).

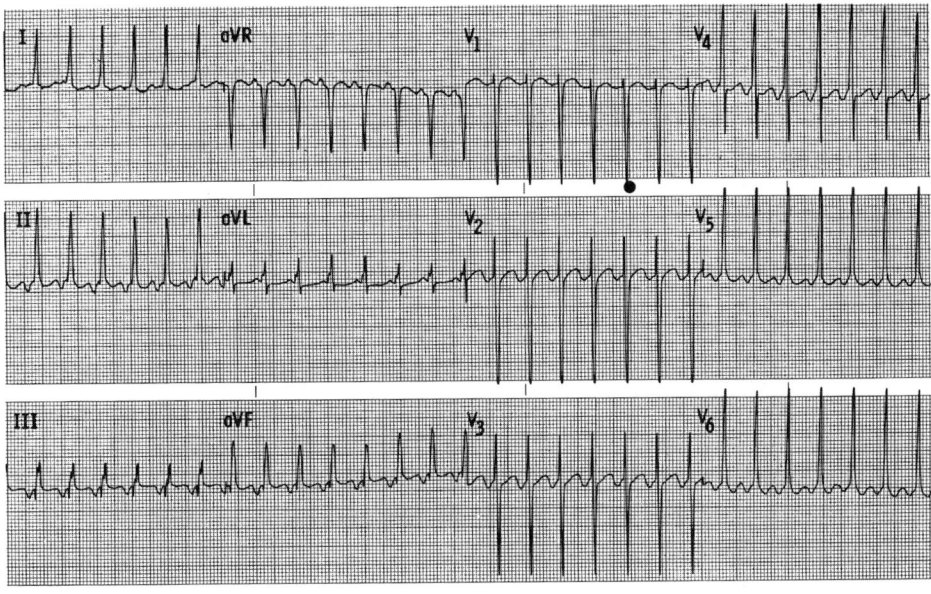

NONPAROXYSMAL ATRIOVENTRICULAR JUNCTIONAL TACHYCARDIA

Definition

Nonparoxysmal AV JT is moderately rapid and regular tachycardia with normal QRS complexes originating from any portion of the AV junctional tissue. The QRS complexes may be preceded by or followed by retrograde P waves.

Diagnostic Criteria (Fig. 9-4)

- Moderately rapid regular tachycardia (rate of 60–130 bpm) with normal QRS complexes.
- Retrograde P waves may be preceded or followed by QRS complexes.
- Regular tachycardia without discernible P waves in some cases.
- Regular tachycardia with independent sinus P waves or other atrial arrhythmias (e.g., AF), causing AV dissociation in some cases.
- Regular tachycardia may show broad or bizarre QRS complexes because of AVC, LBBB, or RBBB.
- Tachycardia is not paroxysmal in nature.

Diagnostic Pearls

Nonparoxysmal AV JT often occurs in the presence of AF or atrial flutter producing complete AV dissociation (Fig. 9-5). The underlying disorder producing this arrhythmia is most commonly digitalis intoxication or acute diaphragmatic (inferior) myocardial infarction. Slow VT is closely simulated when AV JT is associated with AVC, LBBB, or RBBB (see Chapters 6 and 10).

Figure 9-4
Nonparoxysmal atrioventricular junctional tachycardia (rate of 100 bpm).

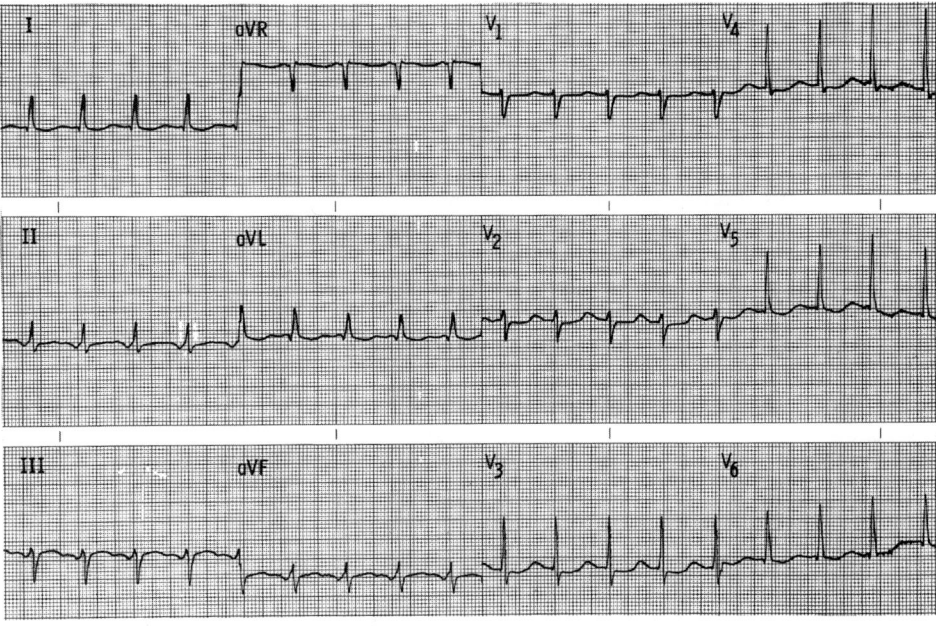

NONPAROXYSMAL ATRIOVENTRICULAR JUNCTIONAL TACHYCARDIA IN THE PRESENCE OF ATRIAL FIBRILLATION

Definition

Nonparoxysmal AV JT in the presence of AF is moderately rapid and regular tachycardia with normal QRS complexes originating from any portion of the AV junction in the presence of AF producing complete AV dissociation.

Diagnostic Criteria (see Fig. 9-5)

- Moderately rapid and regular tachycardia (rate of 60–130 bpm) with normal QRS complexes in the presence of AF producing complete AV dissociation.
- No discernible P waves because of AF waves replacing P waves.
- Regular tachycardia may be associated with broad or bizarre QRS complexes because of AVC, LBBB, or RBBB.

Diagnostic Pearls

Nonparoxysmal AV JT in the presence of AF is most commonly observed in patients with digitalis intoxication. When AV JT is associated with the broad QRS complexes, VT is closely simulated (see Chapters 6 and 10).

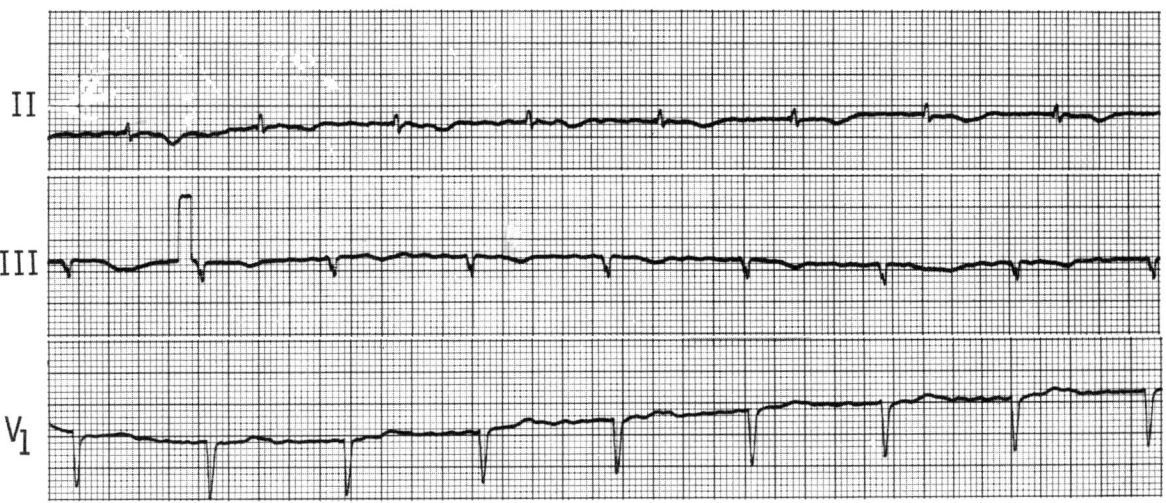

Figure 9-5
Atrial fibrillation with nonparoxysmal atrioventricular junctional tachycardia (rate of 73 bpm) producing complete atrioventricular dissociation as a result of digitalis intoxication.

ATRIOVENTRICULAR JUNCTIONAL ESCAPE RHYTHM

AV JEBs and JER, like AV JPCs, may originate from any location in the AV junctional tissue. AV JEBs may appear singly or consecutively as group beats. When six or more AV JEBs appear consecutively, the term *atrioventricular junctional escape rhythm* is used. AV JEBs or JER appear as a physiologic mechanism and therefore are the most common arrhythmias generated by passive impulse formation.

Under normal circumstances, AV JEBs and JER do not appear because the AV junctional pacemaker is controlled by the sinus node, which produces impulses faster than the AV junction. Thus, the AV junction is continuously depressed by the rapidly discharging sinus impulses. However, AV JEBs or JER appear when the sinus node produces impulses slower than usual (sinus bradycardia) or when the impulse from the sinus node fails to reach the AV

junction, as in sinus arrest, sinoatrial block, or AV block. One or two AV JEBs commonly follow the postectopic pause of APCs, AV JPCs, or VPCs.

AV JEBs or JER may occur in the presence of an ectopic atrial rhythm, including AF, atrial flutter, and tachycardia when the atrial impulses fail to reach the AV junction due to high-degree or complete AV block.

AV JEBs or JER may be preceded by or followed by retrograde P waves, depending on the location of the ectopic pacemaker in the AV junction and the status of the antegrade and retrograde conduction systems. However, more commonly, AV JEBs or JER produce only QRS complexes in the presence of independent atrial activity, thus producing transient or continuous AV dissociation.

The usual rate of AV JER is 45–60 bpm. When the rate of an AV JER exceeds 60 bpm, the mechanism involved is considered to be different from escape rhythm and is termed *nonparoxysmal AV junctional tachycardia.*

Unlike sinus rhythm, AV JER is usually not influenced by maneuvers such as carotid sinus stimulation, respiration, exercise, and so forth.

ATRIOVENTRICULAR JUNCTIONAL ESCAPE RHYTHM

Definition

AV JER is a slow and regular rhythm with normal QRS complexes originating from any location in the AV junctional tissue. The QRS complex may be preceded by or followed by a retrograde P wave.

Diagnostic Criteria (Fig. 9-6)

- Regular rhythm with normal QRS complexes (rate of 40–60 bpm).
- The QRS complexes may be preceded by or followed by a retrograde P waves (inverted P waves in leads II, III, and aVF and upright P waves in lead aVR).
- Regular and slow rhythm with normal QRS complexes without any discernible P waves in some cases.
- Regular and slow rhythm with normal QRS complexes in the presence of independent sinus P waves or any atrial arrhythmias (e.g., AF) producing AV dissociation in some cases.

- The QRS complexes are broad and bizarre when there is preexisting LBBB or RBBB.

Diagnostic Pearls

AV junctional escape rhythm is the most common arrhythmia as a result of passive impulse formation. AV JER often occurs in the presence of marked sinus bradycardia or complete AV block producing AV dissociation (discussed in the section on atrioventricular dissociation). The pure form of AV JER (see Fig. 9-6) is rather uncommon.

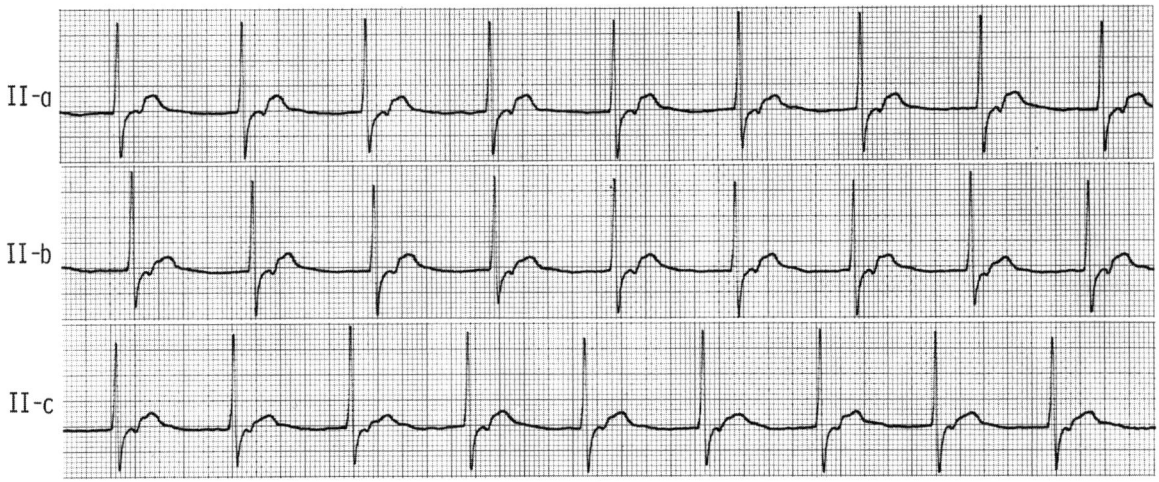

Figure 9-6
Atrioventricular junctional escape rhythm with a rate of 60 bpm. Note that every QRS complex is followed by a retro-grade P wave. Leads II a–c are continuous.

ATRIOVENTRICULAR JUNCTIONAL ESCAPE RHYTHM IN THE PRESENCE OF SINUS BRADYCARDIA

Definition

AV JER in the presence of sinus bradycardia is a slow and regular rhythm with normal QRS complexes in the presence of marked sinus bradycardia producing AV dissociation.

Diagnostic Criteria (Fig. 9-7)

- Regular rhythm with normal QRS complexes (rate of 40–60 bpm) in the presence of marked sinus bradycardia producing complete or incomplete AV dissociation.
- The QRS complexes may be broad and bizarre when there is preexisting LBBB or RBBB.

Diagnostic Pearls

It is important to remember that AV JER often occurs as a physiologic phenomenon when there is marked sinus bradycardia producing AV dissociation (discussed in the section on atrioventricular disassociation). Ventricular escape rhythm will be closely simulated when AV JER is associated with LBBB or RBBB (see Chapter 10).

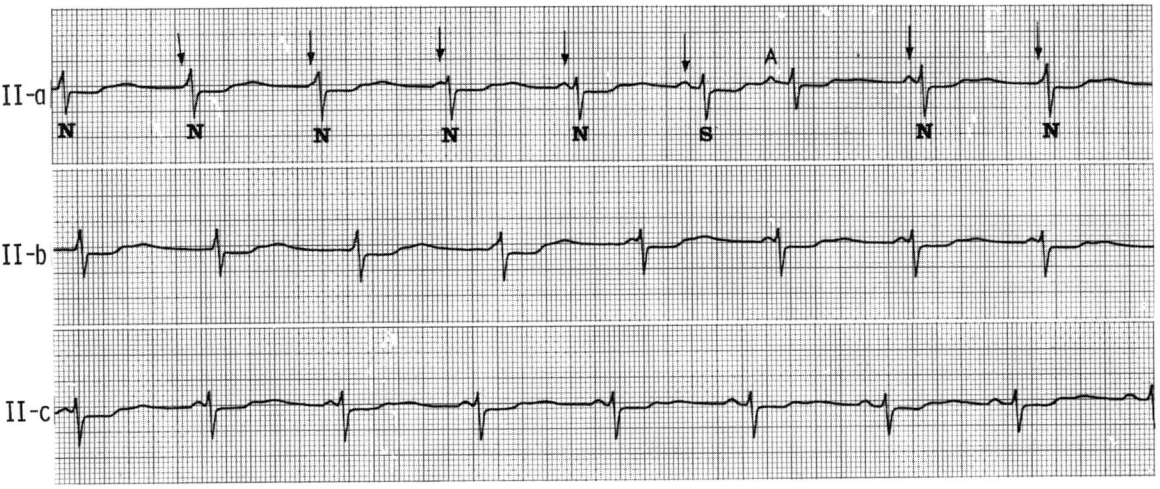

Figure 9-7

Sinus arrhythmia with sinus bradycardia (marked S) and intermittent atrioventricular junctional escape rhythm (marked N) producing incomplete atrioventricular dissociation. Arrows indicate sinus P waves, and leads II a–c are continuous. Note an atrial premature contraction (marked A). Hypokalemia is considered because of the predominant U waves.

SINUS RHYTHM WITH ATRIOVENTRICULAR JUNCTIONAL ESCAPE RHYTHM DUE TO COMPLETE ATRIOVENTRICULAR BLOCK

See Chapter 11.

ATRIAL FIBRILLATION WITH ATRIOVENTRICULAR JUNCTIONAL ESCAPE RHYTHM DUE TO COMPLETE ATRIOVENTRICULAR BLOCK

See Chapter 11.

ATRIOVENTRICULAR DISSOCIATION

By definition, AV dissociation indicates that the atria and ventricles beat independently, so the P waves, AF waves, or atrial flutter waves and the QRS complexes do not have any relationship. The various underlying cardiac arrhythmias produce AV dissociation.

It should be emphasized that AV dissociation is by no means a complete description of the cardiac arrhythmia because it is always a consequence of some other cardiac mechanism.

AV dissociation is diagnosed when the atria and the ventricles beat independently. There are *three basic major rhythm disturbances* that produce AV dissociation. They are (1) slowing or impairment of sinus impulse formation or impairment of the conduction at the sinoatrial junction; (2) acceleration of impulse formation in the AV junction or ventricles; and (3) AV conduction disturbances, including artificial pacemaker-induced ventricular rhythms. In AV dissociation, the atrial mechanism may be AF, atrial flutter, or tachycardia. In rare instances of AV dissociation, both the atria and ventricles are activated independently by two or more different pacemakers in the AV junction to produce double or triple AV JT or JERs. When there are one or more atrial or ventricular fusion beats in AV dissociation, the term *incomplete AV dissociation* is used. If no captured beats exists, *complete AV dissociation* is said to be present.

If the mechanism of AV dissociation is not complete AV block, whenever any chamber is *not* in the refractory state, one of the two pacemakers may activate the entire heart. In other words, the sinus or ectopic atrial pacemaker may control the ventricles when the ventricles are not in a refractory phase. This is termed *ventricular captured beat*. Ventricular captured beat in the presence of AV dissociation merely indicates normally conducted sinus or atrial (i.e., fibrillation) beat. Likewise, an ectopic pacemaker in the AV junction or ventricles or an artificial pacemaker that controls the ventricles may activate the atria in a retrograde fashion when the atria are not in a refractory phase. This phenomenon is termed *atrial captured beat*. It should be noted that the atrial captured beat originating from the AV junction (rarely ventricles) may be followed by a reciprocal beat due to a re-entry phenomenon. Reciprocal beats are discussed in Chapter 13. If the captured impulse in the atria or ventricles simultaneously meets with an impulse from another pacemaker, partial atrial or ventricular captured beats develop. This phenomenon may be referred to as atrial or ventricular fusion beats, respectively. Recognizing captured beats is not difficult because they occur prematurely with a constant P-R or R-P relationship when the atrial mechanism is not fibrillation or atrial flutter. When the underlying atrial mechanism is AF or atrial flutter, in the presence of AV dissociation, ventricular captured beats are actually normally conducted ordinary AF or atrial flutter beats. Often, ventricular captured beats exhibit AVC because of a short coupling interval. Once a captured beat occurs, one pacemaker may control the entire heart either temporarily or continuously. Ventricular captured beats are very common in the presence of underlying AF because AV JT or AV JER often occurs intermittently or periodically. Needless to say, it is impossible for atrial captured beats to occur when the underlying rhythm is AF or atrial flutter, since the atria are constantly activated by one or more rapidly discharging atrial ectopic foci.

Atrial or ventricular captured beats may occur in double or triple AV JTs or JERs when antegrade or retrograde conduction is not completely blocked. For a similar reason, atrial or ventricular fusion beats may be observed in double or triple AV JTs or JERs. In addition, atrial or ventricular captured beats may be observed in artificial pacemaker-induced ventricular rhythm unless there is a complete block in antegrade or retrograde conduction.

In any event, *incomplete AV dissociation* occurs whenever a captured beat (either complete or partial) is present and is named so because the atria and ventricles have some relationship to each other, even though only momentarily. In the presence of intermittent complete AV block, captured beats may intermittently occur; this situation has been called *high-degree block* or *advanced AV block* (see Chapter 11). This is also a form of incomplete AV dissociation.

If there are no captured beats and the atria and ventricles beat independently throughout, it is called *complete AV dissociation*.

ATRIOVENTRICULAR DISSOCIATION DUE TO ATRIOVENTRICULAR JUNCTIONAL TACHYCARDIA IN THE PRESENCE OF SINUS RHYTHM

Definition

AV dissociation due to AV JT in the presence of sinus rhythm is an independent regular tachycardia with normal QRS complexes in the presence of sinus rhythm in the atria producing complete or incomplete AV dissociation.

Diagnostic Criteria (Fig. 9-8)

- Regular tachycardia with normal QRS complexes in the presence of independent sinus rhythm in the atria (upright P waves in leads II, III, and aVF and inverted P waves in lead aVR) producing AV dissociation.
- AV JT may be paroxysmal (rate of 160–250 bpm) or nonparoxysmal (rate of 70–130 bpm).
- The QRS complexes may be bizarre or broad because of AVC, LBBB, or RBBB.

- There may or may not be ventricular or atrial captured beats (discussed earlier).

Diagnostic Pearls

AV JT, particularly the nonparoxysmal form, often occurs in the presence of independent sinus rhythm in the atria producing complete or incomplete AV dissociation. Thus, the atrial mechanism must be recognized and diagnosed properly when AV JT is observed.

Figure 9-8
Sinus rhythm with intermittent nonparoxysmal atrioventricular junctional tachycardia (rate of 75 bpm) producing incomplete atrioventricular dissociation. Arrows indicate sinus P waves. Note a ventricular captured beat (normally conducted sinus beat, the last beat in the rhythm strip).

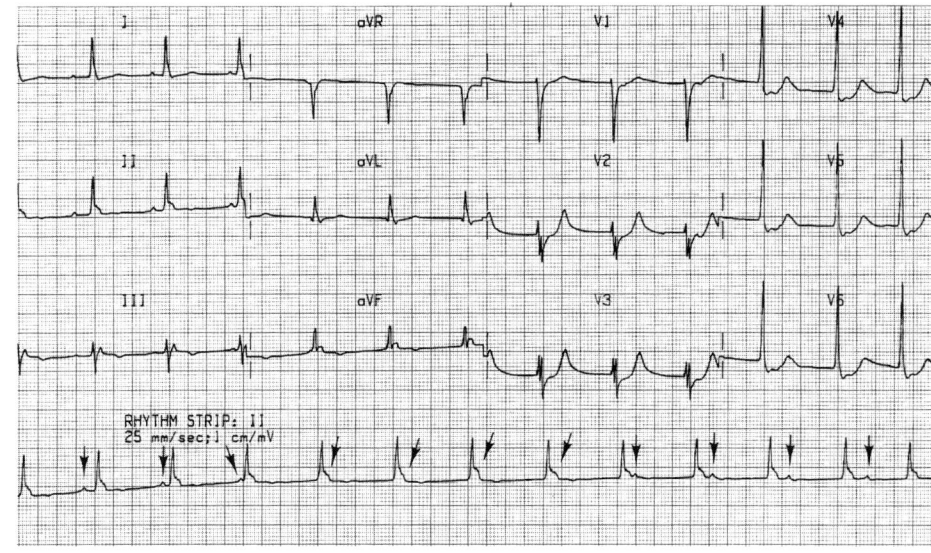

ATRIOVENTRICULAR DISSOCIATION DUE TO ATRIOVENTRICULAR JUNCTIONAL TACHYCARDIA IN THE PRESENCE OF ATRIAL FIBRILLATION

Definition

AV dissociation due to AV JT in the presence of AF is an independent regular tachycardia with normal QRS complexes in the presence of AF producing complete or incomplete AV dissociation.

Diagnostic Criteria (Fig. 9-9)

- Regular tachycardia with normal QRS complexes in the presence of independent AF producing AV dissociation.
- In most cases, nonparoxysmal AV JT (rate: 70–130 bpm) coexists with independent AF.
- The QRS complexes may be broad because of LBBB or RBBB.

Diagnostic Pearls

When nonparoxysmal AV JT is recognized, the underlying atrial mechanism is commonly AF producing AV dissociation. The underlying disorder responsible for the production of this arrhythmia is most commonly digitalis intoxication.

Figure 9-9
Atrial fibrillation with non-paroxysmal atrioventricular junctional tachycardia (rate of 105 bpm) producing complete atrioventricular dissociation. This patient is known to have had chronic atrial fibrillation for many years.

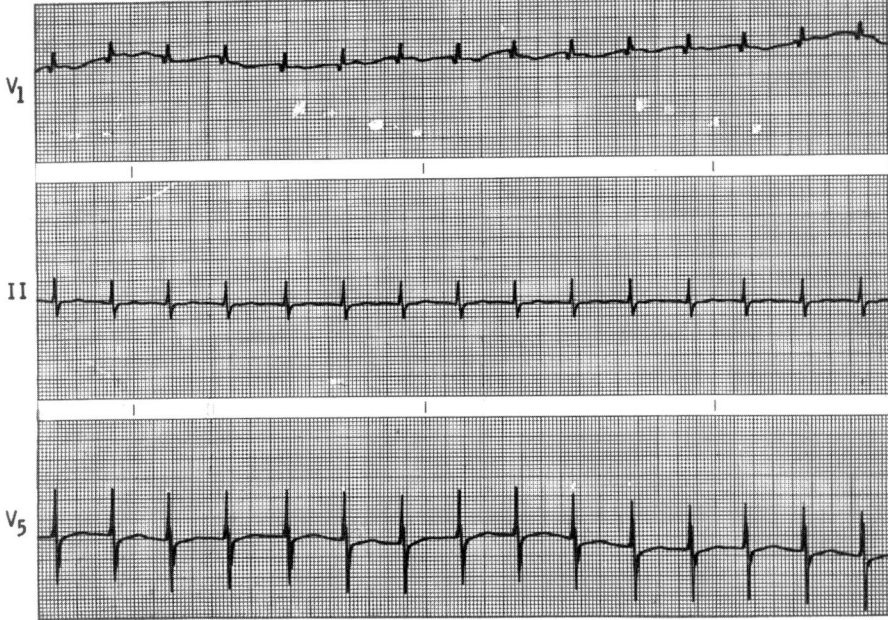

ATRIOVENTRICULAR DISSOCIATION DUE TO DOUBLE OR TRIPLE ATRIOVENTRICULAR JUNCTIONAL RHYTHMS OR TACHYCARDIAS

See Chapter 13.

RECIPROCAL BEATS AND RECIPROCATING TACHYCARDIA

See Chapter 13.

10

Ventricular Arrhythmias

Ventricular arrhythmias may be generated by either *active* or *passive* impulse formation. A relatively uncommon ventricular arrhythmia is produced by a parasystolic mechanism (see Chapter 13). Active impulse formation from a ventricular focus may produce a ventricular premature contraction (VPC), ventricular tachycardia (VT), ventricular flutter, and ventricular fibrillation (VF). These ventricular arrhythmias occur regardless of the underlying cardiac rhythm. Passive impulse formation of the ventricles, on the other hand, occurs when the atrioventricular (AV) junction fails to produce an impulse passively in spite of the fact that atrial impulses are unable to reach the ventricles (common-

ly due to high-degree or complete AV nodal block) in the expected time or when the AV block is distal to the AV node (infranodal block). The rhythm generated by passive impulse formation by the ventricles is termed *ventricular escape rhythm* (VER) or *idioventricular rhythm.*

Ventricular arrhythmias, regardless of the fundamental mechanism, may originate from any location in the ventricles. The configuration of the QRS complex in ventricular arrhythmias is greatly influenced by the location of the ectopic focus. The configuration may be almost normal and resemble a sinus beat or may be so bizarre that the duration of the QRS complex may exceed 0.16 second. Various electrocardiographic findings supporting ventricular ectopy are summarized in Table 6-2.

The most common ventricular arrhythmia and, in fact, the most common ectopic beats encountered in human hearts are, without doubt, VPCs. Since VPCs may be observed in almost every individual some time during his or her life, even without demonstrable heart disease, the occasional occurrence of this arrhythmia is insignificant clinically. Generally, the numbers of VPCs increase with age and are rare in children. Frequent VPCs, particularly multifocal ones, are almost always found in diseased hearts and are commonly due to digitalis intoxication, acute myocardial infarction (MI), or advanced congestive heart failure.

Ventricular tachyarrhythmias, including VT, ventricular flutter, and VF, are almost always found in serious heart disease and often are fatal unless immediately treated. These arrhythmias are frequently initiated by an isolated VPC, particularly one that is multifocal in origin. It is commonly observed that VT may transform to ventricular flutter and VF or vice versa in the same patient.

The relatively new terms *sustained VT* and *nonsustained VT* have been used in the recent literature. The term *nonsustained VT* is used when VT persists up to 29 sec-

onds, whereas the term *sustained VT* is used when VT persists more than 29 seconds.

Various ventricular arrhythmias are summarized as follows.

1. VPCs
   a. VPC with full compensatory pause
   b. Interpolated VPC
   c. VPC followed by an atrial echo beat
   d. Multifocal VPCs
   e. Grouped VPCs
2. VT
   a. Paroxysmal VT (sustained or nonsustained)
   b. Accelerated idioventricular rhythm (nonparoxysmal VT)
   c. Parasystolic VT
   d. Torsade de pointes (multiformed VT)
3. Ventricular flutter-fibrillation
   a. Ventricular flutter
   b. VF
   c. Chaotic ventricular rhythm
4. VER (idioventricular rhythm)
5. Ventricular parasystole

VENTRICULAR PREMATURE CONTRACTIONS

VPCs are the most common cardiac arrhythmia and may be observed in practically every individual some time during his or her life. This arrhythmia is uncommon in children, but its incidence increases with age, even without demonstrable heart disease. Although VPCs are commonly found in healthy adults, especially after excessive ingestion of coffee or tea, heavy smoking, or emotional excitement, the frequent occurrence of this arrhythmia, particularly when it is multifocal in origin, nearly always indicates organic heart disease.

VPCs may originate from a single focus or from multiple foci anywhere in the ventricles. They may occur rarely, occasionally, or frequently, and regularly or irregularly. There may be two or more consecutive VPCs that may lead to VT, ventricular flutter, or VF. Any underlying cardiac rhythm may be present concomitantly with VPCs. This arrhythmia is almost always followed by a full compensatory pause; interpolated VPCs are only occasionally observed, especially when the basic cardiac rhythm is slow. The term *ventricular group beats* is used when two to five VPCs occur consecutively. The term *VT* is used when six or more VPCs occur consecutively.

VPCs are diagnosed when a wide and bizarre QRS complex appears prematurely without a preceding ectopic P wave. A full compensatory pause almost always follows this arrhythmia. VPCs may occur every other beat (ventricular bigeminy), every third beat (ventricular trigeminy), or every fourth beat (ventricular quadrigeminy) in the presence of any underlying cardiac rhythm (e.g., sinus rhythm, atrial fibrillation [AF], or atrial flutter).

VPC is almost always followed by a full compensatory pause (meaning that the sinus P-P cycle is not disturbed), but VPC may be interpolated. On rare occasions, VPC may be followed by a retrograde P wave (atrial echo beat).

VENTRICULAR PREMATURE CONTRACTION

Definition

VPC is the premature occurrence of a bizarre and broad QRS complex originating from any position of the ventricles.

Diagnostic Criteria (Fig. 10-1)

- Premature occurrence of a bizarre and broad QRS complex not preceded by a premature P wave.
- Full compensatory pause after a bizarre and broad QRS complex in nearly all cases.
- The sinus P-P cycle is not disturbed by a VPC in nearly all cases.
- Occasionally, a VPC may be interpolated (discussed in the next section; Fig. 10-2).
- On rare occasions, a VPC may be followed by a retrograde P wave (atrial echo beat).
- VPC is always followed by a long pause in the presence of AF or atrial flutter.

Diagnostic Pearls

Atrial premature contractions with aberrant ventricular conduction (AVC) or bundle branch block closely mimics a VPC. However, a premature P wave preceding a bizarre beat excludes the possibility of a VPC. When the underlying rhythm is AF or atrial flutter, a VPC is always followed by a long ventricular pause (important finding to distinguish VPC from AVC in AF). It is extremely important to remember that the sinus P-P cycle is *not* disturbed by a VPC in nearly all cases.

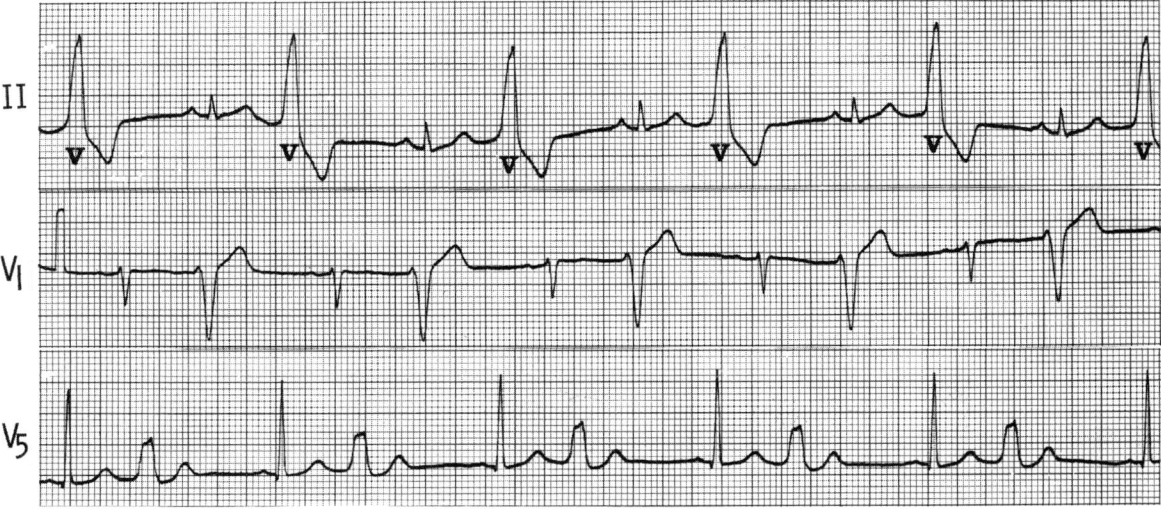

Figure 10-1
Sinus rhythm with frequent ventricular premature contractions (marked V) producing ventricular bigeminy.

INTERPOLATED VENTRICULAR PREMATURE CONTRACTION

Definition

Interpolated VPC is a VPC sandwiched between two consecutively occurring sinus beats without pause.

Diagnostic Criteria (see Fig. 10-2)

- VPC sandwiched between two consecutively occurring sinus beats.
- The R-R interval of two consecutively occurring sinus beats that contains an interpolated VPC is slightly (at times, significantly) longer than the basic sinus P-P (or R-R) cycle.
- The above-mentioned electrocardiographic finding is due to concealed ventriculoatrial conduction of the ectopic ventricular impulse, which leads to a longer P-R interval of the sinus beat immediately following an interpolated VPC.
- The sinus P-P cycle is not disturbed by an interpolated VPC.

Diagnostic Pearls

Interpolated VPC tends to occur when the underlying rhythm is relatively slow sinus bradycardia. In addition, interpolated VPC is more common in healthy individuals than in patients with cardiac disease. Interpolated VPC is a true extra heartbeat because the underlying sinus rhythm continues without missing any QRS complex of the sinus origin.

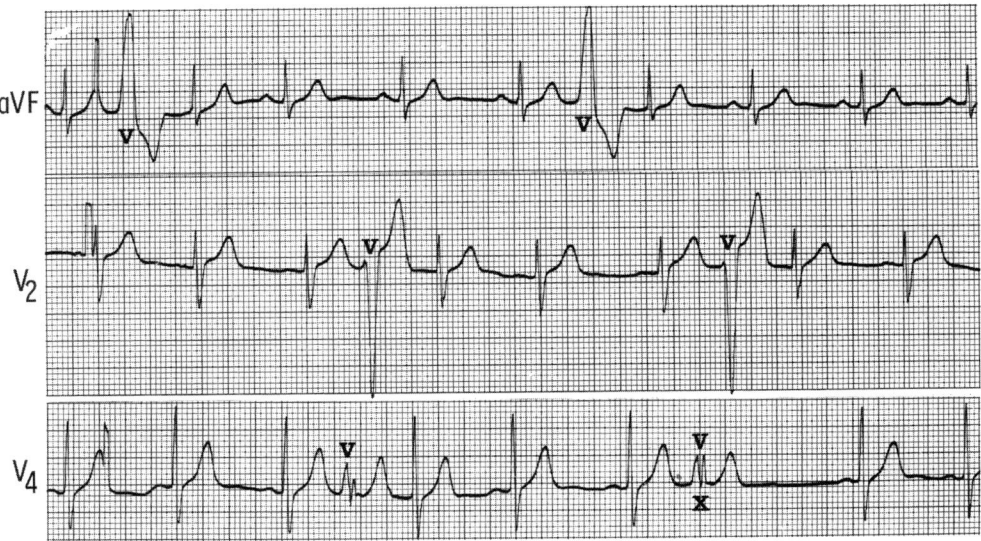

Figure 10-2
Sinus rhythm with interpolated ventricular premature contractions (marked V) and an ordinary ventricular premature contraction (marked X).

MULTIFOCAL VENTRICULAR PREMATURE CONTRACTIONS

Definition

Multifocal VPCs are VPCs originating from two or more locations in the ventricles.

Diagnostic Criteria (Fig. 10-3)

- VPCs originating from two or more foci in the ventricles and producing two or more different QRS configurations
- Constant or varying coupling intervals
- Full compensatory pause following a VPC in sinus rhythm
- Long ventricular pause following a VPC in AF or atrial flutter

Diagnostic Pearls

Multifocal VPCs usually occur among older adults with diseased hearts. In addition, multifocal VPCs are frequently observed in advanced digitalis intoxication, particularly in the presence of underlying AF.

Figure 10-3
Sinus rhythm with multifocal ventricular premature contractions. The Holter monitor ECG rhythm strips A–D are not continuous.

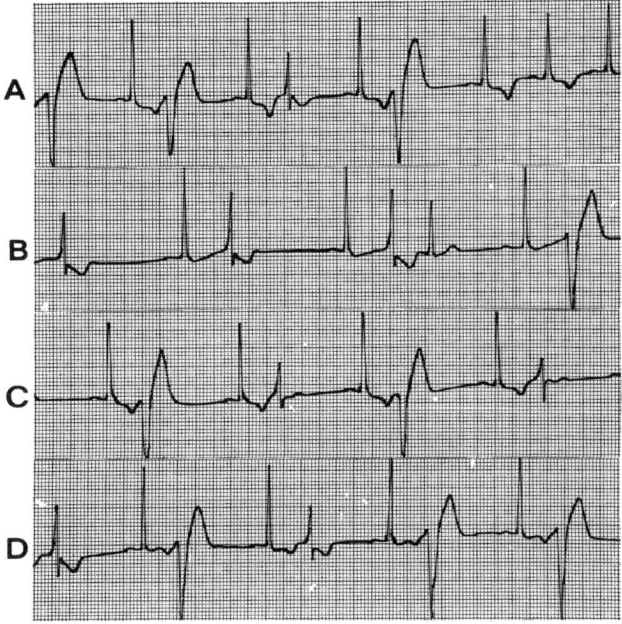

GROUPED VENTRICULAR PREMATURE CONTRACTIONS

Definition

Grouped VPCs are two to five consecutively occurring VPCs.

Diagnostic Criteria (Fig. 10-4)

- Two to five consecutively occurring VPCs.
- The configuration of the VPC may be identical or may vary.
- Interectopic intervals (R-R interval between consecutively occurring VPCs) may be constant but more commonly vary.
- Grouped VPCs are usually followed by a long ventricular pause.
- Underlying cardiac rhythm may be sinus or ectopic (e.g., AF).

Diagnostic Pearls

Grouped VPCs should be distinguished from consecutively occurring AVC. A long ventricular pause following bizarre and broad QRS complexes supports the diagnosis of grouped VPCs, particularly when the underlying rhythm is AF (see Fig. 6-6). Various electrocardiographic findings that support ventricular ectopy are summarized in Table 6-2.

Figure 10-4
*Sinus rhythm
(marked S) with
grouped ventricular
premature contrac-
tions (marked V).
Note occasional
ventricular fusion
beats (marked FB).
Leads II a–c are
not continuous.*

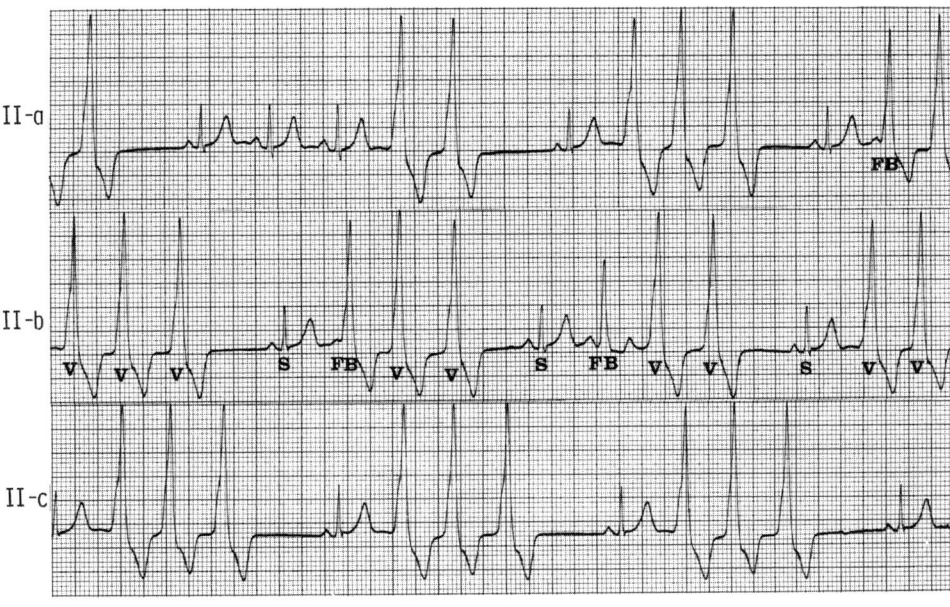

VENTRICULAR TACHYCARDIA

The term *VT* is used when six or more consecutive VPCs occur. VT, like isolated VPCs, may originate from any ventricular location. Since cardiac impulses originating from a ventricular focus are transmitted in an abnormal fashion, the QRS complex in VT is usually bizarre and wide (≥ 0.12 second). VT may occur transiently as a short paroxysm, or it may persist for a long time, as long as the underlying cause is not corrected. Between bouts of VT, one or more sinus beats or isolated VPCs may occur intermittently. The atrial mechanism is often sinus, but it may be an ectopic rhythm such as AF, atrial flutter, or tachycardia, although identifying the atrial mechanism is often difficult.

By and large, there are three forms of VT. The most common form is, needless to say, paroxysmal VT, which is often paroxysmal in nature and usually has rapid rates (180–250 beats per minute [bpm]) similar to those in paroxysmal atrial or AV junctional tachycardia. The less common form is nonparoxysmal VT (idioventricular tachycardia or accelerated ventricular rhythm), which is analogous to nonparoxysmal AV junctional tachycardia. Nonparoxysmal VT is almost always found in acute MI (usually during the first 24–72 hours) and has a relatively slow rate (70–130 bpm). This form of VT is considered to be produced by an acceleration of the impulse formation of idioventricular pacemaker. A rare form of VT is considered to be generated by a parasystolic mechanism; its usual rates are similar to those of nonparoxysmal VT (see Chapter 13). The R-R intervals may be precisely regular, but it is not uncommon to observe a slight irregularity. VT is commonly unifocal, but it may originate from two or more independent ventricular foci. VT is nearly always found in patients with advanced organic heart disease. Ventricular flutter or VF may follow VT, and the outcome is frequently fatal.

Relatively new terms, *nonsustained VT* and *sustained VT,* have been introduced in the literature. *Nonsustained VT* is used when VT lasts 29 seconds or less, whereas *sustained VT* means that VT persists for long period of time (>29 seconds).

Torsade de pointes is a special kind of multiformed VT that is discussed later in this chapter.

NONSUSTAINED VENTRICULAR TACHYCARDIA

Definition

Nonsustained VT is six or more consecutively occurring VPCs lasting up to 29 seconds.

Diagnostic Criteria (Fig. 10-5)

- Six or more consecutively occurring VPCs lasting up to 29 seconds.
- Ventricular rate of 140–180 bpm (in some cases, the rate may be faster or slower than the usual rate ranges).
- Consecutively occurring VPCs may be unifocal or multifocal.
- The interectopic intervals (VT cycle) are often not constant.
- Nonsustained VT often occurs intermittently.
- The underlying rhythm may be sinus or any ectopic rhythm (e.g., AF).

Diagnostic Pearls

A short episode of nonsustained VT should be distinguished from consecutively occurring AVC, particularly in the presence of underlying AF (see Fig. 6-6). A lack of a pause following consecutively occurring bizarre beats excludes the possibility of nonsustained VT. Various electrocardiographic findings that support ventricular ectopies are summarized in Table 6-2. Nonsustained VT becomes sustained VT when the patient's clinical condition further deteriorates.

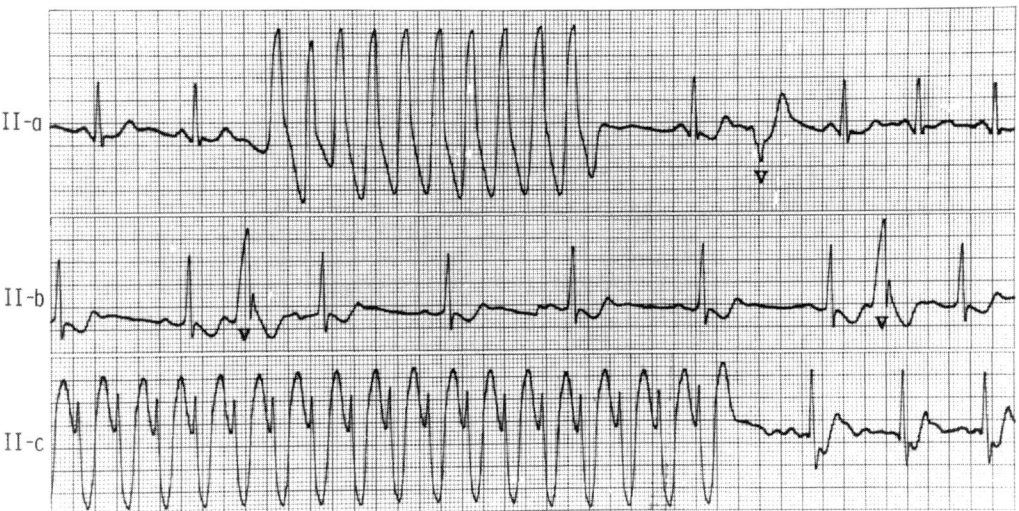

Figure 10-5
Sinus rhythm with multifocal ventricular premature contractions (marked V) and intermittent nonsustained ventricular tachycardia (rate of 155–166 bpm) originating from two foci. Note that all ventricular premature contractions are interpolated.

SUSTAINED VENTRICULAR TACHYCARDIA

Definition

Sustained VT is VT lasting longer than 29 seconds.

Diagnostic Criteria (Fig. 10-6)

- Consecutively occurring VPCs (VT) lasting longer than 29 seconds.
- Ventricular rate of 140–180 bpm (in some cases, the rate may be faster or slower than the usual rate ranges).
- VT may be unifocal or multifocal (the QRS complexes may be uniformed or multiformed).
- VT cycle is usually regular, but it may be slightly irregular during an early phase of the paroxysm.
- VT cycle is often irregular when the tachycardia is multifocal in origin.
- VT may occur in the presence of underlying sinus rhythm or any ectopic rhythm (e.g., AF).

Diagnostic Pearls

Differential diagnosis between sustained VT and any form of supraventricular tachycardia with bizarre or broad QRS complexes (due to left bundle branch block [LBBB], right bundle branch block [RBBB], or AVC) is often difficult. The proper diagnostic approach has been described in Chapter 6. One important clue to diagnose VT is to recognize the identical QRS configuration of an isolated VPC and VT, as the same ectopic focus in the ventricles is capable of producing VPCs as well as VT in the same patient. Various electrocardiographic findings that support ventricular ectopies are summarized in Table 6-2.

Figure 10-6
Sustained ventricular tachycardia with a rate of 187 bpm. Note that the QRS configurations of the ventricular premature contractions and ventricular tachycardia are identical.

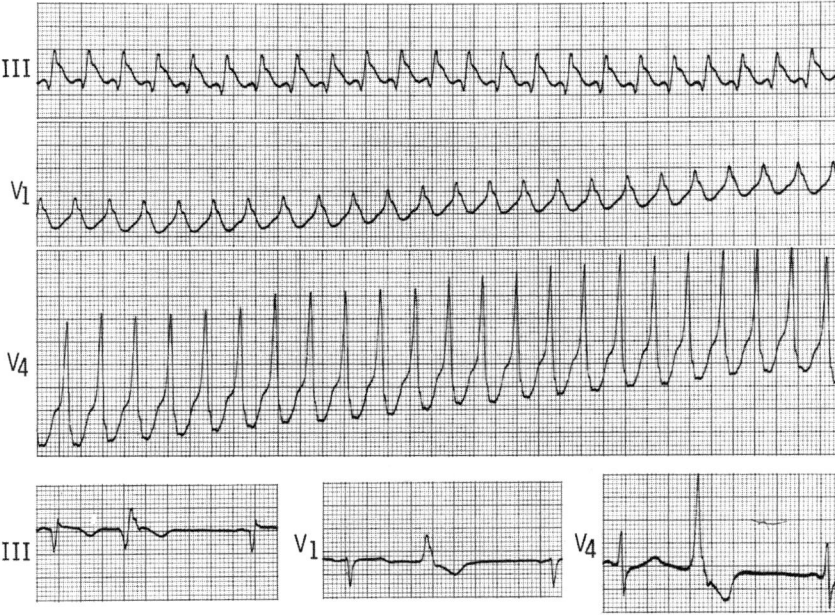

BIDIRECTIONAL VENTRICULAR TACHYCARDIA

Definition

Bidirectional VT is VT with two different QRS complexes alternating on every other beat.

Diagnostic Criteria (Fig. 10-7)

- VT having different QRS configurations that alternate on every other beat.
- The ventricular rate of 140–180 bpm (in some cases, the rate may be faster or slower than the usual rate ranges).
- The R-R intervals (ventricular cycles) are precisely regular in unifocal bidirectional VT.
- Two different R-R intervals (ventricular cycles) alternate in bifocal bidirectional VT.
- The underlying atrial mechanism is almost always an ectopic rhythm (e.g., AF, atrial flutter, or tachycardia), leading to AV dissociation.

Diagnostic Pearls

At a glance, bidirectional VT is obvious in most cases because it has two different bizarre QRS complexes alternating throughout. It is important to remember that the atrial mechanism is nearly always ectopic (e.g., AF, atrial flutter, or tachycardia). The most common underlying cause of bidirectional VT is advanced digitalis intoxication; the prognosis is grave.

Figure 10-7
Atrial fibrillation with bidirectional ventricular tachycardia with a rate of 156 bpm producing complete atrioventricular dissociation as a result of far-advanced digitalis intoxication.

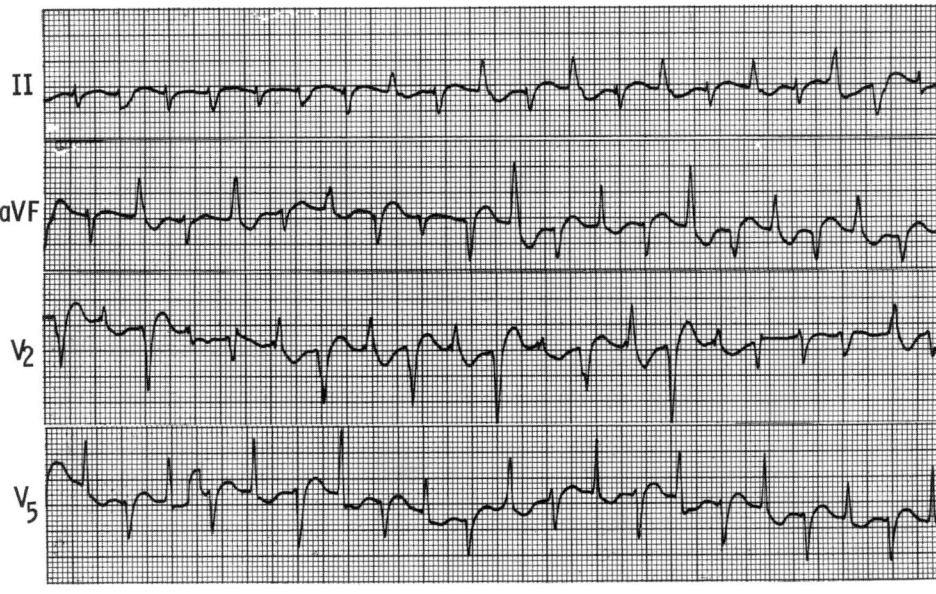

ACCELERATED IDIOVENTRICULAR RHYTHM

Definition

Accelerated idioventricular rhythm (AIVR) is six or more consecutively occurring VPCs with a slow ventricular rate (the usual rate is 70–130 bpm). AIVR is often called other terms such as *idioventricular tachycardia*, *nonparoxysmal VT*, or *slow VT*.

Diagnostic Criteria (Fig. 10-8)

- Six or more consecutively occurring VPCs with a relatively slow ventricular rate (average rate of 70–130 bpm).
- The QRS complex configuration is uniform in most cases, but it may vary.
- The ventricular, cycle is regular in most cases, but it may be irregular, especially when AIVR is short in duration.
- AIVR may occur in the presence of underlying sinus rhythm or any ectopic atrial rhythm (e.g., AF, atrial flutter, tachycardia).

Diagnostic Pearls

When AIVR occurs intermittently with a short paroxysm, the electrocardiographic finding may mimic intermittent LBBB or RBBB. Remember that the ventricular ectopy is *not* preceded by any premature P wave. AIVR is often observed immediately after cardiac surgery and is self-limited in most cases.

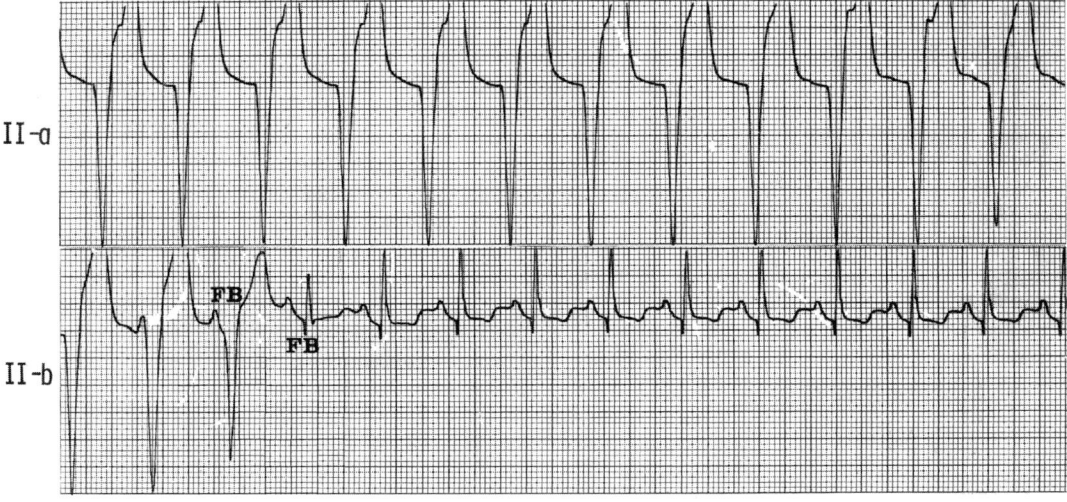

Figure 10-8
Sinus rhythm with intermittent accelerated idioventricular rhythm (rate of 98 bpm). Note occasional ventricular fusion beats (marked FB). Leads II a and b are continuous.

TORSADE DE POINTES

Torsade de pointes is an atypical VT that occurs most frequently during quinidine therapy but may be induced by other etiologic factors. It is important to recognize this atypical VT—because its clinical significance, therapeutic approach, and rather unique QRS morphology during the tachycardia—are considerably different from those of ordinary VT. The term *torsade de pointes* was popularized by Dessertenne when the arrhythmia was described for the first time in 1966. Characteristically, torsade de pointes is manifested by a long Q-T interval, polymorphous QRS complexes with varying R-R intervals, and fluctuating QRS axes. As a rule, VT is initiated by a VPC occurring relatively late during ventricular repolarization, but the arrhythmia is often terminated spontaneously.

It has been shown repeatedly that the conventional mode of therapy for this VT may not only be ineffective but also even hazardous in most cases. Isoproterenol infusion is the usually recommended initial therapy for torsade de pointes, primarily because the drug shortens the ventricular repolarization time. When isoproterenol is ineffective or contraindicated, however, ventricular pacing is considered to be a safe and reliable method for the treatment of this arrhythmia.

Torsade de pointes frequently causes recurrent episodes of syncope or near-syncope, and its occurrence is considered to be the most serious complication of quinidine therapy. In addition, torsade de pointes has been reported during other antiarrhythmic drug therapies (e.g., procainamide and disopyramide therapy). Furthermore, the arrhythmia may also occur in cases of electrolyte disturbances, congenital Q-T syndrome, and coronary artery disease, even in the absence of any antiarrhythmic drug effect. Possible causes of torsade de pointes are summarized in Table 10-1.

It can be said that the vulnerable period of the ventricles is prolonged proportionally to the duration of the T wave. Since the prolonged Q-T interval responsible for the production of torsade de pointes is invariably associated with markedly broad T wave, any cardiac impulse (commonly VPCs) may easily provoke VT and VF (the R-on-T phenomenon), even if a ventricular ectopic beat occurs during the late portion of the cardiac cycle. As a matter of fact, torsade de pointes often transforms to VF in many cases. Hence, in reality, this arrhythmia is prefibrillatory multiformed VT.

Various electrocardiographic manifestations of torsade de pointes are summarized as follows:

Table 10-1. Possible causes of torsade de pointes

Drug-induced causes
    Antiarrhythmic drugs
        Quinidine, procainamide, disopyramide, ajmaline, amiodarone, and lidocaine
    Other drugs
        Phenylamine, phenothiazines, tricyclic antidepressant drugs
Non–drug-induced causes
    Congenital Q-T prolongation syndrome
        Jervell and Lange-Nielsen syndrome
        Romano-Ward syndrome
    Electrolyte disturbances
        Hypokalemia
        Hypomagnesemia
    Intrinsic cardiac diseases
        Myocardial ischemia and infarction
        Myocarditis
        Bradyarrhythmias
           Marked sinus bradycardia (e.g., sick sinus syndrome)
           Advanced or complete atrioventricular block
    Mitral valve prolapse syndrome

Non–drug-induced causes *(continued)*
    Liquid protein diets
    Central nervous system disorders (e.g., subarachnoid hemorrhage)
    Hypothermia

1. During sinus rhythm (at times, ectopic rhythms such as AF), the Q-T interval is markedly prolonged (often >0.60 second) and has very broad T waves.
2. The arrhythmia is often initiated by a VPC with a long coupling interval and the R-on-T phenomenon.
3. The arrhythmia consists of large and bizarre multiformed QRS complexes with a frequency of 100–180 bpm (at times, as rapid as 200–300 bpm).
4. The amplitude and direction of the QRS complexes frequently vary from beat to beat, leading to a picture of a torsion around an isoelectric line. Consequently, the French name torsade de pointes ("torsion of points") was given to describe the arrhythmia.
5. The arrhythmia may terminate spontaneously and may repeat itself after several seconds or minutes. On the other hand, the arrhythmia often transforms to VF; and sudden death may occur.

TORSADE DE POINTES

Definition

Torsade de pointes is multiformed VT initiated by VPCs with prolonged Q-T intervals and broad T waves.

Diagnostic Criteria (Fig. 10-9)

- Multiformed VT initiated by a VPC with the R-on-T phenomenon (the QRS complex of a VPC superimposed on the top of the T wave of the preceding beat) in the presence of a prolonged Q-T interval with a broad T wave.
- Multiformed VT is usually irregular, with components of ventricular flutter and/or VF.
- The ventricular rate is 140–180 bpm (the rate may be faster or slower than this range).
- The broad T waves may be upright or inverted.
- The underlying cardiac rhythm may be sinus or any atrial mechanism (e.g., AF, atrial flutter, or tachycardia).
- Multiformed VT often transforms to VF.

Diagnostic Pearls

Torsade de pointes is generally easy to diagnose by recognizing VT of various forms initiated by a VPC in the setting of markedly prolonged Q-T intervals having broad T waves. However, certain artifacts may mimic torsade de pointes (see Figs. 6-1 and 6-2). The most common underlying cause responsible for the production of this arrhythmia is quinidine toxicity.

Figure 10-9
Leads II a–e are continuous. The rhythm is multiformed ventricular tachycardia initiated by frequent ventricular premature contractions (marked V) with R-on-T phenomenon as a result of prolonged Q-T interval with broad T waves due to quinidine (torsade de pointes).

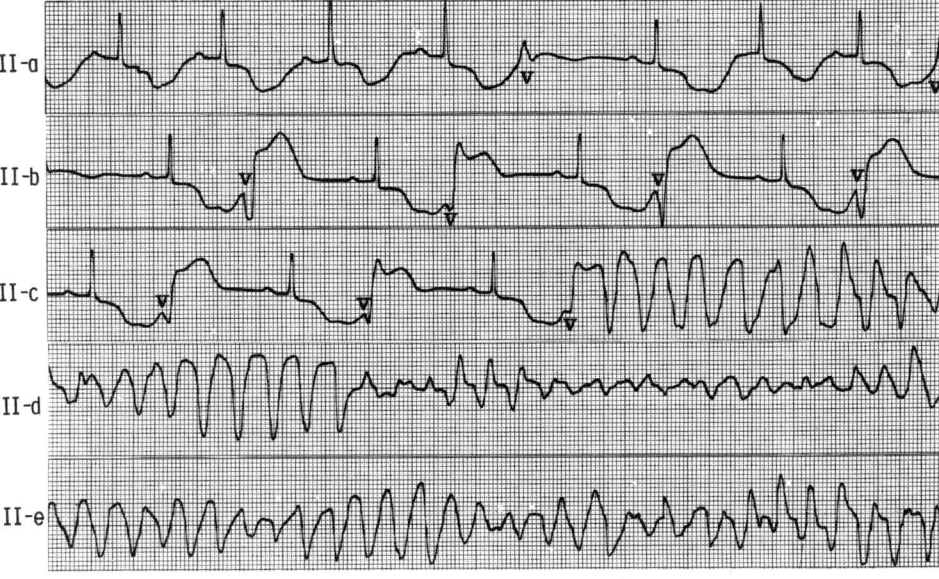

VENTRICULAR FLUTTER
AND FIBRILLATION

Ventricular flutter and VF are the worst cardiac arrhythmias encountered in the human heart. They are the most common causes of sudden death and are particularly associated with acute MI. When ventricular flutter or VF occurs in acute MI, sudden death frequently results even before symptoms or anatomic alteration of the myocardium develops. Ventricular flutter and VF often coexist or transform from one to the other; a pure form of ventricular flutter is relatively uncommon. Because of the frequent association of ventricular flutter and VF, the mixed form is called *ventricular flutter-fibrillation*, which is analogous to atrial flutter-fibrillation.

In both ventricular flutter and VF, the distinction between the QRS complex, the S-T segments, and T waves is absent. Instead, a regular and consecutive undulation occurs in ventricular flutter, whereas a grossly irregular undulation of varying amplitude is present in VF.

VENTRICULAR FLUTTER

Definition

Ventricular flutter is a regularly occurring undulation (wave form) originating from any portion of the ventricles.

Diagnostic Criteria (Fig. 10-10)

- Regularly occurring undulation (wave form) with no boundary between the QRS complexes, S-T segments, and T waves, leading to a continuous loop.
- The usual rate is 140–180 bpm (the rate may be faster or slower than the usual rate range in some cases).
- No discernible P waves or any other atrial activities.
- Ventricular flutter often transforms from or to VF or VT, and at times to unstable VER or ventricular standstill, leading to chaotic ventricular rhythm (discussed in the section on chaotic ventricular rhythm).

Diagnostic Pearls

Ventricular flutter is easily recognized by most readers because of its characteristic electrocardiographic finding (regularly occurring undulation without any boundary between the QRS complex, S-T segment, and T wave). However, ventricular flutter should be distinguished from various artifacts (see Figs. 6-1 and 6-2).

Figure 10-10
Ventricular flutter with a rate of 215 bpm.

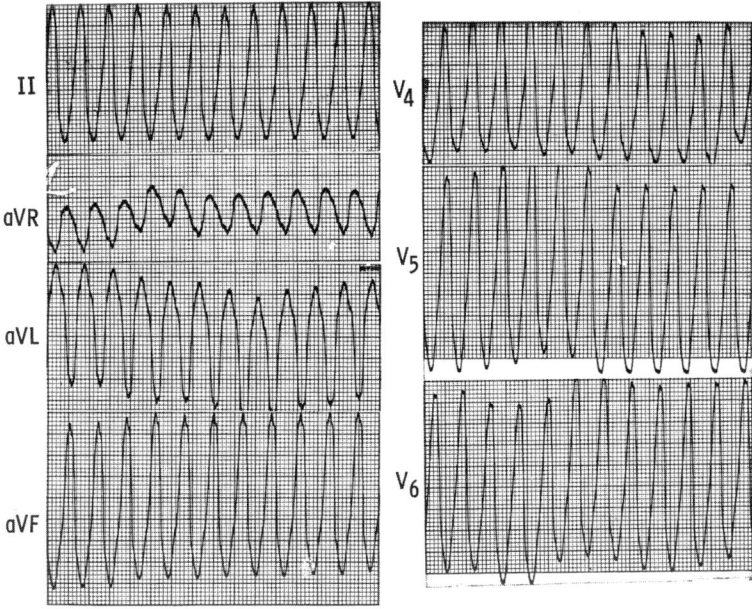

VENTRICULAR FIBRILLATION

Definition

VF is very rapid, chaotic, and grossly irregular multiformed electrocardiographic complexes of various amplitudes originating anywhere in the ventricles.

Diagnostic Criteria (Fig. 10-11)

- Very rapid, chaotic, and grossly irregular multiformed electrocardiographic complexes with various amplitudes.
- No discernible P waves or any other atrial activities.
- The exact ventricular rate is impossible to determine, but it is usually faster than 140–180 bpm.
- No discernible S-T segment, T wave, or clear-cut QRS complex.
- VF is often preceded or followed by VT, ventricular flutter, unstable VER, or ventricular standstill, leading to chaotic ventricular rhythm (discussed in the section on chaotic ventricular rhythm).

Diagnostic Pearls

VF is easy to recognize because of its characteristic electrocardiographic finding, which usually occurs in patients with advanced heart disease. However, various artifacts may produce a similar electrocardiographic finding that mimics VF (see Figs. 6-1 and 6-2).

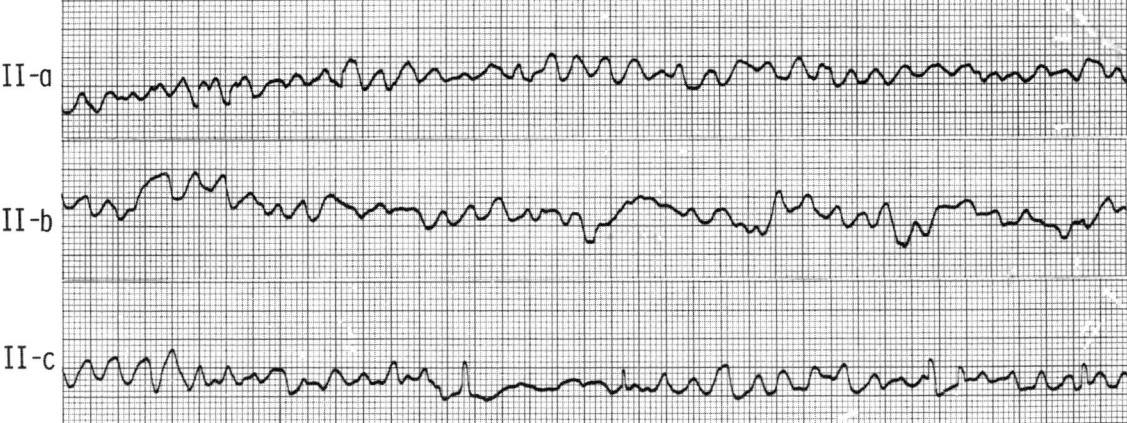

Figure 10-11
Ventricular fibrillation. Leads II a–c are not continuous.

CHAOTIC VENTRICULAR RHYTHM

The term *chaotic rhythm* has been used to designate multifocal ventricular rhythms with extremely unstable mechanisms. Thus, chaotic rhythm often consists of a period of VT, VF, or ventricular flutter; multifocal VPCs; high-degree or complete AV block; VER (idioventricular rhythm); and ventricular standstill. By precise definition, each portion of the electrographic tracing usually shows a specific cardiac arrhythmia (e.g., VT or idioventricular rhythm). However, at times, some part of the chaotic rhythm cannot be described specifically, particularly immediately before death. In the dying heart, the ventricles may be controlled by two or more ventricular foci. For example, a portion of the ventricles may have VF or ventricular flutter, whereas the remaining portion of the ventricles may have VER. In this circumstance, the term *ventricular dissociation* is used. In a practical sense, whenever the term *chaotic rhythm* is used, the predominant cardiac rhythm consists of ventricular flutter, VF, and VER.

CHAOTIC VENTRICULAR RHYTHM

Definition

Chaotic ventricular rhythm is a multifocal ventricular rhythm consisting of periods of grouped VPCs, VT, VF, ventricular flutter, VER, and ventricular standstill.

Diagnostic Criteria (Fig. 10-12)

- Various multifocal and multiformed ventricular rhythms as described above.
- The predominant cardiac rhythms consist of ventricular flutter, VF, and unstable VER.
- The underlying atrial mechanism is often AF with advanced AV block.
- Ventricular dissociation and ventricular standstill are the usual final events in dying hearts.

Diagnostic Pearls

Chaotic ventricular rhythm is usually observed in the dying hearts of patients with advanced heart disease. The major components of the cardiac rhythms consist of VT, ventricular flutter, VF, and ventricular standstill, leading to ventricular dissociation, very slow and unstable ventricular escape rhythm, and, finally, ventricular standstill.

Figure 10-12
Chaotic ventricular rhythm consisting of areas of ventricular tachycardia, ventricular flutter, and ventricular escape rhythm arising from different foci.

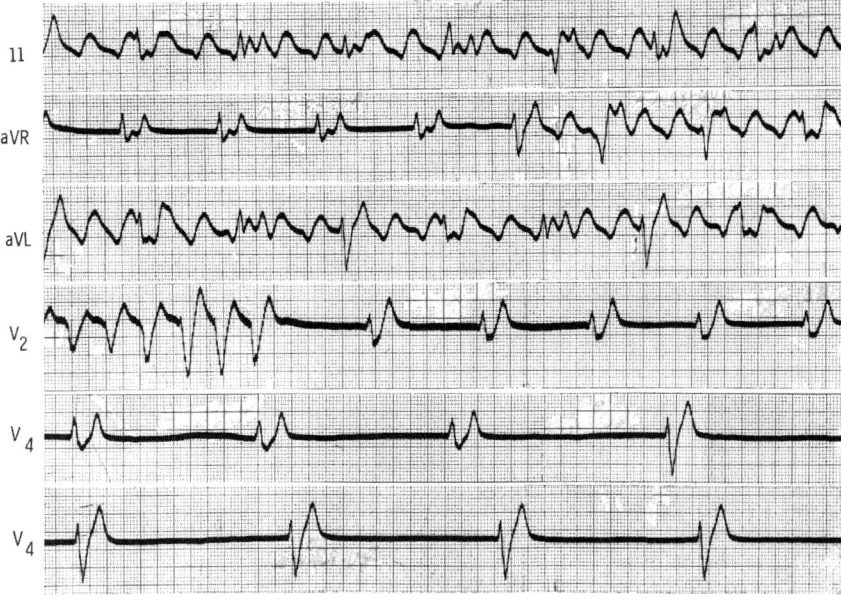

VENTRICULAR ESCAPE RHYTHM

Ventricular escape (idioventricular) beats and rhythm, like VPCs and VT, may originate from any location in the ventricles. Ventricular escape beats (VEBs) may appear singly or consecutively as group beats. When six or more consecutive VEBs appear, the term *VER* is used. VEBs or VER are generated by passive impulse formation in the ventricles when the AV junction is unable to produce escape impulses despite the fact that the sinus or atrial impulses do not reach the AV junction in the expected time or when the site of complete AV block is distal to the His bundle.

Under normal circumstances, like AV junctional escape rhythm, VER does not appear because these subsidiary pacemakers are controlled by the sinus node, which has a faster inherent rate. Thus, the AV junctional pacemakers and the ventricular pacemakers are continuously depressed by the rapidly discharging sinus impulses. The most common cause of VER is complete infranodal AV block, often resulting from bilateral bundle branch block (BBBB). Less commonly, VEBs or VER may occur following sinus arrest (pause) or sinoatrial (SA) block when the AV junction is unable to produce escape impulses. VEBs or VER may occur in the presence of an ectopic atrial rhythm, including AF, atrial flutter, and tachycardia, when the atrial impulses fail to reach the ventricles due to high-degree or complete infranodal AV block, frequently resulting from BBBB. Not uncommonly, VER may occur without the presence of definite atrial activity in the terminal stages of advanced heart disease. Extremely rarely, VEBs or VER may be followed by a retrograde P wave when the impulses from the ventricular ectopic focus activate the atria in a retrograde fashion. The usual rate of VER is 30–40 bpm but may be as slow as 15–20 bpm. This arrhythmia is nearly always found in advanced heart disease, especially in elderly individuals, and is often a terminal cardiac arrhythmia.

VENTRICULAR ESCAPE RHYTHM

Definition

VER is a slow and regular escape rhythm originating from any location in the ventricles.

Diagnostic Criteria (Fig. 10-13)

- Regular and slow rhythm with broad QRS complexes (QRS interval is ≥0.12 second in most cases).
- The usual ventricular rate is 20–40 bpm (the rate may be slower or faster than the usual rate range).
- The underlying cardiac rhythm is advanced or complete AV block in most cases (see Chapter 11).
- In rare cases, the broad QRS complex may be followed by a retrograde P wave.
- The underlying atrial mechanism may be sinus or ectopic (e.g., AF).

Diagnostic Pearls

The pure form of VER is rather unusual, and in most cases, VER is observed as a result of advanced or complete AV block (see Chapter 11). AV junctional escape rhythm with LBBB or RBBB closely mimics VER. Under this circumstance, it is important to confirm the preexisting LBBB or RBBB by reviewing previous electrocardiographic tracings.

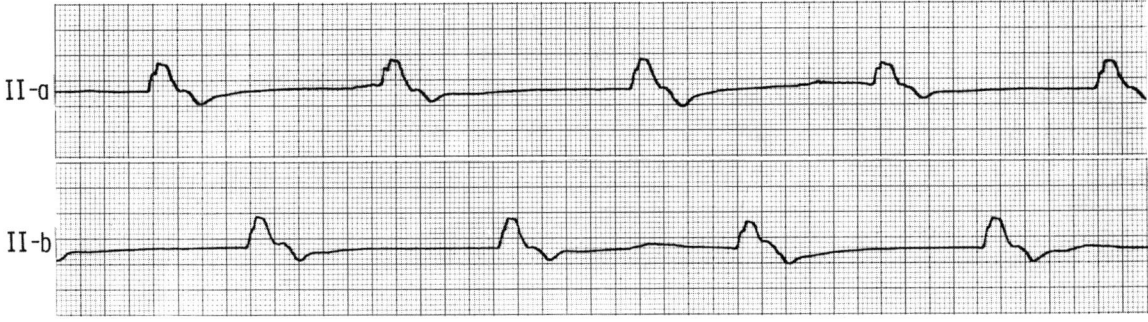

Figure 10-13
Ventricular escape rhythm with a rate of 30 bpm. Lead II a and b are continuous.

VENTRICULAR STANDSTILL

Ventricular standstill (arrest), like atrial standstill (arrest), is usually the consequence of some other cardiac arrhythmia. The term *ventricular standstill* is used when no QRS complex is observed for a few seconds or longer. Ventricular standstill may occur in the presence of any atrial activity (sinus or ectopic), but both atrial and ventricular activity may be absent altogether. Ventricular standstill results when a subsidiary pacemaker fails to produce an escape impulse during sinus arrest or SA block. Sinus arrest often follows after spontaneous termination of an ectopic tachycardia or even after a single ectopic beat because of the depression of the pacemaking function in the sinus node. In this circumstances, ventricular standstill frequently results because the subsidiary pacemaker also may not produce an escape impulse at the expected time. Ventricular standstill may be produced by carotid sinus stimulation during supraventricular tachyarrhythmias. Carotid sinus syncope is often manifested by a long ventricular standstill. In addition, post-tachyarrhythmia ventricular pause is extremely common following the termination of atrial, AV junctional, or ventricular tachyarrhythmias either by drugs or direct current shock. Not uncommonly, ventricular standstill may result in advanced or complete AV block when concealed AV conduction occurs, leading to suppression of a subsidiary pacemaker. On rare occasions, ventricular standstill may occur suddenly during sinus rhythm. In the dying heart, needless to say, ventricular standstill eventually results either following VT, ventricular flutter or VF, or slow VER.

VENTRICULAR STANDSTILL (ARREST)

Definition

No QRS complex for a few seconds or longer.

Diagnostic Criteria (Fig. 10-14)

- No QRS complex for a few seconds or longer regardless of the underlying cardiac rhythm.
- Ventricular standstill may occur abruptly without preceding any ectopic beats or ectopic tachyarrhythmia during sinus rhythm.
- Ventricular standstill often occurs following termination of various ectopic tachyarrhythmias.
- Ventricular standstill frequently occurs following sinus arrest or SA block in patients with advanced sick sinus syndrome.
- Ventricular standstill often occurs in elderly patients with sick sinus syndrome during chronic AF or atrial flutter with advanced AV block.

Diagnostic Pearls

Ventricular standstill is *not* a primary cardiac rhythm disorder in most cases, and it often follows prolonged sinus arrest, SA block, and AF with advanced AV block in patients with advanced sick sinus syndrome. In addition, ventricular standstill often occurs on termination of various ectopic tachyarrhythmias.

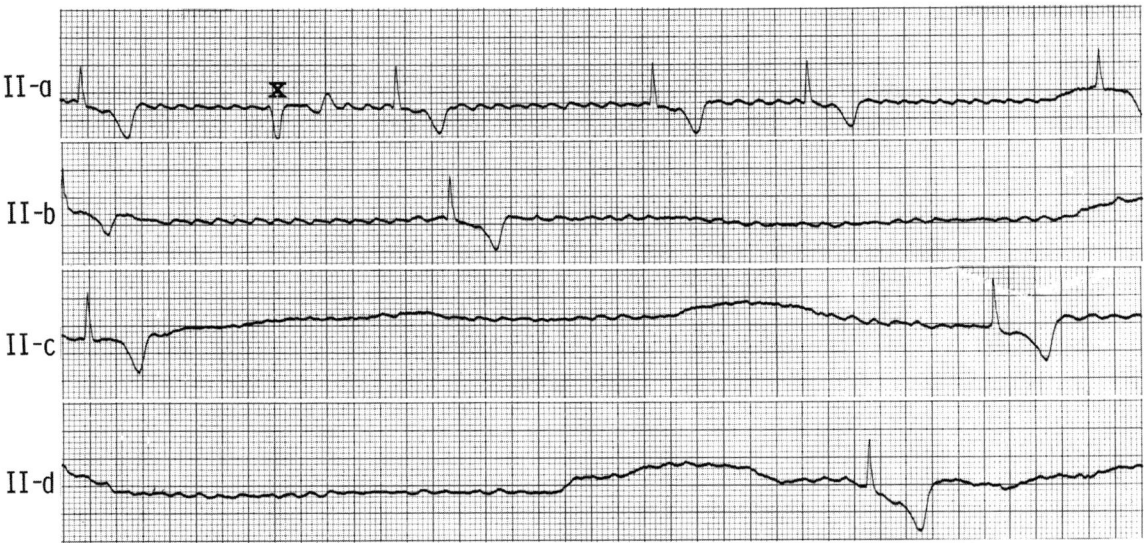

Figure 10-14
Atrial fibrillation with advanced atrioventricular block and areas of ventricular standstill. Note a ventricular escape beat (marked X). Leads II a–d are not continuous.

VENTRICULAR PARASYSTOLE

Ventricular parasystole is a rather uncommon ventricular arrhythmia. The configuration of the QRS complex in ventricular parasystole is essentially the same as that of an ordinary VPC, but the former produces an independent ventricular rhythm in the presence of any underlying rhythm. A detailed description of ventricular parasystole is found in Chapter 13.

11

Atrioventricular Block

Conduction disturbances may occur anywhere in the heart and are ordinarily expressed as a *heart block*. In general, impaired conduction is divided into five categories according to the location of the block:

1. Sinoatrial block (conduction disturbances at the sinoatrial junctional tissues)
2. Intra-atrial block (conduction disturbance within the atria)
3. Atrioventricular (AV) block (conduction disturbance at the AV junctional tissue)
4. Intra-His block (conduction disturbance within the His bundle)

5. Intraventricular block (conduction disturbance within the ventricles or bundle branch system)

Among these conduction disturbances, AV block and intraventricular block are commonly observed and may be associated with a block anywhere else in the heart. Although a precise definition of AV block is a conduction disturbance occurring at the AV junction, the term *heart block* has been used loosely to designate AV block.

AV block is characterized by an abnormally prolonged AV conduction time (P-R interval) or failure of conduction of one or more atrial impulses (either sinus or ectopic) due to a prolonged refractory period in the AV junctional tissue. Thus, true AV block must be distinguished from functional AV block, which occurs as a physiologic mechanism. For example, when a sinus P wave that falls outside the Q-T interval of the preceding ventricular beat fails to conduct to the ventricles or conducts slowly (P-R interval of ≥0.21 second), a true AV block is said to be present. Atrial flutter with a 2:1 AV conduction (see Fig. 8-7), on the other hand, commonly occurs due to a functional rather than a true AV block because the AV junctional tissue is unable to respond to the rapid atrial rate due to its longer refractory period. For a similar reason, the P wave of the atrial premature contraction (APC) often fails to conduct to the ventricles when the P wave appears soon after the QRS complex of the preceding beat. The P-R interval of an APC becomes prolonged when the P wave falls in the second half of the Q-T interval of the preceding beat. These alterations of the AV conduction in an APC are functional (physiologic) and therefore *not* a manifestation of a true AV block.

It has been shown that the normal absolute refractory period of the AV junctional tissue corresponds approximately to the initial half of the Q-T interval and that the relative refractory period corresponds to the second half of the Q-T interval. In general, the duration of the refractory period of the AV junction is directly related to the length of the preceding cardiac cycle. Thus, it can be said that the longer the preceding cycle length, the longer the duration of the refractory period of the beat following that cycle, and the shorter the preceding cycle, the shorter the duration of the refractory period. This electrophysiologic finding is termed *Ashman's phenomenon*.

AV block is divided into two major categories—namely, incomplete (partial) and complete AV block. Incomplete AV block includes first-, second-, and advanced (high-degree) AV block. AV block may occur transiently, intermittently, or permanently, and the type and the degree of AV block may change from time to time, even in the same individual. In general, the following classification of AV block is used according to the degree of the AV conduction disturbance.

AV block may be classified according to the degree of AV block (Table 11-1) or according to the site of an AV block (Table 11-2).

1. *First-degree AV block* is characterized by a prolonged P-R interval (≥0.21 second in adults and ≥0.18 second in children) in which every atrial impulse reaches the ventricles.

Table 11-1. Classifications of atrioventricular block according to the degree of the block

First-degree AV block
Second-degree AV block
   Wenckebach AV block: AV nodal block (Mobitz type I
     AV block)
   Mobitz type II AV block: Infranodal block
   2:1 AV block
Advanced (high-degree) AV block
Complete (third-degree) AV block

Table 11-2. Classifications of atrioventricular block according to the site of the block

AV nodal block (intranodal block)
Infranodal block
   Intra-His block
   Infra-His block

2. *Second-degree AV block* is diagnosed when some of the atrial impulses fail to reach the ventricles so that QRS complexes are unexpectedly dropped. AV conduction ratios are used to compare the number of impulses conducted to the atria to those conducted to the ventricles. For instance, 4:3 AV block indicates that for every four atrial impulses, three are conducted to the ventricles.

    There are two types of second-degree AV block. The common type is called Wenckebach (Mobitz type I) second-degree AV block. In this type, the P-R interval of each successively conducted beat lengthens progressively until a P wave is not followed by a QRS complex (blocked P wave). The uncommon type is characterized by the occurrence of a blocked P wave and otherwise constant P-R intervals in all conducted beats (Mobitz type II AV block). AV conduction ratios may be 3:2, 4:3, 5:4, 6:5, and so forth in either Mobitz type I or II AV block. The AV ratio may be fixed or vary throughout the tracing. When every other atrial impulse is blocked, 2:1 AV block is diagnosed. It should be noted that Mobitz type I (Wenckebach) AV block represents AV nodal block, whereas Mobitz type II AV block is infranodal block (usually a manifestation of incomplete trifascicular block).

3. *Advanced (or high-degree) AV block* is diagnosed when a blocked P wave occurs in more than a 2:1 AV con-

duction ratio. Thus, 3:1, 4:1, 5:1, and 6:1 AV blocks belong in this category. AV conduction ratios of the even numbers, such as 4:1 or 6:1 AV block, are much more common than those of the odd numbers, such as 3:1 or 5:1 AV block. In advanced AV block, AV junctional escape beats (JEBs) (less commonly ventricular escape beats [VEBs]) frequently appear as a physiologic mechanism, leading to incomplete AV dissociation.

4. *Complete (third-degree) AV block* indicates that none of the atrial impulses are conducted to the ventricles. Consequently, in almost every case, AV junctional escape rhythm (JER) or rarely, ventricular escape rhythm (VER) appears to control the ventricles. In complete AV block, atrial and ventricular activities are independent, leading to complete AV dissociation (see Chapter 9). Complete AV block may be due to a block in the AV node (AV nodal block), in the His bundle (intra-His block), or in the bilateral bundle branches (infra-His block).

It has been pointed out that Mobitz type II AV block is due to partial bilateral bundle branch block (BBBB) and frequently is a precursor of complete AV (infranodal) block. An AV conduction disturbance is frequently bidirectional, but it may be unidirectional. For example, antegrade AV conduction may be impaired in the presence of normal retrograde ventriculoatrial conduction or vice versa.

For proper diagnosis of AV block, it is essential to understand the exact mechanism of Wenckebach (Mobitz type I) AV block fully. Diagrammatic representation of Wenckebach AV block is illustrated in Fig. 11-1. Note the characteristic features of Wenckebach AV block, consisting of a progressive lengthening of the P-R intervals with a progressive shortening of the R-R intervals (ventricular cycles) until a blocked P wave occurs. When the AV conduction ratios remain constant, the cardiac rhythm characteristically produces a regular irregularity of the ventricular cycles. It can be said that a full understanding of Wenckebach AV block is the most important basic electrocardiographic knowledge needed to be able to interpret various cardiac arrhythmias correctly.

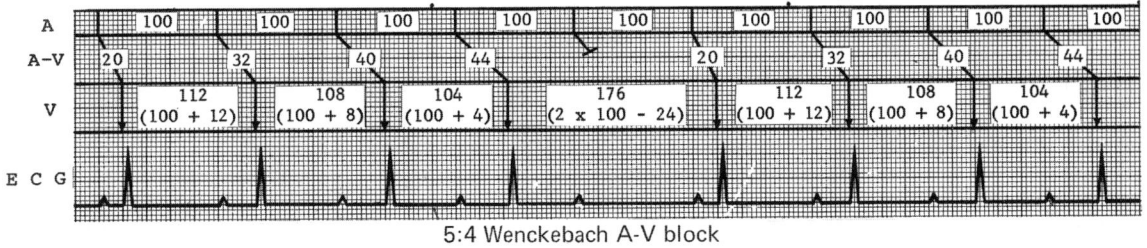

5:4 Wenckebach A-V block

Figure 11-1

Mobitz type I (Wenckebach) atrioventricular block. The numbers represent hundredths of a second. The numbers in the upper row represent the atrial cycle (P-P interval) with a rate of 60 bpm. The numbers within the oblique lines at atrioventricular level indicate the A-V conduction time (P-R interval). The progressive lengthening of the P-R intervals is apparent until a blocked atrial impulse (dropped P wave) occurs. Following this blocked atrial impulse, the P-R interval shortens to its original value (0.20 second), and the sequence is repeated. The numbers in the lower row represent the duration of successive ventricular cycles. The progressive shortening of the ventricular cycle length (R-R interval) is due to the progressive increment of atrioventricular conduction before the blocked atrial impulse and the decrement immediately following the blocked P wave. The numbers in parentheses in the lower row indicate the degree of increment or decrement in the ventricular cycle length.

FIRST-DEGREE ATRIOVENTRICULAR BLOCK

Definition

First-degree atrioventricular block is the prolongation of the P-R interval due to an increased relative refractory period in the AV junction (increased in the AV junction in nearly all cases). Rarely, the prolonged P-R interval may be due to an increased relative refractory period in the His bundle or both bundle branches.

Diagnostic Criteria (Fig. 11-2)

- Prolonged P-R interval of 0.21 second or more in adults.
- Prolonged P-R interval of 0.19 second or more in children.
- Constant P-R interval.
- The QRS complex may be normal or broad (pre-existing left bundle branch block [LBBB] or right bundle branch block [RBBB]).

Diagnostic Pearls

It should be noted that all P waves are conducted to the QRS complexes with constant and prolonged P-R intervals. By and large, markedly prolonged P-R intervals often progress to Wenckebach AV block.

Figure 11-2
Sinus rhythm with first-degree atrioventricular lock. Arrows indicate sinus P waves.

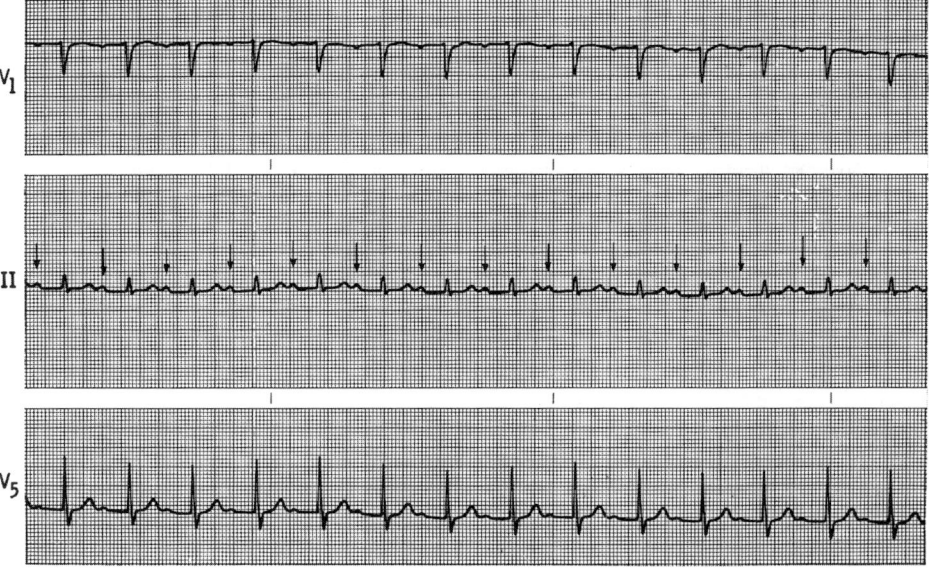

WENCKEBACH (MOBITZ TYPE I) ATRIOVENTRICULAR BLOCK

Definition

Wenckebach (Mobitz type I) AV block is characterized by a progressive increment of the P-R intervals as a result of a progressive increment of the refractory period in the AV junction until a blocked P wave occurs. Wenckebach AV block nearly always represents AV nodal block.

Diagnostic Criteria (Fig. 11-3)

- Progressive increment of the P-R intervals until a blocked P wave occurs.
- Progressive shortening of the R-R intervals (ventricular cycles) until a blocked P wave occurs.
- The AV conduction ratios may be constant or variable.
- The longest R-R interval is shorter than two cycles of the P-P interval.
- Regular irregularity of the R-R intervals (ventricular cycles) when the AV conduction ratio is fixed.

Diagnostic Pearls

A possibility of Wenckebach AV block should always be considered when the cardiac rhythm reveals a regular irregularity of cardiac cycle. Likewise, Wenckebach AV block is a strong possibility when the cardiac rhythm demonstrates grouped QRS complexes that are followed by pauses. Clinically, the most common cause of Wenckebach AV block is acute diaphragmatic (inferior) myocardial infarction.

Figure 11-3
Sinus rhythm with 5:4 Wenckebach atrioventricular block. Note a progressive lengthening of the P-R intervals until a blocked P wave occurs.

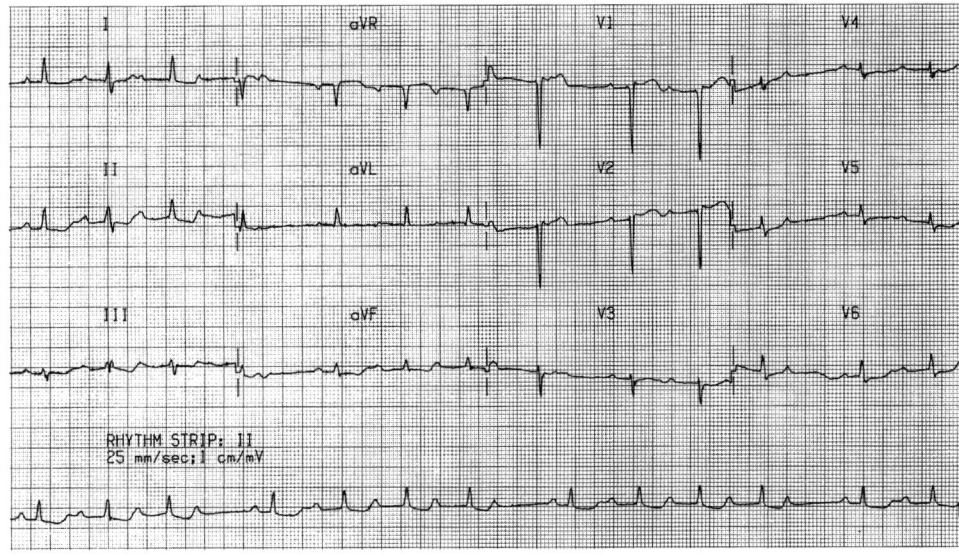

ATRIAL FLUTTER WITH WENCKEBACH (MOBITZ TYPE I) ATRIOVENTRICULAR BLOCK

Definition

Atrial flutter with Wenckebach (Mobitz type I) AV block is characterized by a progressive increment of F-R intervals as a result of a progressive increment of the refractory period in the AV junction until a pause occurs. Wenckebach AV block almost always represents AV nodal block.

Diagnostic Criteria (Fig. 11-4)

- Progressive increment of the F-R intervals until a pause occurs.
- Progressive shortening of the R-R intervals (ventricular cycles) until a pause occurs.
- The AV conduction ratio may be constant or variable.
- Regular irregularity of the R-R intervals (ventricular cycles) when the AV conduction ratio is fixed.
- When 2:1 and 4:1 AV conduction ratios alternate, pseudo-ventricular bigeminy is produced, and the long R-R inter-val is shorter than four atrial flutter cycles, whereas the short R-R interval is longer than two atrial flutter cycles.

Diagnostic Pearls

When the atrial mechanism is atrial flutter, Wenckebach AV block is often unrecognized by many inexperienced readers. Wenckebach AV block should be considered immediately when the ventricular group beats are followed by a pause in atrial flutter.

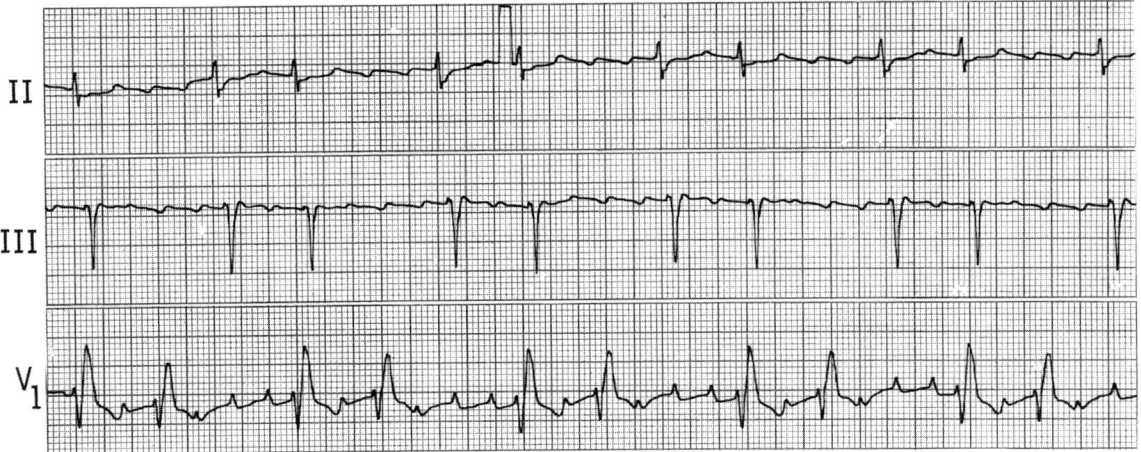

Figure 11-4
Atrial flutter with Wenckebach atrioventricular block. Note that 2:1 and 4:1 atrioventricular conduction ratios alternate.
The long R-R interval is shorter than four flutter cycles, whereas the short R-R interval is longer than two flutter cycles.

MOBITZ TYPE II ATRIOVENTRICULAR BLOCK

Definition

Mobitz type II AV block is the periodic or intermittent occurrence of blocked P waves without Wenckebach phenomenon. Mobitz type II AV block represents infranodal block and is a form of incomplete BBBB (see Table 4-2).

Diagnostic Criteria (Fig. 11-5)

- Periodic or intermittent occurrence of blocked P waves without Wenckebach phenomenon.
- Constant P-R intervals in all conducted beats.
- The R-R interval including the blocked P wave is two times the P-P interval.
- Regular irregularity of the R-R cycles when the AV conduction ratio is constant.
- Common association with hemiblocks, LBBB, RBBB, or bifascicular block (BFB).

Diagnostic Pearls

It is extremely important to remember that Mobitz type II AV block is nearly always associated with the underlying hemiblocks, RBBB, LBBB, or BFB because Mobitz type II AV block is a form of incomplete BBBB. Mobitz type II AV block often progresses to a more advanced form of BBBB, and a permanent artificial pacemaker is frequently indicated in this circumstance.

Figure 11-5
Sinus rhythm with Mobitz type II atrioventricular block. Arrows indicate sinus P waves, and a blocked P wave is marked X. Note that the P-R intervals are constant in all conducted beats. The diagnosis of bifascicular block consisting of right bundle branch block and left anterior hemiblock is readily made. In addition, a possibility of posterolateral myocardial infarction is considered.

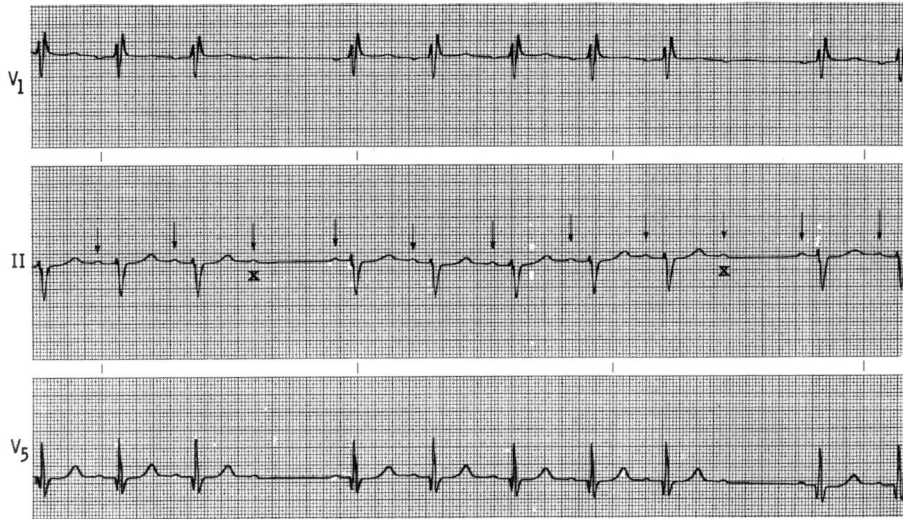

2:1 ATRIOVENTRICULAR BLOCK WITH NORMAL QRS COMPLEXES

Definition

Every other P wave is conducted to the ventricles and the QRS complexes are normal. AV block in this case represents a variant of Wenckebach AV block in nearly all cases. The block represents AV nodal block.

Diagnostic Criteria (Fig. 11-6)

- Every other P wave is not conducted to the ventricles.
- The QRS complexes are normal in all conducted beats.
- The P-R intervals of all conducted beats are constant.
- The R-R intervals (the ventricular cycles) are two times the P-P cycles.
- Typical Wenckebach AV block (see Fig. 11-3) may occur intermittently in the same electrocardiographic tracing.

Diagnostic Pearls

Sinus rhythm with 2:1 AV block is often misdiagnosed as marked sinus bradycardia when every other blocked P wave is *not* recognized. The reason for this error is that many inexperienced readers fail to recognize blocked P waves, which are frequently superimposed on the T waves of the preceding beats. Careful observation is essential to identify the blocked P waves, which may *not* be readily visible.

Figure 11-6
Sinus rhythm with 2:1 atrioventricular block (most likely atrioventricular nodal block). Arrows indicate P waves.

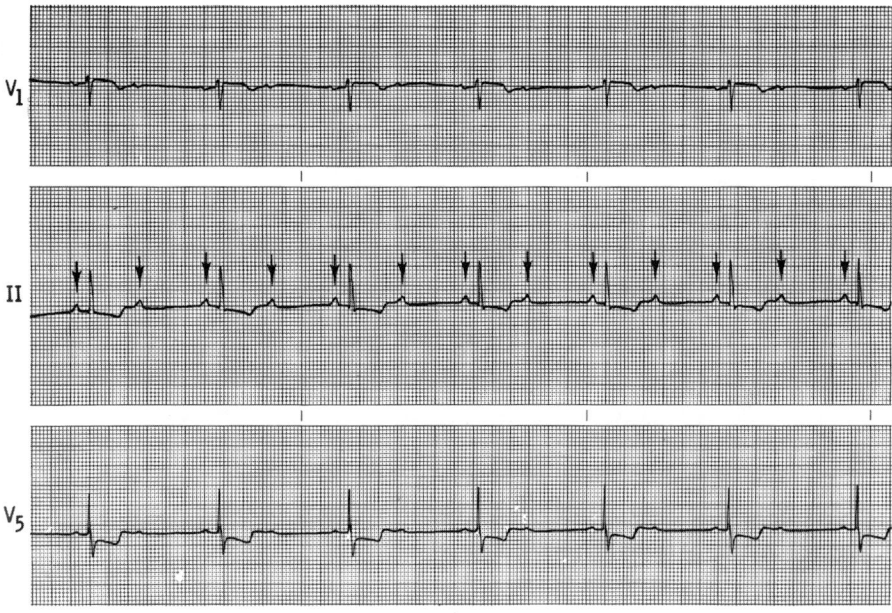

2:1 ATRIOVENTRICULAR BLOCK WITH BROAD QRS COMPLEXES

Definition

Every other P wave is *not* conducted to the ventricles and the QRS complexes are broad and bizarre because of underlying RBBB, LBBB, or BFB. This AV block is a variant of Mobitz type II AV block (see Fig. 11-5), thus representing infranodal block in nearly all cases.

Diagnostic Criteria (Fig. 11-7)

- Every other P wave is *not* conducted to the ventricles.
- The QRS complexes are broad because of underlying RBBB, LBBB, or BFB.
- On rare occasions, the QRS complexes demonstrate left anterior hemiblock or left posterior hemiblock.
- The P-R intervals of all conducted beats are constant.
- The R-R intervals (ventricular cycles) are two times the P-P cycles.
- Typical Mobitz type II AV block may occur intermittently in the same electrocardiographic tracing.

Diagnostic Pearls

Sinus rhythm with 2:1 AV block is often misdiagnosed as marked sinus bradycardia when the blocked P waves are *not* recognized. In addition, erroneous diagnosis of complete AV block with VER may be entertained because of slow ventricular rhythm with broad QRS complexes. Every reader should try to recognize every other P wave with constant P-R intervals in all conducted beats to make the correct diagnosis.

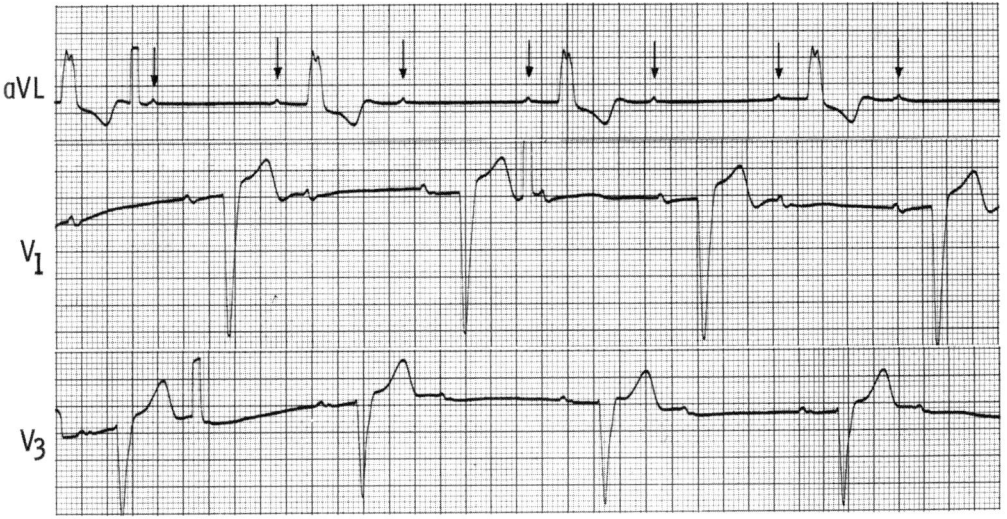

Figure 11-7
Sinus rhythm with 2:1 atrioventricular block associated with left bundle branch block. The atrioventricular block most likely represents an infranodal block. Arrows indicate P waves.

SINUS RHYTHM WITH ADVANCED (HIGH-DEGREE) ATRIOVENTRICULAR BLOCK

Definition

Sinus rhythm with advanced (high-degree) AV block is a sinus rhythm with a 3:1 or higher AV block. The block may be an AV nodal block or infranodal block.

Diagnostic Criteria (Fig. 11-8)

- Sinus rhythm with a 3:1 or higher AV block.
- The QRS complexes are normal or broad (because of preexisting LBBB or RBBB).
- One or more AV junctional (less commonly ventricular) escape beats often occur, leading to incomplete AV dissociation.
- AV conduction ratio may be constant or variable.

Diagnostic Pearls

When the AV block is far advanced and AV JEBs frequently occur, a certain portion of the electrocardiographic tracing often demonstrates complete AV block. Some authors use the term *almost complete AV block* to designate the far-advanced AV block. When the AV conduction ratio is constant (e.g., 3:1 or 4:1 AV block), the cardiac rhythm superficially mimics a markedly slow sinus bradycardia. Again, recognizing every P wave is essential to make the correct diagnosis.

Figure 11-8
Sinus rhythm with intermittent atrioventricular junctional escape rhythm (rate: 45 bpm) due to advanced atrioventricular block as a result of acute diaphragmatic mycoardial infarction. Note a ventricular captured beat (the last beat).

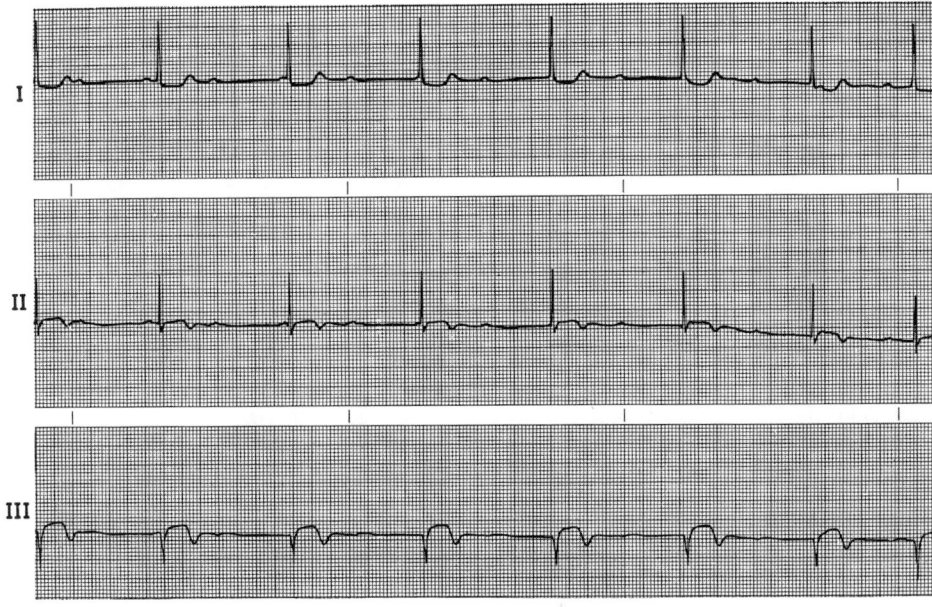

ATRIAL FIBRILLATION WITH ADVANCED ATRIOVENTRICULAR BLOCK

Definition

Atrial fibrillation (AF) with advanced AV block is AF with slow ventricular response (ventricular rate ≤80 beats per minute [bpm]) as a result of advanced AV block.

Diagnostic Criteria (Fig. 11-9)

- AF with slow ventricular response (rate of ≤80 bpm)
- One or more AV junctional (less commonly ventricular) escape beats occur, leading to incomplete AV dissociation.
- The QRS complexes may be normal or broad (because of LBBB or RBBB).
- The R-R intervals are usually irregular but may be constant in certain areas because of intermittent escape beats.

Diagnostic Pearls

AF with advanced AV block may be misinterpreted as other forms of bradyarrhythmias. Remember that a pure form of AF always produces very rapid ventricular rates (range of 120–200 bpm). Therefore, advanced AV block should be considered when AF exhibits slow ventricular rate (<80 bpm).

Figure 11-9
AF with advanced atrioventricular block producing occasional atrioventricular junctional escape beats (rate: 42 bpm), and frequent ventricular premature contractions with group beats (two in a row). The Holter monitor ECG rhythm strips A to D are not continuous.

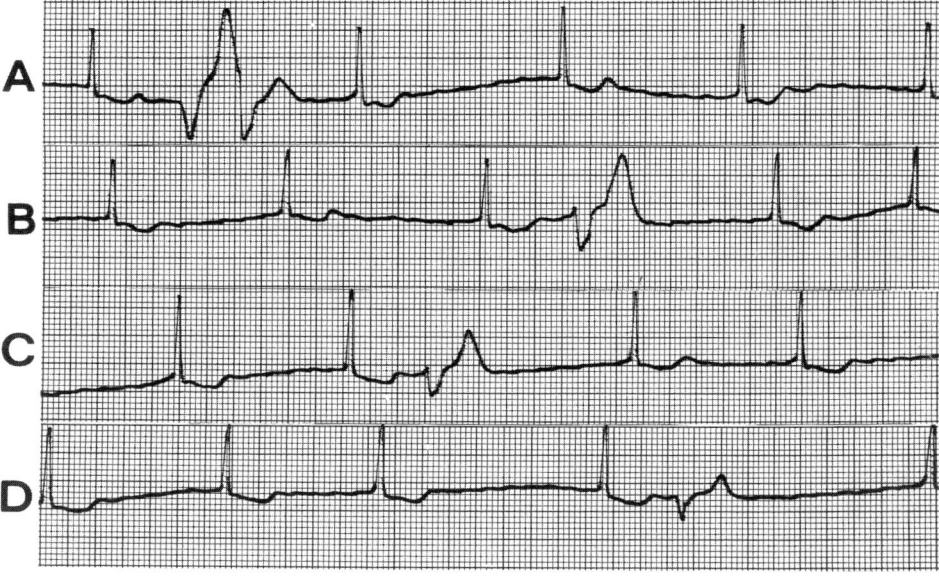

SINUS RHYTHM WITH ATRIOVENTRICULAR JUNCTIONAL ESCAPE RHYTHM DUE TO COMPLETE ATRIOVENTRICULAR BLOCK

Definition

Sinus rhythm with AV JER due to complete AV block is a sinus rhythm in the atria with independent AV JER in the ventricles as a result of complete AV block. In this case, the block represents AV nodal block.

Diagnostic Criteria (Fig. 11-10)

- Independent P waves of sinus origin and the QRS complexes of AV junctional origin due to complete AV block in the AV junction.
- The QRS complexes are normal in most cases.
- The QRS complexes may be broad when there is pre-existing LBBB, RBBB, or BFB.
- The ventricular rate is 40–60 bpm (<40 bpm in some cases).
- The R-R intervals (ventricular cycles) are constant.

- Ventriculophasic sinus arrhythmia in 30% (discussed in the section on ventriculophasic sinus arrhythmia).

Diagnostic Pearls

Complete AV block should be distinguished from other bradyarrhythmias. Independent atrial and ventricular activities confirm the diagnosis of complete AV block. The term *advanced AV block* is used even when there is only a single ventricular captured beat (normally conducted beat).

Figure 11-10
Sinus rhythm with AV JER (ventricular rate: 38 bpm) due to complete AV block. Arrows indicate P waves.

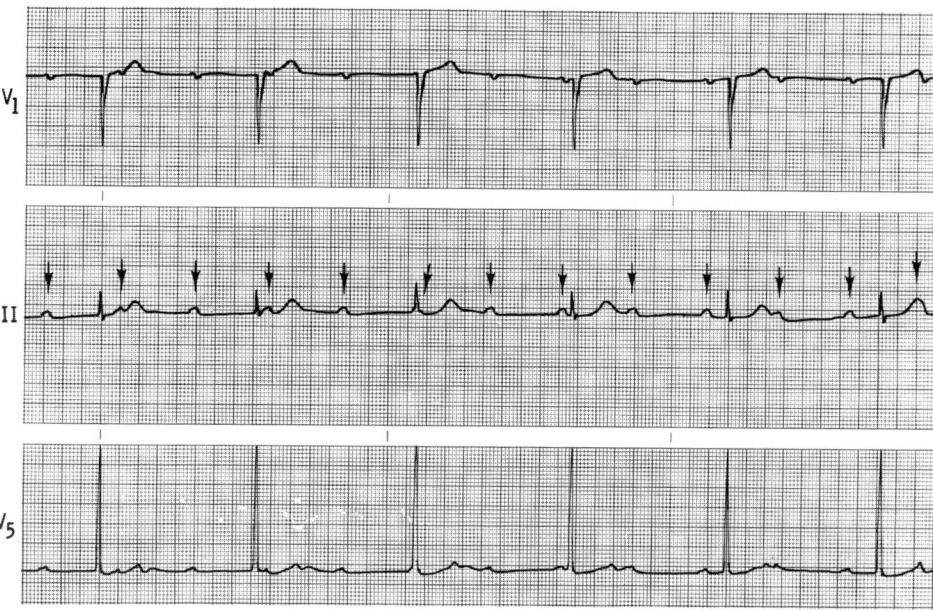

ATRIAL FIBRILLATION WITH COMPLETE ATRIOVENTRICULAR BLOCK

Definition

AF with complete AV block is AF in the atria with independent AV junctional (less commonly ventricular) escape rhythm as a result of complete AV block.

Diagnostic Criteria (Fig. 11-11)

- AF with independent QRS complexes due to complete AV block.
- The QRS complexes are normal when AV JER is present in the ventricles (AV nodal block).
- The QRS complexes are broad when there is preexisting LBBB, RBBB, or BFB in AV JER or VER is present in the ventricles (infranodal block).
- The ventricular rates in AV JER and VER range from 40 to 60 bpm and from 30 to 50 bpm, respectively.
- The R-R intervals (ventricular cycles) are constant.

Diagnostic Pearls

Even when the atrial mechanism is not discernible, the atrial activity is usually AF. AF with complete AV block should be distinguished from many other forms of bradyarrhythmias. The underlying disorder in the production of AF with complete AV block is commonly advanced sick sinus syndrome.

Figure 11-11
AF with atrioventricular junctional escape rhythm (rate: 40 bpm) due to complete atrioventricular block.

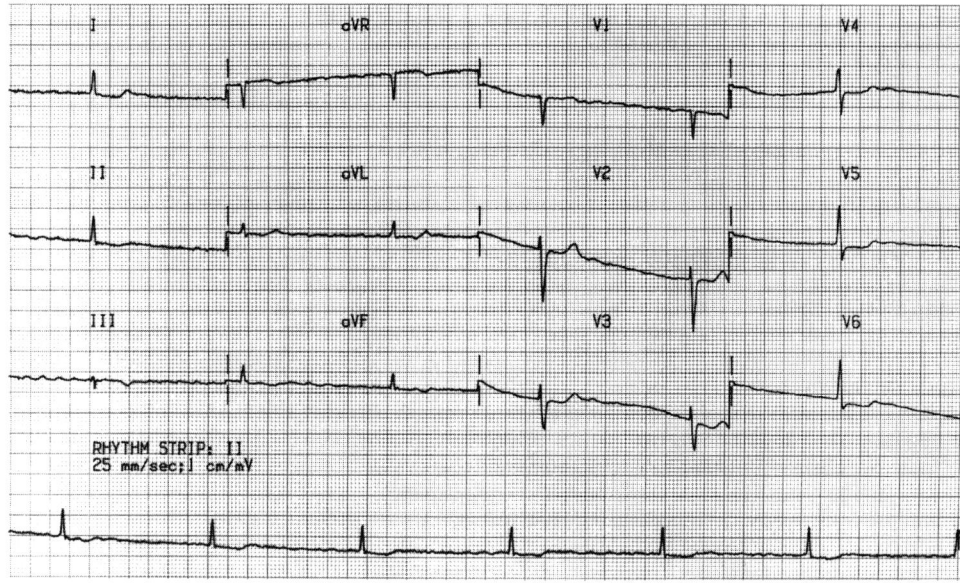

SINUS RHYTHM WITH VENTRICULAR ESCAPE RHYTHM DUE TO COMPLETE ATRIOVENTRICULAR BLOCK

Definition

Sinus rhythm with VER due to complete AV block is a sinus rhythm in the atria with independent VER (idioventricular rhythm) as a result of complete AV block. In this case, the block represents infranodal block.

Diagnostic Criteria (Fig. 11-12)

- Independent P waves of sinus origin and the broad QRS complexes of ventricular origin due to a block below the AV node (usually distal to the His bundle).
- The QRS complexes are usually very broad and bizarre.
- Ventricular rate is 30–50 bpm (<30 bpm in some cases).
- The R-R intervals (the ventricular cycles) are constant unless the rhythm progressively deteriorates to ventricular standstill.
- Ventriculophasic sinus arrhythmia in 30% (discussed in the section on ventriculophasic sinus arrhythmia).

- Sinus rhythm with ventricular escape rhythm often represents complete BBBB (see Chapter 4).

Diagnostic Pearls

VER is readily recognized by most readers because the cardiac rhythm characteristically demonstrates a very slow and regular ventricular rhythm with very broad QRS complexes. The rhythm should be distinguished from all other forms of bradyarrhythmias, such as markedly slow sinus bradycardia or AV JER with preexisting RBBB or LBBB (see Chapters 7 and 9).

Figure 11-12
Sinus rhythm with ventricular escape rhythm (rate: 33 bpm) due to complete atrioventricular block. Arrows indicate P waves.

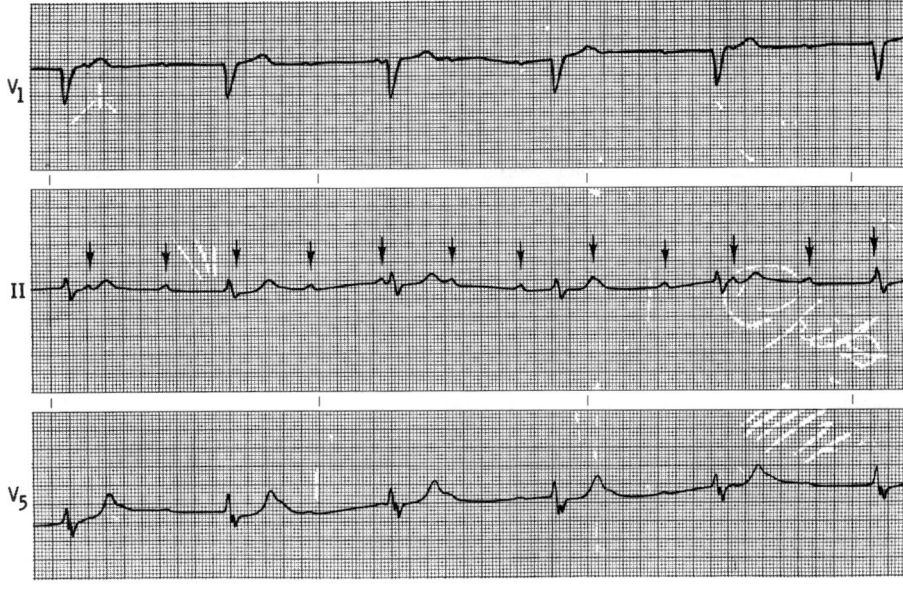

VENTRICULOPHASIC SINUS ARRHYTHMIA

Definition

Ventriculophasic sinus arrhythmia is characterized by a P-P interval that includes a QRS complex shorter than the P-P interval without a QRS complex in the presence of complete AV block.

Diagnostic Criteria (Fig. 11-13)

- In the presence of complete AV block, a P-P interval (P waves of sinus origin) that includes a QRS complex shorter than the P-P interval without a QRS complex.
- In rare cases, a reverse phenomenon may occur.
- Ventriculophasic sinus arrhythmia may be observed in the presence of second-degree AV block, artificial pacemaker-induced ventricular rhythm, and a ventricular premature contraction (VPC) with a full compensatory pause (a P-P interval that includes a VPC shorter than the P-P interval without a VPC).

Diagnostic Pearls

Ventriculophasic sinus arrhythmia is observed in approximately 30% of cases of complete AV block. The exact mechanism responsible for the development of ventriculophasic sinus arrhythmia is not clearly understood, but it seems to be due to some mechanical or hemodynamic mechanism. Ventriculophasic sinus arrhythmia per se is insignificant clinically.

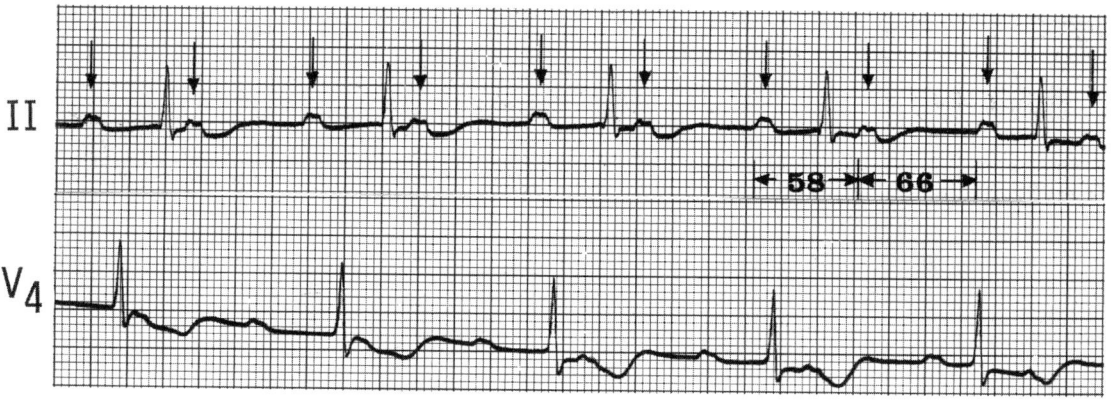

Figure 11-13
Sinus rhythm with atrioventricular junctional escape rhythm (rate: 48 bpm) due to complete atrioventricular block, associated with ventriculophasic sinus arrhythmia. Note that the P-P interval, which includes a QRS complex, is shorter than the P-P interval without a QRS complex. The numbers represent hundredths of a second. Arrows indicate P waves.

12

Wolff-Parkinson-White Syndrome (Ventricular Pre-Excitation Syndrome)

The primary reason every physician should be fully familiar with Wolff-Parkinson-White (WPW) syndrome is the frequent occurrence of various ectopic tachyarrhythmias. In addition, the electrocardiographic findings in WPW syndrome may closely resemble many other electrocardiographic abnormalities that are frequently misinterpreted in daily practice.

WPW syndrome was first recognized as a clinical entity by three physicians—Wolff, Parkinson, and White—in 1930. Electrocardiographic findings that were found to be characteristic of this syndrome were described by Wilson in 1915 and Wedd in 1921.

Since WPW syndrome is a congenital cardiac anomaly, other congenital anomalies (cardiac or noncardiac) often coexist with the syndrome.

WPW syndrome has been known as a benign syndrome. There are no subjective manifestations or hemodynamic alterations in this syndrome as long as there is no ectopic tachyarrhythmia. The tachyarrhythmias may occur at any time and may begin at birth or during infancy, childhood, or adult life. Sixty to 70% of the cases of WPW syndrome have been encountered in healthy individuals without organic heart disease.

For some reason, many physicians, including cardiologists, often fail to recognize WPW syndrome. In addition to the frequent occurrence of various tachyarrhythmias, WPW syndrome mimics other electrocardiographic abnormalities, including myocardial infarction (MI), right bundle branch block (RBBB), left bundle branch block (LBBB), hemiblocks, right ventricular hypertrophy (RVH), and left ventricular hypertrophy (LVH). Ventricular tachycardia (VT) is closely simulated when WPW syndrome is associated with a very rapid supraventricular tachyarrhythmia (e.g., atrial fibrillation [AF]) with anomalous conduction. False-positive exercise electrocardiographic test results are very common occurrences in individuals with WPW syndrome.

Probably the most important clinical significance of WPW syndrome is a danger of provoking VT or ventricular fibrillation (VF) after administering digitalis or verapamil when treating various supraventricular tachyarrhythmias, particularly AF. The reason for this is that digitalis and verapamil may enhance the conduction via an accessory pathway, leading to a faster ventricular rate. The faster ventricular rate may further provoke VT or VF and even sudden death. Thus, digitalis and verapamil are contraindicated in the treatment of various supraventricular tachyarrhythmias with anomalous conduction.

The true incidence of WPW syndrome is difficult to assess, but it has been estimated to be between 0.15% and 0.20% in the general population. The syndrome occurs more frequently in men than in women, with an incidence of 54–70% in men.

DIAGNOSTIC CRITERIA

WPW syndrome can be diagnosed by a 12-lead electrocardiogram (ECG), an electrophysiologic study (EPS), or vectorcardiogram (VCG).

Electrocardiographic Findings

- The typical electrocardiographic findings include a short P-R interval and a prolonged QRS interval due to a delta wave (initial slurring of the QRS complex, Fig. 12-1).

- Recognizing the delta wave is a key point in diagnosing the syndrome. In some cases of WPW syndrome, however, the delta wave may not be obvious.
- In proven WPW syndrome, the P-R interval may be longer than 0.12 second, and the QRS interval may be narrower than 0.10 second.
- The actual values of the P-R and QRS intervals in WPW syndrome are greatly influenced by the pre-existing values of these intervals.
- The term *Lown-Ganong-Levine (LGL) syndrome* has been used when the ECG shows a short P-R interval and narrow QRS complex without a clear-cut delta wave associated with recurrent tachyarrhythmias. LGL syndrome is considered to be a variant of WPW syndrome.
- The term *concealed bypass tract* has been mentioned often in recent literature. It refers to the presence of a bypass tract incapable of anterograde atrioventricular (AV) conduction. The impulses, however, can conduct retrogradely from ventricles to the atria. In this case, a 12-lead ECG fails to reveal any evidence of WPW syndrome. During reciprocating tachycardia, ventriculoatri-al (VA) conduction often shows delayed VA activation in this circumstance.
- It should be emphasized that many normal individuals may have a short P-R interval, particularly during stressful situations. Obviously, this isolated electrocardiographic finding is usually meaningless.

Vectorcardiographic Findings

A unique finding in WPW syndrome is the initial conduction delay of the QRS sÊ loop, which can be readily recognized by any physician familiar with VCGs.

Findings from Electrophysiologic Studies

In equivocal cases of WPW syndrome, a His bundle ECG may be necessary to confirm the diagnosis. In the His bundle ECG of WPW syndrome, the H-V interval is shorter than normal. The His bundle potential may occur simultaneously with the ventricular deflection or may occur even later than the onset of the ventricular deflection. These findings are thought to occur because of premature activation of a portion of the ventricles via anomalous conduction.

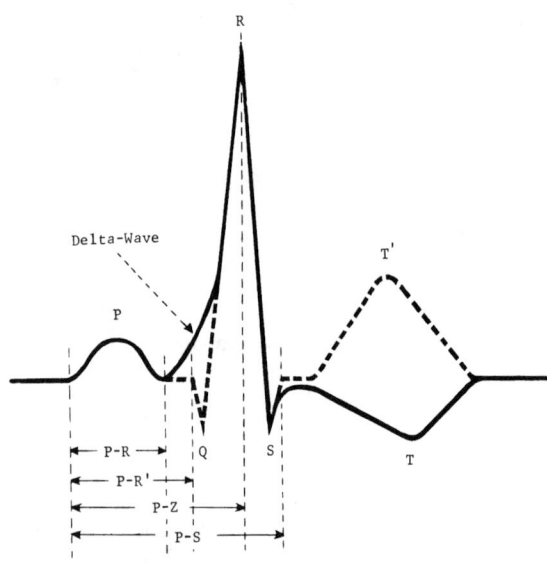

Figure 12-1

The uninterrupted line indicates anomalous conduction in Wolff-Parkinson-White (WPW) syndrome; the dotted line indicates normal conduction. P-R and P-R′ intervals are atrioventricular conduction times in WPW syndrome and normal conduction, respectively. The P-R interval is shorter than the P-R′ interval due to the presence of a delta wave. Note that intervals P-Z and P-S are constant during anomalous and normal conduction. The T wave in WPW syndrome is inverted because of secondary T wave changes.

CLASSIFICATION

The WPW syndrome has been traditionally classified into two types, A and B, depending on the direction of the delta wave. This classification is an oversimplification, however, because many cases of WPW syndrome do not belong to either type A or B. The direction of the delta wave is primarily influenced by the location of the accessory pathway.

Type A Wolff-Parkinson-White Syndrome

- In type A WPW syndrome, the delta wave is directed anteriorly (commonly to the right and less commonly to the left).
- In general, lead V_1 shows R, RS, Rs, RSr', and Rsr' patterns, whereas leads V_5 and V_6 show Rs or R deflection.
- Superficially, type A WPW syndrome resembles RBBB, RVH, or posterior MI.
- When the QRS complexes in all precordial leads are upright, a type A WPW syndrome should be considered as the first diagnostic possibility.
- In type A WPW syndrome, a premature activation occurs in the left ventricle.

Type B WPW Syndrome

- In type B WPW syndrome, the delta wave is directed posteriorly (commonly to the left and less commonly to the right).
- Thus, the left precordial leads (leads I, aVL, and V_{4-6}) show tall R waves with delta waves, whereas leads V_{1-2} show negative QRS complexes (Q-S waves) with delta waves.
- The electrocardiographic findings in type B WPW syndrome may closely resemble LBBB and LVH.

- At times, a pseudo–anteroseptal MI is produced in type B WPW syndrome.
- In type B, a premature activation takes place in the right ventricle.

In both type A and B WPW syndrome, the delta wave is often directed inferiorly. This electrocardiographic finding commonly produces Q-S or Q waves in leads II, III, and aVF that closely simulate diaphragmatic (inferior) MI.

TACHYARRHYTHMIAS

The most significant clinical aspect of the WPW syndrome is, needless to say, the frequent occurrence of supraventricular tachyarrhythmias. The incidence of tachyarrhythmias in WPW syndrome has been reported to be 40–80%. The mechanisms of reciprocating tachycardia are illustrated in Figures 12-2 and 12-3. The most common tachyarrhythmia in WPW syndrome is reciprocating tachycardia.

Recently, the *procainamide test* has been performed at various medical centers to determine the degree of risk when dealing with patients with WPW syndrome who have fre-

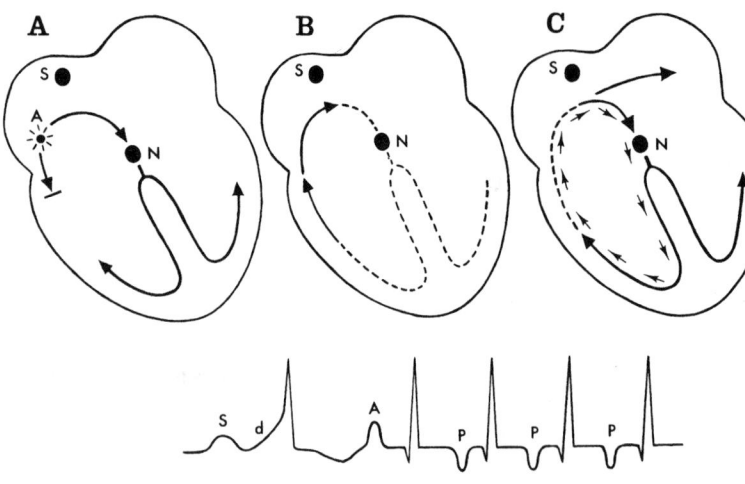

Figure 12-2

The mechanism of a reciprocating tachycardia with a normal QRS complex in the Wolff-Parkinson-White syndrome. In A, the atrial premature impulse (marked A) is conducted to the atrioventricular node (marked N), but the atrial premature impulse is blocked in the anomalous pathway. The atrial premature impulse is then conducted to both ventricles by way of a bundle branch system. In B, the atrial premature impulse is conducted to the atria in retrograde fashion to produce an inverted P wave. In C, the impulse is conducted in a clockwise fashion, producing a reciprocating (re-entry) cycle; the same cycle may repeat indefinitely. Note that the QRS complex during the tachycardia is normal. (S = sinus node; d = delta wave; P = inverted P wave.)

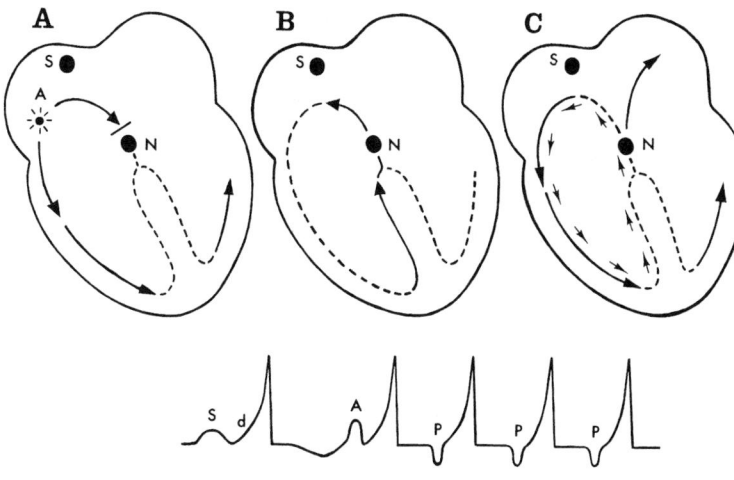

Figure 12-3
Reciprocating tachycardia with anomalous conduction in the Wolff-Parkinson-White syndrome. The re-entry cycle is counterclockwise, which is exactly the reverse direction of that shown in Figure 12-2.

quent tachyarrhythmias. This is particularly true when the patient suffers from AF with very rapid ventricular response.

It has been suggested that the rapid infusion of procainamide, 10 mg/kg IV given over 5 minutes, will produce a complete block over an accessory pathway in patients whose bypass tracts have relatively long refractory periods (>270 msec) and would be able to conduct at only relatively slow or moderately rapid rates during AF. In this circumstance, the refractory period refers to the ability of the accessory pathway to successfully conduct an atrial premature beat. Thus, it can be said that the shorter the refractory period, the greater the likelihood of rapid conduction via an accessory pathway in AF or atrial flutter. In this test, when the QRS complex reveals normalization without a delta wave abruptly during the procainamide infusion of 10 mg/kg or less, there is generally minimal risk of developing rapid anomalous AV conduction even if AF or atrial flutter occurs. Therefore, the possibility of sudden death will be very small in this circumstance.

It should be noted that the procainamide test is virtually useless when the delta wave is *not* obvious during anomalous AV conduction because a normalization of the QRS complex will be difficult or almost impossible to document during the test. The procainamide test may produce complications, including marked hypotension and AV block of varying degrees.

Reciprocating Tachycardia

- Reciprocating tachycardia (the usual rate is 140–250 beats per minute [bpm]) is found in the majority of cases (75–80% of all tachyarrhythmias).
- This type of tachycardia had been called paroxysmal atrial tachycardia until recently.
- At present, the term *reciprocating* or *re-entrant* tachycardia is more commonly used because the tachycardia is considered to be due to a re-entry phenomenon (see Figs. 12-2 and 12-3). The term *circus movement* tachycardia has been frequently used in European literature to designate the same finding.
- In reciprocating tachycardia, the QRS complex is usually normal (narrow). A broad QRS complex due to anomalous conduction is much less common.

Atrial Flutter and Atrial Fibrillation

- Atrial flutter and AF are rather uncommon in WPW syndrome; their incidence constitutes only 20–25% of all tachyarrhythmias.

- Among these two rhythm disorders, atrial flutter is extremely rare.
- The QRS complexes during AF or flutter in the WPW syndrome are extremely bizarre and broad in most cases.
- Broad and bizarre QRS complexes are observed in this circumstance because of anomalous AV conduction due to the nature of WPW syndrome itself plus aberrant ventricular conduction due to a very rapid ventricular rate (ventricular rate of 250–300 bpm).
- VT or even VF is closely simulated when atrial flutter or AF with anomalous AV conduction occurs.
- In WPW syndrome, atrial flutter often exhibits 1:1 AV conduction, which results in an extremely rapid ventricular rate.
- It should be remembered that atrial flutter or AF in WPW syndrome may lead to VT or VF and even sudden death, especially following the administration of digitalis or verapamil.

Ventricular Tachyarrhythmias

- Although the occurrence of VT has previously been reported in WPW syndrome, AF or atrial flutter with anomalous AV conduction has simply been misinterpreted in most, if not all cases.
- On the other hand, a true incidence of VF has been reported in WPW syndrome recently.
- Sudden death in the WPW syndrome is most likely due to VF following atrial flutter or AF with extremely rapid ventricular response, especially after the administration of digitalis or verapamil.

Other Arrhythmias

In addition to the above-mentioned tachyarrhythmias, various other arrhythmias, such as ventricular premature contractions (VPCs), AV dissociation, ventricular parasystole, or atrial parasystole, may simply coexist with WPW syndrome.

OTHER CLINICAL SIGNIFICANCE

In addition to recognizing the frequent association of various supraventricular tachyarrhythmias, recognizing WPW syndrome is extremely important because the QRS complex in WPW syndrome often resembles various other electro-cardiographic findings.

- The diagnosis of diaphragmatic (inferior) MI is frequently made erroneously in cases of WPW syndrome (either type A or B), because of Q or Q-S waves in leads II, III, and aVF. This electrocardiographic finding is observed when the delta wave is directed inferiorly.
- Type B WPW syndrome may closely resemble anterior or anteroseptal MI.
- Because of the broad QRS complexes due to the delta waves in WPW syndrome, LBBB or RBBB is closely simulated.
- Type A WPW syndrome may also be misdiagnosed as true posterior MI or RVH because of the tall R waves in leads V_{1-3}.
- At times, a pseudolateral MI is produced in WPW syndrome.
- It is also common to observe tall R waves in leads I, aVL, and V_{4-6} with the secondary S-T and T wave changes in type B WPW syndrome. This electrocardiographic finding demonstrates a pseudo-LVH.
- When the WPW syndrome is observed intermittently, the electrocardiographic finding resembles VPCs or even short runs of VT.
- Recently, it has been demonstrated that a false-positive exercise electrocardiographic test is common in the WPW syndrome, especially in type B. Therefore, no significant diagnostic value is obtained from exercise electrocardiographic test results when the patient is known to have WPW syndrome.

DISORDERS ASSOCIATED WITH WOLFF-PARKINSON-WHITE SYNDROME

- It has been demonstrated that patients with WPW syndrome often suffer from some form of psychoneurotic disorders and hyperthyroidism. The direct relationship between these disorders and WPW syndrome is unknown, however.
- Some patients with AF in WPW syndrome not uncommonly suffer from rheumatic heart disease.
- Congenital cardiac anomalies frequently associated with WPW syndrome include Ebstein's anomaly, atrial septal defect, idiopathic hypertrophic subaortic stenosis, and mitral valve prolapse syndrome.
- Occasionally, WPW syndrome may coexist with other abnormalities, including true MI, LBBB, or RBBB.

MECHANISMS: ELECTROPHYSIOLOGIC STUDIES

Recently, EPSs have been performed frequently in patients with WPW syndrome for diagnostic and therapeutic purposes, especially in dealing with high-risk patients. The indications and roles of EPS in WPW syndrome are summarized in Tables 12-1 and 12-2.

Reciprocating Tachycardia

- Electrophysiologic and pathologic studies suggest that the WPW syndrome occurs because of a premature activation of a portion of the ventricles as a result of an anomalous AV conduction via an accessory pathway directly from the atria to the ventricles.
- The remaining portion of the ventricular activation results from varying degree fusion of transmission via both the normal AV conduction system and the accessory pathway. In the majority of cases of WPW syndrome, the anomalous AV conduction is considered to occur through the Kent bundle.
- On the other hand, a normal P-R interval with a delta wave may result from slow conduction via the Kent bundle or conduction via the Mahaim tract.
- Conduction through the James bundle, an AV nodal bypass tract, has been considered to be responsible for the LGL syndrome.
- An important role of the His bundle ECG is to provide information so that the physician can diagnose WPW syndrome accurately and understand the exact mechanisms of tachyarrhythmias associated with the syndrome.
- In an equivocal case, a physician can confirm the diagnosis of WPW syndrome using the His bundle ECG and by recognizing a shorter-than-normal H-V interval, the simultaneous occurrence of His bundle deflection and ventricular deflection, or even the occurrence of ventricular deflection preceding the His bundle potential.
- Electrophysiologic properties of both normal and anomalous AV pathways in patients with WPW syndrome can be examined by the His bundle recordings and atrial stimulation.
- The P-delta interval represents the duration of the anomalous pathway conduction time, whereas the A-H interval (simultaneously recorded) indicates normal AV conduction time.

Table 12-1. Indications for an electrophysiologic study in Wolff-Parkinson-White (WPW) syndrome

An electrophysiologic study in WPW syndrome is indicated for the following:

When the diagnosis of WPW syndrome is equivocal in suspected individuals with tachyarrhythmias

In patients with known WPW syndrome and a family history of premature sudden death

In patients with asymptomatic WPW syndrome with high-risk occupations or activities

Before cardiac surgery (for other reasons) in patients with WPW syndrome

For the proper selection of antiarrhythmic drug(s) in patients with WPW syndrome that is associated with significant tachyarrhythmias

In patients considered for nondrug therapy (e.g., antitachycardia pacing or surgery) because of life-threatening or drug-resistant tachyarrhythmias

- The configuration of the QRS complex in WPW syndrome depends on the degree of fusion in ventricular activation between the impulse conducted via the anomalous conduction and the normal AV conduction. The QRS complex is relatively narrow when the P-delta and A-H intervals are similar in duration, whereas the QRS contour is markedly bizarre when the A-H interval is long and the P-delta interval is short.

- Refractory periods of both normal and anomalous pathways can be determined using the extrastimulus technique. It has been demonstrated recently that supraventricular tachycardia in WPW syndrome represents reciprocating tachycardia due to a re-entry phenomenon.

- The reason for the re-entry is that the marked discrepancy between the refractory periods in the normal and anomalous pathways predisposes to the initiation of the reciprocating tachycardia. Diagrammatic illustrations regarding the mechanisms of reciprocating tachycardia in this syndrome are found in Figures 12-2 and 12-3.

- Once re-entry is established, the impulse may be conducted antegradely to the ventricles via the normal pathway and retrogradely to the atria via the anomalous

Table 12-2. Roles of electrophysiologic studies in Wolff-Parkinson-White syndrome

Confirm the diagnosis of Wolff-Parkinson-White syndrome
Localize accessory pathway(s) by mapping
Determine the mechanisms of tachyarrhythmias:
  Reciprocating tachycardia (orthodromic or antidromic)
  Atrial fibrillation or atrial flutter
Determine the following:
  Shortest R-R interval in atrial fibrillation
  Refractory period of accessory pathways (bypass tracts)
  Ease of atrial fibrillation induction and duration of atrial fibrillation
Determine the effect of isoproterenol infusion on the following:
  Initiation of tachyarrhythmia(s)
  Refractory period of accessory pathway(s)
  Shortest R-R interval during anomalous conduction
Evaluate the efficacy of treatment with the following:
  Antiarrhythmic agents
  Antitachycardia devices
  Catheter ablation
  Antiarrhythmic surgery

pathway (see Fig. 12-2). In this case, the QRS configuration during the tachycardia is normal.

- On the other hand, the re-entry impulse may be conducted antegradely to the ventricles via the anomalous pathway and retrogradely to the atria via the normal pathway. In this circumstance, the QRS complex during the tachycardia is bizarre (see Fig. 12-3).
- Clinically, the majority of cases with reciprocating tachycardia in WPW syndrome show normal QRS complexes because the re-entry cycle is carried out via antegrade normal AV conduction with retrograde anomalous conduction (see Figs. 12-2 and 12-3).
- The direction of the re-entry cycles depends on the availability of either the normal or the anomalous pathway, whichever is in a nonrefractory period. Namely, a premature impulse (commonly atrial and less commonly AV junctional or ventricular) will be blocked in a pathway that is refractory, whereas it will be conducted antegradely in another pathway that is nonrefractory. The re-entry impulse then will be conducted to the atria in retrograde fashion via the pathway that was previously refractory (see Figs. 12-2 and 12-3).
- The re-entry cycles may repeat once, twice, or even indefinitely. Reciprocating tachycardia is often terminated by a properly timed atrial premature beat (either spontaneous or induced).
- Multiple accessory pathways in WPW syndrome have been reported by this author previously, and the His bundle electrocardiographic analysis on double accessory pathways has been described recently.

Atrial Fibrillation and Atrial Flutter

- The exact mechanism responsible for the initiation of AF in WPW syndrome is not clearly understood.
- It is considered that AF is triggered by the re-entry impulse, which stimulates the atria during the atrial vulnerable period.
- In AF or atrial flutter in WPW syndrome, the rapid atrial impulses may be conducted to the ventricles via normal or accessory pathways, whichever is nonrefractory.
- The QRS complexes during AF or atrial flutter in this syndrome are frequently bizarre and wide because of anomalous conduction plus the common occurrence of aberrant ventricular conduction due to an extremely rapid ventricular rate.

- According to EPS results, patients whose R-R intervals (ventricular cycles) are shortest during AF with an anomalous AV conduction range of 210–250 msec belong to high-risk groups. In other words, many patients with short R-R intervals develop serious symptoms (e.g., syncope or near-syncope) that may lead to life-threatening ventricular tachyarrhythmias and even sudden death. The short refractory period (<270 msec) of the bypass tract is shown to have a similar clinical significance.

PREVENTION AND TREATMENT OF TACHYARRHYTHMIAS

Needless to say, no treatment is indicated when WPW syndrome is not associated with tachyarrhythmias. Similarly, a transient arrhythmia with a short duration also requires no therapy. It should be noted, however, that an EPS is strongly recommended even in asymptomatic WPW syndrome if there is a family history of premature cardiac death or if the individual is going to participate in any type of high-risk occupations or physical activities (see Table 12-1). According to the EPS results, prophylactic drug therapy may be indicated in some cases under these circumstances. Paroxysmal reciprocating tachycardia in WPW syndrome is often terminated by vagal maneuvers such as carotid sinus stimulation or Valsalva maneuvers. On the other hand, many patients with tachyarrhythmias in WPW syndrome require various antiarrhythmic agents (Table 12-3) either acutely or as a long-term maintenance therapy. In urgent situations, especially in AF or atrial flutter with extremely rapid ventricular response, direct current shock may be needed. When tachyarrhythmias become refractory, an artificial pacemaker or even surgical therapy should be considered.

The His bundle ECG has provided significant contributions to the drug therapy for various tachyarrhythmias in the WPW syndrome. The drug of choice can be determined specifically according to the electrophysiologic properties of various antiarrhythmic agents for a given tachyarrhythmia in the WPW syndrome (see Table 12-3). Procainamide and quinidine are found to be very effective in the treatment of various supraventricular tachyarrhythmias (particularly AF) with anomalous conduction in WPW syndrome because these drugs very effectively depress the conduction via the anomalous pathway (see Table 12-3). Namely, these agents primarily produce a lengthening of the effective

Table 12-3. Effects of drugs on refractory periods in normal and anomalous pathways

Drug	Effect on atrioventricular node	Effect on accessory pathway
Adenosine		0
Propranolol		0
Digitalis		∅
Lidocaine	0	
Quinidine	∅	
Procainamide	0	
Phenytoin	∅	Variable
Amiodarone		
Ajmaline	0	
Verapamil		Variable

 = increase in refractory period; ∅ = decrease in refractory period; 0 = no change in refractory period.

refractory period in the accessory pathway (see Table 12-3). In addition, quinidine is considered to be very effective because it is capable of suppressing atrial (less commonly AV junctional or ventricular) premature beats, which commonly initiate the paroxysmal reciprocating tachycardia in WPW syndrome.

It has been shown that adenosine (intravenous injection) is extremely effective in terminating reciprocating tachycardia with normal QRS complexes in WPW syndrome (see Table 12-3) because the drug suppresses the conduction in the normal AV conduction system. Thus, adenosine is considered to be the drug of choice in this circumstance. For preventing reciprocating tachycardia with normal QRS complexes in WPW syndrome, beta-blocking agents (e.g., propranolol) are highly recommended.

The danger of provoking VT or VF after administering digitalis or verapamil in the treatment of various tachyarrhythmias with anomalous conduction in WPW syndrome has been repeatedly emphasized because these agents enhance the conduction via an accessory pathway so that the clinical situation deteriorates further.

WOLFF-PARKINSON-WHITE SYNDROME TYPE A

Definition

WPW syndrome type A is characterized by a short P-R interval with a broad QRS complex due to a delta wave (initial slurring of the QRS complex) that is directed anteriorly and either inferiorly or superiorly.

Diagnostic Criteria (Fig. 12-4)

- Short P-R interval (usually <0.12 second) with a broad QRS complex (usually >0.10 second) due to a delta wave.
- The delta wave is directed anteriorly and either inferiorly or superiorly.
- The QRS complexes are often upright (positive) in all precordial leads.
- A pseudo–inferior-posterior MI pattern is often produced.
- Various supraventricular tachyarrhythmias often occur.

Diagnostic Pearls

Recognizing a delta wave is a key point in diagnosing WPW syndrome. Type A WPW syndrome should be considered as a first diagnostic possibility when dealing with any electrocardiographic tracing showing upright (positive) QRS complexes in all precordial leads. The delta waves are pronounced in leads V_{1-3} in type A WPW syndrome. Type A WPW syndrome superficially mimics RBBB.

Figure 12-4
Sinus rhythm with type A Wolff-Parkinson-White syndrome. Diaphragmatic and posterior myocardial infarction are superficially simulated. Figures 12-4 and 12-8 were obtained from the same patient (a 24-year-old man) on different occasions.

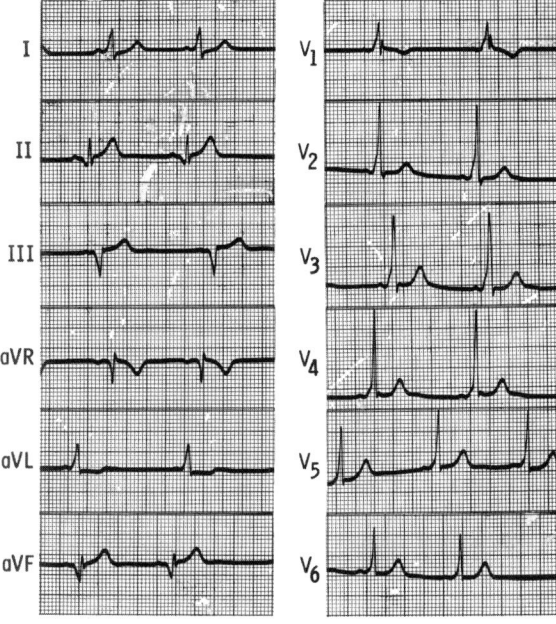

WOLFF-PARKINSON-WHITE SYNDROME TYPE B

Definition

WPW syndrome type B is characterized by a short P-R interval with a broad QRS complex due to a delta wave (initial slurring of the QRS complex) that is directed posteriorly and either inferiorly or superiorly.

Diagnostic Criteria (Fig. 12-5)

- Short P-R interval (usually <0.12 second) with a broad QRS complex (usually >0.10 second) due to a delta wave.
- The delta wave is directed posteriorly and either inferiorly or superiorly.
- The QRS complexes in leads V_{1-3} usually disclose Q-S waves or rS complexes, whereas leads V_{4-6} show tall and broad QRS complexes.
- Type B WPW syndrome often produces pseudo–inferior MI and pseudo–anteroseptal or anterior MI.
- Various supraventricular tachyarrhythmias often occur.

Diagnostic Pearls

Again, recognizing a delta wave is a key point in diagnosing WPW syndrome. The delta waves are pronounced in leads I, aVL, and V_{4-6} in type B WPW syndrome. Type B WPW syndrome superficially mimics LBBB.

Figure 12-5
Sinus arrhythmia with type B Wolff-Parkinson-White syndrome. Pseudo–anteroseptal myocardial infarction is produced.

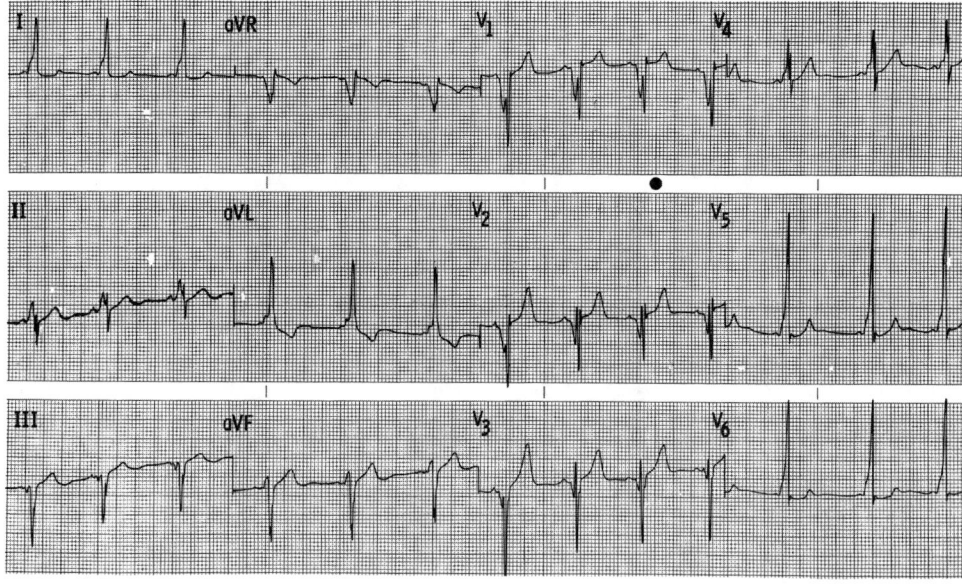

INTERMITTENT WOLFF-PARKINSON-WHITE SYNDROME

Definition

In intermittent WPW syndrome, the cardiac impulses from the sinus node are conducted to the ventricles via an accessory pathway (bypass tract) only intermittently.

Diagnostic Criteria (Fig. 12-6)

- A delta wave occurs only intermittently so that the remaining QRS complexes are normal.
- Intermittent WPW syndrome may occur in both types A and B.
- Some QRS complexes show the characteristic features of ventricular fusion beats when the cardiac impulses are conducted to the ventricles via an accessory pathway (bypass tract) and the normal AV conduction system simultaneously.
- Various supraventricular tachyarrhythmias are less common in intermittent WPW syndrome.

Diagnostic Pearls

Intermittent WPW syndrome superficially resembles VPCs or even a short episode of VT. Again, recognizing a delta wave is a key issue in correctly diagnosing WPW syndrome.

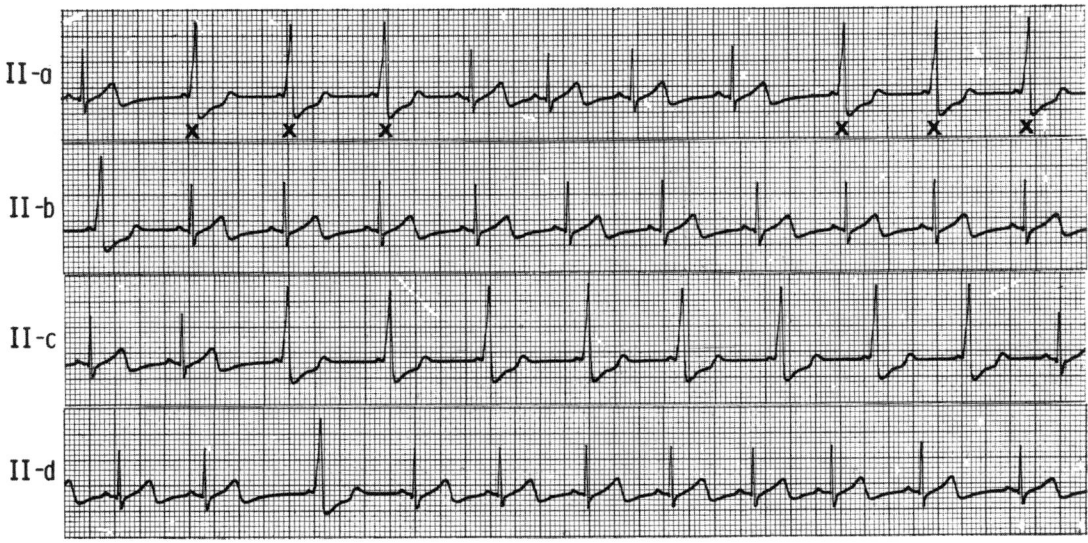

Figure 12-6
Sinus arrhythmia with intermittent Wolff-Parkinson-White syndrome (marked X). Leads II a–d are continuous.

RECIPROCATING TACHYCARDIA IN WOLFF-PARKINSON-WHITE SYNDROME

Definition

Reciprocating tachycardia in WPW syndrome is a regular tachycardia due to a re-entry mechanism (see Figs. 12-2 and 12-3) in WPW syndrome.

Diagnostic Criteria (Fig. 12-7)

- Regular tachycardia due to a re-entry mechanism (discussed previously) in WPW syndrome.
- The QRS complexes may be followed by retrograde P waves, but the P waves are often not discernible.
- The ventricular rates range from 140 to 250 bpm (at times, <140 bpm).
- The QRS complexes may be normal (see Fig. 12-2) or broad (see Fig. 12-3), depending on the direction of the re-entry cycle.

Diagnostic Pearls

WPW syndrome should always be considered as the underlying disorder when any individual (particularly young adults and children) develops a regular tachycardia with normal or broad QRS complexes. In a practical sense, retrograde P waves are *not* easily demonstrable in reciprocating tachycardia in WPW syndrome.

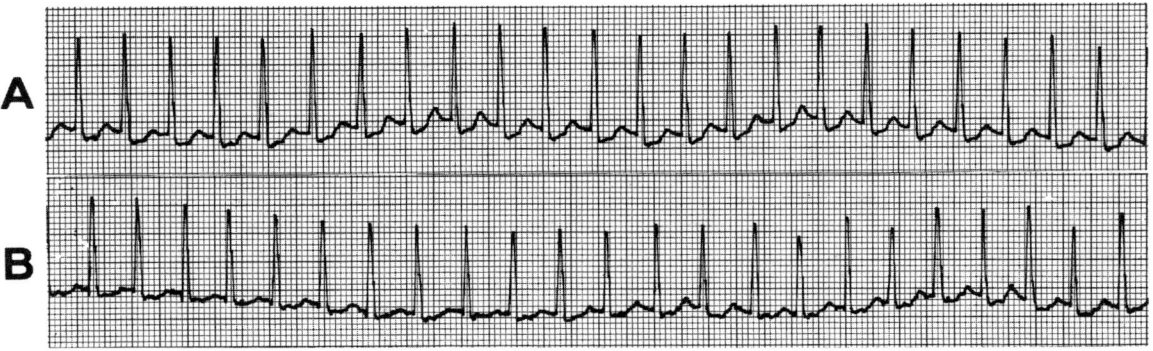

Figure 12-7
Reciprocating tachycardia (rate of 187 bpm) due to Wolff-Parkinson-White syndrome. The rhythm strips A and B are not continuous.

ATRIAL FIBRILLATION IN WOLFF-PARKINSON-WHITE SYNDROME

Definition

AF in WPW syndrome is AF with a very rapid ventricular response in WPW syndrome. The QRS complexes are usually extremely broad and bizarre.

Diagnostic Criteria (Fig. 12-8)

- AF (see Fig. 8-10) with a very rapid ventricular response (rate of 140–300 bpm).
- The QRS complexes are extremely broad and bizarre in most cases because the atrial impulses are conducted to the ventricles very rapidly via an accessory pathway (bypass tract).
- The QRS complexes are normal intermittently when the atrial impulses are conducted to the ventricles via a normal AV conduction system.
- AF may occur in both types A and B WPW syndrome, but it seems to occur more frequently in type A.
- An additional factor that produces extremely bizarre QRS complexes in AF in this circumstance is consecutively occurring aberrant ventricular conduction (see Fig. 6-6) because of a very rapid ventricular rate.

Diagnostic Pearls

WPW syndrome should always be considered first as an underlying disorder in any individuals (particularly young adults and children) who develop AF. This is particularly true when the ventricular rate is very rapid (>300 bpm) and the QRS complexes are extremely broad. VT is closely simulated, but grossly irregular ventricular cycles confirm the diagnosis of AF. By and large, when the ventricular rate is near 300 bpm in AF with broad QRS complexes, the diagnosis of WPW syndrome is certain.

Figure 12-8
Atrial fibrillation with anomalous atrioventricular conduction due to type A Wolff-Parkinson-White syndrome (rate of 200–280 bpm).

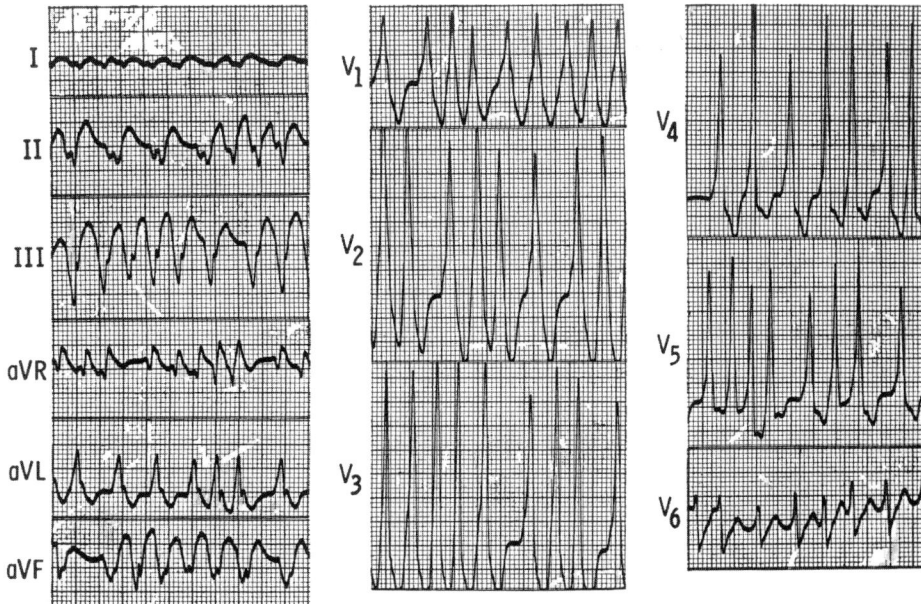

WOLFF-PARKINSON-WHITE SYNDROME ASSOCIATED WITH BUNDLE BRANCH BLOCK

Definition

WPW syndrome associated with bundle branch block is a combination of WPW syndrome (defined previously; see Figs. 12-4 and 12-5) and LBBB or RBBB (defined previously; see Figs. 4-4 and 4-5).

Diagnostic Criteria

To make the diagnosis of WPW associated with bundle branch block, the following must be present (Fig. 12-9):

• Diagnostic criteria of WPW syndrome (see Figs. 12-4 and 12-5)
• Diagnostic criteria of LBBB (see Fig. 4-5) or RBBB (see Fig. 4-4)

Diagnostic Pearls

Because of two coexisting electrocardiographic abnormalities responsible for the production of broad QRS complexes (see Table 6-1), the QRS complexes tend to be extremely bizarre and broad. Remember that the initial portion of the QRS complex is broad because of a delta wave in WPW syndrome, whereas the last portion of the QRS complex is broad because of LBBB or RBBB. When two electrocardiographic abnormalities causing broad QRS complexes are present, inexperienced readers often fail to recognize one of two electrocardiographic findings (usually WPW syndrome).

Figure 12-9
Atrial flutter with a 2:1 atrioventricular conduction and type A Wolff-Parkinson-White syndrome associated with right bundle branch block. Note frequent ventricular premature contractions (the third, eighth, and thirteenth beats).

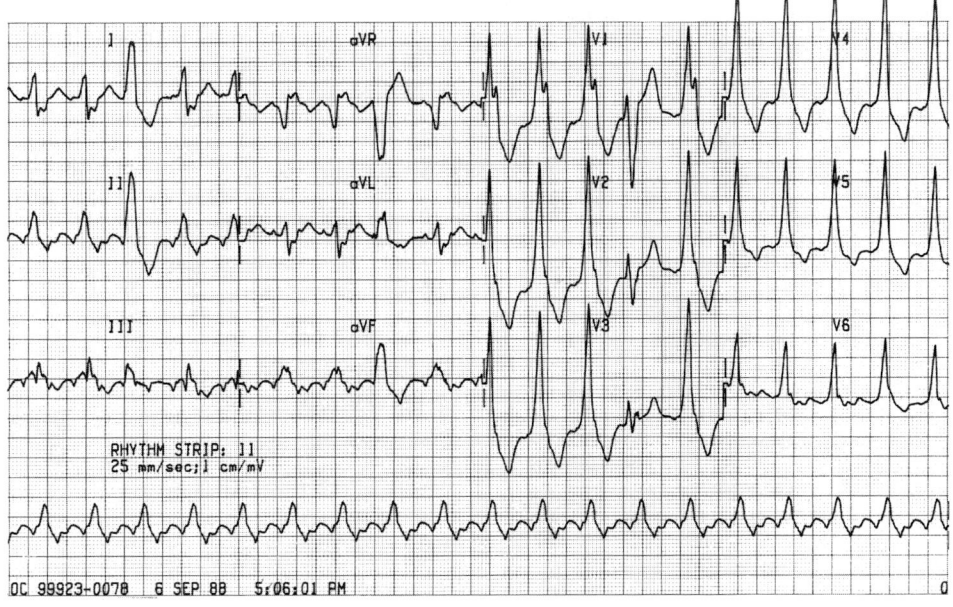

WOLFF-PARKINSON-WHITE SYNDROME ASSOCIATED WITH MYOCARDIAL INFARCTION

Definition

WPW syndrome associated with MI is a combination of WPW syndrome (defined previously; see Figs. 12-4 and 12-5) and MI (defined previously; see Figs. 5-8 through 5-15).

Diagnostic Criteria (Fig. 12-10)

- Diagnostic criteria of WPW syndrome (see Figs. 12-4 and 12-5)
- Occurrence of new pathologic Q waves in the involved electrocardiographic leads facing the MI
- Development of a new S-T segment and/or T wave abnormalities (usually an S-T segment elevation with inverted T waves) to replace the preexisting S-T segment and/or T wave abnormalities in WPW syndrome

Diagnostic Pearls

When two electrocardiographic abnormalities coexist, recognizing both electrocardiographic findings is not always easy. Every reader should pay particular attention to the newly developed primarily S-T segment and/or T wave changes in the presence of WPW syndrome. Nevertheless, the diagnosis of old MI is often difficult or at times even impossible when there is a coexisting WPW syndrome because both abnormalities can cause abnormal Q waves.

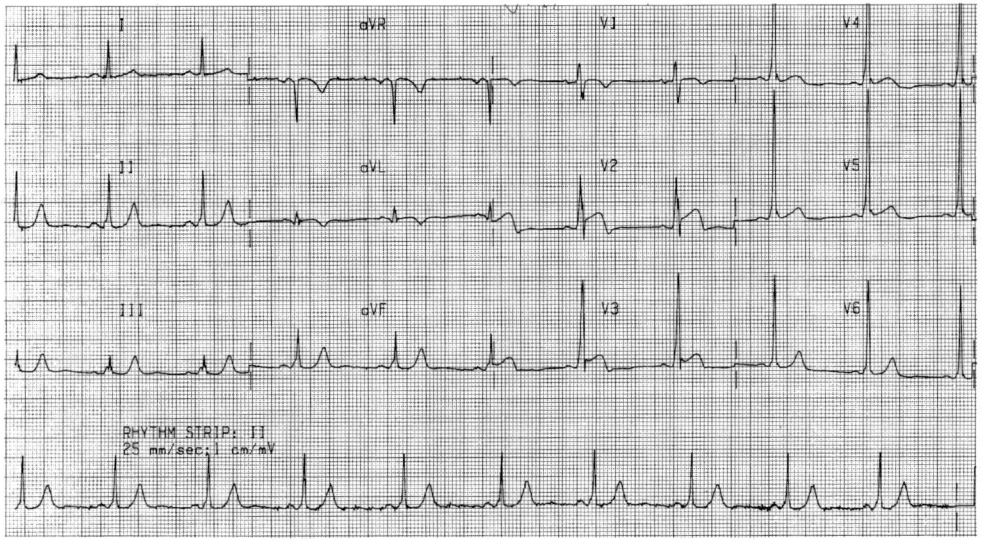

Figure 12-10   *Wolff-Parkinson-White syndrome associated with acute anteroseptal subepicardial injury and ischemia—an early finding of acute anteroseptal myocardial infarction.*

13

Uncommon Arrhythmias and Electrocardiographic Abnormalities

Relatively uncommon cardiac arrhythmias and electrocardiographic abnormalities are summarized in Table 13-1.

RECIPROCAL BEATS AND RHYTHM (ECHO BEATS AND RHYTHM)

Reciprocal beats and rhythm (echo beats and rhythm) are considered to be generated by a specific form of re-entry phenomenon. This arrhythmia nearly always arises from atri-

oventricular (AV) junctional tachycardia (JT) or junctional escape rhythms (JERs). In addition, an echo beat often occurs following the longest P-R or R-P interval during Wenckebach AV or ventriculoatrial (VA) block. It is extremely unusual to observe reciprocal beats in the presence of normal sinus rhythm without AV conduction disturbance. Occasionally, reciprocal beats may be initiated by AV junctional premature contractions (JPCs) or ventricular premature contractions (VPCs). Rarely, atrial premature contractions (APCs) and even sinus beats may be followed by reciprocal beats.

Table 13-1. Uncommon arrhythmias and electrocardiographic abnormalities

Reciprocal beats rhythm	Electrical alternans
Parasystole	Ventricular electrical alternans
Ventricular parasystole	Atrial electrical alternans
Atrial parasystole	Repolarization electrical alternans
AV junctional parasystole	Combined electrical alternans
Fascicular parasystole	Fascicular beats, rhythm, and tachycardia
Multifocal parasystole	Multifocal AV junctional tachycardias and rhythms
Dissociation	
Atrial dissociation	
Ventricular dissociation	
Slow atrial rhythm	
Left atrial rhythm	
Right atrial rhythm	
Coronary sinus rhythm	
Coronary nodal rhythm	
Aberrant atrial conduction (Chung's phenomenon)	

AV = atrioventricular.

A reciprocal beat is diagnosed when a retrograde P wave is noted to be "sandwiched" between two closely spaced QRS complexes, the first of which originates from an ectopic focus (commonly the AV node). As a result, the QRS complex following the retrograde P wave appears earlier than the usual R-R cycle of the basic rhythm.

The fundamental mechanism (Fig. 13-1) responsible for the genesis of reciprocal beats is considered to be due to a specific form of a *re-entry phenomenon* occurring in the AV junctional tissue. One assumes that there is a longitudinal dissociation present in the AV junctional fibers, which have different degrees of depressed conductivity. Thus, some of the longitudinal fibers are more markedly depressed than others. Consequently, unidirectional block of retrograde conduction occurs in the more depressed fibers in addition to a generalized delay in retrograde conduction in all of the AV junctional fibers. The impulse originating from the AV node is conducted in both directions—namely, to the ventricles (antegrade) and toward the atria (retrograde). The retrograde impulse soon reaches the depressed AV junctional fibers. The retrograde impulse is completely blocked in the more depressed fibers and conducted at a slower speed than usual in a retrograde fashion in the remaining, less depressed fibers. The R-P interval in a reciprocal beat is consequently prolonged (>0.20 second) because of the delayed retrograde conduction. In the meantime, the more depressed longitudinal fibers, which were previously refractory to the retrograde impulse, recover their conductivity. As a result, the retrograde impulse splits

before reaching the atria. One impulse continues in a retrograde direction to the atria, and another retraces its steps in an antegrade direction toward the AV node. In other words, the antegrade impulses traverse down the now responsive longitudinal fibers that were previously refractory. When the time required (the R-R interval, including the sandwiched P wave) for the retrograde conduction of the AV nodal impulse (R-P interval) and the subsequent antegrade conduction of the re-entry impulse (P-R interval), is sufficient for the ventricles to recover from their initial response to the AV nodal impulse, a second ventricular complex—namely, the *reciprocal beat*—results.

PARASYSTOLE

Parasystole consists of the simultaneous activity of two (rarely more) independent impulse-forming centers, one of which is "protected" from the other, each competing to activate the atria, ventricles, or both. The parasystolic pacemaker may be located anywhere in the heart but is commonly located in the ventricles, less commonly in the AV junction, and rarely in the atria. The incidence of parasystole is 0.13%, in this author's

Figure 13-1

Mechanism of reciprocal beats. The genesis of a reciprocal beat is considered to be due to a specific form of re-entry phenomenon occurring in the atrioventricular junctional tissues. It is assumed that there is a longitudinal dissociation present in the atrioventricular junctional fibers, which have different degrees of depressed conductivity. Thus, some of the longitudinal fibers (closely hatched area) are more depressed than others (widely hatched area). Consequently, unidirectional block of retrograde conduction in the more depressed fibers and a generalized delay in retrograde conduction in the whole of the atrioventricular junctional fibers occur. The impulse originating from the atrioventricular node is conducted in both directions, to the ventricles (V = antegrade) and toward the atria (A = retrograde). The retrograde impulse soon reaches the depressed atrioventricular junction fibers. The retrograde impulse is completely blocked at the more depressed fibers (closely hatched area) and conducted at a slower speed than usual in a retrograde fashion in the remaining less depressed fibers (widely hatched area). In the meantime, the more depressed longitudinal fibers (closely hatched area), which were previously refractory to the retrograde impulse, recover their conductivity. As a result, the retrograde impulse splits before reaching the atria (marked A). One impulse continues in a retrograde direction to the atria, and another retraces its steps in an antegrade direction toward the atrioventricular node. When the time required (the R-R interval, which includes the "sandwiched" P wave) for the retrograde conduction of the atrioventricular nodal impulse (R-P interval) and the subsequent antegrade conduction of the re-entry impulse (P-R interval) are sufficient for the ventricles to recover from their initial response to the atrioventricular nodal impulse, a second ventricular complex, the reciprocal beat, results.

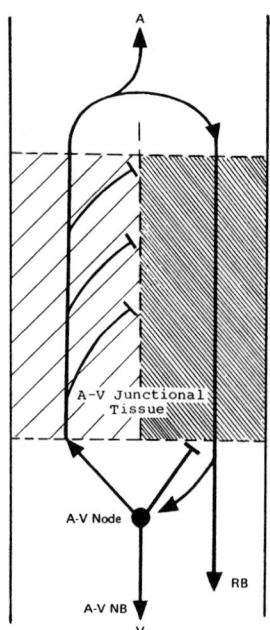

Figure 13-2
Mechanism of parasystole. The theories of protection block and exit block in parasystole are illustrated. The parasystolic pacemaker is assumed to be located in the center of the diagram. Exit block is considered to be present when the parasystolic impulses are blocked by the outer ring. This is a form of unidirectional block. Conversely, the inner ring (protection block) prevents the transmission of the impulses from the outside. Protection block is another form of unidirectional block and is in the reverse direction of exit block. The parasystolic rhythm will be abolished when the exit block occurs. Consecutive parasystolic beats can appear, or the parasystole may even become the dominant rhythm when the protection block ensues.

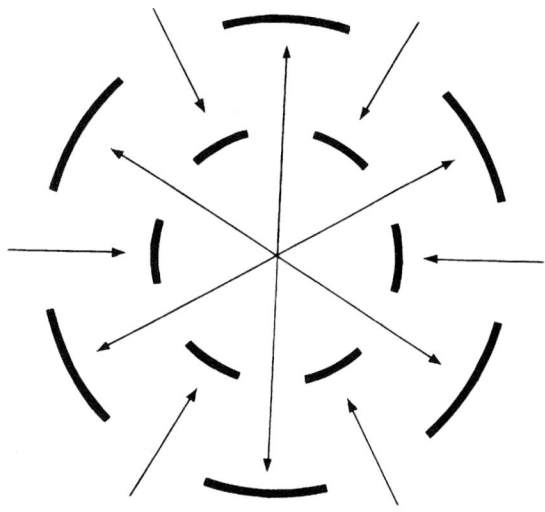

experience. Ventricular parasystole has been encountered much more frequently than supraventricular parasystole.

The mechanism of parasystole is described as follows (Fig. 13-2). Protection block (entrance block) and exit block are forms of unidirectional block in the heart. It is generally agreed that the parasystolic center, regardless of its location, is protected by a unidirectional block from the transmission of impulses originating from any basic rhythm (protection block). If a continuous protection block ensues, the parasystolic pacemaker will act as the dominant pacemaker and produce a continuous parasystolic rhythm or even a parasystolic tachycardia. The exit block, which is in the direction opposite the protection block, prevents the outward transmission of the parasystolic impulses. If there is an occasional exit block, the parasystolic beats appear intermittently, whereas if the exit block is continuous, the parasystolic rhythm will disappear. Exit block must be assumed to occur when the parasystolic rhythm is calculated to be rapid and the ectopic heart action it causes is slow in spite of the nonrefractory phase of the basic rhythm. The ectopic rate of parasystolic tachycardia ranging from 70 to 150 beats per minute [bpm], which is frequently encountered clinically, may be caused by a 2:1 or 3:1 exit block, with the parasystolic rate actually being much faster.

ATRIAL DISSOCIATION

Atrial dissociation, characterized by two sets of independent P waves, has been produced experimentally and also has been found in human hearts.

Various clinical studies unequivocally showed the existence of atrial dissociation, and it became a unique electrocardiographic entity. For instance, transitional electrocardiographic changes from normal sinus rhythm to unilateral atrial fibrillation that were followed by uncomplicated atrial fibrillation were observed in the same patient. Another patient demonstrated transitional changes from sinus rhythm to unilateral atrial flutter, followed by uncomplicated atrial flutter. An extremely rare instance of atrial dissociation was manifested by unilateral atrial tachycardia in the presence of sinus rhythm, and finally the sinus activity ceased in spite of continuous activity of the ectopic atrial rhythm. These clinical observations provided further evidence for the true occurrence of this rare and interesting cardiac arrhythmia in the human heart.

Atrial dissociation is characterized by the presence of a unilateral ectopic atrial rhythm independent of the basic rhythm (sinus or ectopic). None of the impulses of the unilateral atrial rhythm are conducted to the ventricles. The unilateral atrial rhythm is commonly a slow rhythm, but occasionally it may be a tachycardia, flutter, or fibrillation.

The mechanism responsible for the production of atrial dissociation is as follows: It may be assumed that an ectopic atrial focus controls either a part or all of the atria, probably because of intra-atrial block, so that none of the sinus beats interfere with the ectopic atrial rhythm and the ectopic atrial rhythm does not disturb the basis rhythm. None of the ectopic P waves are conducted to the ventricles, indicating that the blocked zone is located in the supranodal area rather than indicating that the ectopic P waves are not strong enough to produce conduction to the ventricles. The phenomenon of atrial dissociation has been attributed to dissociation of a part of the atrial myocardium with ectopic impulse formation and protective entrance and exit block or dynamic bidirectional block. If there were no blocks, the ectopic P wave should conduct to the ventricles whenever the AV junctional tissues are nonrefractory.

Atrial dissociation is almost always observed in patients with far-advanced heart disease.

CORONARY SINUS RHYTHM

When cardiac impulses originate from the atria near the orifice of the coronary sinus vein, the beats produced, called coronary sinus beats, are very similar to so-called upper AV junctional beats. When the six or more consecutive beats appear, the terms *coronary sinus rhythm* and *coronary sinus tachycardia* are used, depending on the heart rate. Coronary sinus beats or rhythm are encountered as natural phenomena and also are produced by artificial pacemakers.

In coronary sinus beats, the atria are activated in a retrograde fashion, since the site of the pacemaker is in the caudal portion of the atria. Consequently, the P waves are inverted in leads II, III, and aVF and upright in lead aVR. Rarely, the P wave may be isoelectric or biphasic in lead aVR. Coronary sinus impulses traverse the entire length of the AV junctional tissue before reaching the ventricles. As a result, the P-R intervals in coronary sinus beats are longer than 0.12 second. Thus, coronary sinus beats show all the features of upper AV junctional beats, except that the P-R interval in coronary sinus beats is longer than 0.12 second. The only differential point between a coronary sinus beat and an upper AV junctional beat is that the P-R interval is longer than 0.12 second in the coronary sinus beats and 0.12 second or shorter in upper AV junctional beats. It should be emphasized, however, that the P-R interval may be longer than 0.12 second in an upper AV junctional beat when there is delayed antegrade AV conduction, leading to findings identical to those of coronary sinus beats. Therefore, the diagnosis of coronary sinus beats cannot be made with certainty.

The P-R interval of the coronary sinus beat may be longer than 0.20 second when significant antegrade conduction delay exists, or it may be shorter than 0.12 second when there is a retrograde conduction defect, leading to findings identical to an upper AV junctional beat. Consequently, differentiation between a coronary sinus beat and an upper AV junctional beat is far from absolute.

Differential diagnosis between a coronary sinus beat and a left atrial beat is difficult because both arrhythmias produce retrograde P waves with a P-R interval of more than 0.12 second. Left atrial beats, however, possess characteristic diagnostic features (e.g., inverted P waves in leads I or V_6 with the "dome and dart" P wave in lead V_1).

CORONARY NODAL RHYTHM

Not uncommonly, the P-P interval may be shorter than 0.12 second, but with the diagnostic features for sinus rhythm present. This type of electrocardiographic finding often occurs during sinus tachycardia, particularly in anxious people, psychiatric patients, and individuals with hyperthyroidism. It may occur even when the rate is slower than 100 bpm. A short P-R interval with a normal QRS complex and a normal P axis has been called coronary nodal rhythm by some investigators.

In coronary nodal rhythm, the P-R interval is between 0.02 and 0.10 second, with upright P waves in leads I and II and a normal QRS complex. It has been suggested that the impulse most likely originates from the region closest to the tail portion of the sinus node; therefore, the mode of impulse propagation is similar to that of ordinary sinus rhythm. Accelerated AV conduction of the sinus impulse via an accessory pathway between the atria and ventricles also is considered to be the mechanism responsible for a short P-R interval and a normal axis of the P wave. Coronary nodal rhythm has been produced experimentally and also found clinically in various conditions. Coronary nodal rhythm has been observed in cases of hyperthyroidism, schizophrenia, welding gas poisoning, atrial infarction, and pulmonary diseases and in hyperexcitable and emotionally disturbed individuals. Recently, two patients were found to have the characteristic electrocardiographic findings of coronary nodal rhythm following open heart surgery.

A short P-R interval with a normal P axis or slight left axis deviation of the P wave is most likely a variant of sinus rhythm rather than coronary nodal rhythm. A relatively short P-R interval might be caused by increased sympathetic tone in some subjects. It should also be noted that some short P-R intervals may not be true P-R intervals (called a P-R distance rather than P-R interval when the P wave and QRS complex are not related) when there is AV dissociation. This occurs when atrial and ventricular complexes are very close to one another but actually independent. In this circumstance, the false appearance of a short P-R interval is observed, particularly when a limited length of electrocardiographic strip is available.

SLOW ATRIAL RHYTHM

Clinically, almost all atrial arrhythmias represent some form of atrial tachyarrhythmias (e.g., atrial tachycardia, fibrillation, flutter). On rare occasions, however, an ectopic atrial mechanism with a slow rhythm, which does not belong to any of the above-mentioned atrial arrhythmias, may be observed clinically and in experimental studies. The slow atrial rhythm may originate from the left or right atrium, but a slow atrial rhythm originating from the right atrium is much less common than from the left. The slow atrial rhythm may represent atrial escape rhythm or slow atrial tachycardia, which may be analogous to nonparoxysmal AV JT.

In left atrial rhythm, the P waves are almost always inverted in leads II and aVF. Lead III also often shows inverted P waves. The P waves are nearly always upright in lead aVR, but rarely they may be biphasic or isoelectric. More reliable findings in left atrial rhythm include inverted P waves in leads I and V_6 and upright P waves (without negative component) in lead V_1 (dome and dart P wave).

A slow right atrial rhythm is much rarer than left atrial rhythm. Right atrial rhythm is impossible to diagnose with certainty unless it occurs alternately or periodically in the presence of sinus rhythm. This is because the axis of the ectopic P wave in right atrial rhythm is very similar to that of sinus rhythm. A P wave with retrograde conduction never occurs in right atrial rhythm.

The clinical significance of slow ectopic atrial rhythm is not understood clearly, but it has been observed in apparently healthy individuals as well as in patients with diseased hearts.

Slow atrial rhythm may be considered to be *atrial escape rhythm*, which is analogous to AV JER. Thus, the atrial escape rhythm is expected to occur when the sinus rhythm slows down and the AV junction fails to produce the escape impulses. In addition, atrial escape rhythm may be observed in various other bradyarrhythmias and after any postectopic pause. However, for an unknown reason, atrial escape rhythm is encountered only on rare occasions in our daily practice.

ABERRANT ATRIAL CONDUCTION (CHUNG'S PHENOMENON)

Occasionally, the P wave of the sinus beat immediately following an APC may have a bizarre configuration that is different from the P wave of an APC or of sinus origin. This is termed *aberrant atrial conduction* and is analogous to aberrant ventricular conduction. Less commonly, aberrant atrial conduction may be observed immediately following AV JPCs or VPCs. Aberrant atrial conduction rarely occurs immediately following atrial, AV junctional, or ventricular parasystolic beats.

Aberrant atrial conduction usually involves the P wave of only one sinus beat immediately following an ectopic beat. On rare occasions, however, aberrant atrial conduction may occur in two or more consecutive sinus beats. When this occurs, aberrant atrial conduction is much more marked in the first sinus P wave than in the second.

The exact mechanism involved in the production of aberrant atrial conduction is not clearly understood, but it most likely occurs because the refractory period of the atria is altered immediately following an ectopic impulse.

Aberrant atrial conduction must be differentiated from a wandering atrial pacemaker, an AV junctional escape beat following a postectopic pause, coexisting multifocal premature contractions, and various artifacts.

The clinical significance of aberrant atrial conduction is again uncertain because of its rare occurrence, but all cases of aberrant atrial conduction observed by this author were found in patients with diseased hearts. Thus, the clinical significance of aberrant atrial conduction may not be the same as in aberrant ventricular conduction.

ELECTRICAL ALTERNANS

Electrical alternans is a relatively rare electrocardiographic phenomenon, the presence of which is considered almost always to be indicative of organic heart disease. Very rarely it has been found in the absence of cardiac disease when the heart rate was rapid.

Electrical alternans is defined as alternating P, QRS, or T complexes or a combination of these occurring with regular rhythm and with constant intervals between the complexes. The complexes in electrical alternans should originate from one pacemaker and should not have any relationship to respiration or any other periodic extracardiac phenomena. On rare occasions, electrical alternans may be observed in atrial fibrillation; in this case, the R-R intervals naturally vary.

The most common form of electrical alternans involves QRS complexes alone and is termed *ventricular electrical alternans*. The occurrence of total (atrial and ventricular) electrical alternans is much less frequent. Extremely rarely, electrical alternans may involve only the S-T segment or T waves and even U waves. Isolated atrial electrical alternans is equally rare.

A 2:1 electrical alternans is a common alternating ratio; a 3:1 alternating ratio is a rare occurrence. Alternating ratios of 4:1, 4:2, 5:3, 5:2, 5:1, and so on may be observed extremely rarely.

When electrical alternans is associated with a relatively slow heart rate, most patients suffer from advanced congestive heart failure, pericardial effusion, or both. The exact mechanism of electrical alternans is not clearly understood, however.

VENTRICULAR DISSOCIATION

The term *ventricular dissociation* is used when the ventricles are independently activated by two or more foci in the ventricles. Thus, a portion of the ventricles may independently show ventricular tachycardia or ventricular fibrillation in the presence of a slow ventricular escape rhythm. Another example of ventricular dissociation may be double or triple ventricular escape rhythms that occur independently. As expected, ventricular dissociation always occurs in terminally ill patients with advanced heart disease. Ventricular dissociation represents various forms of chaotic ventricular rhythm (see Fig. 10-10) and is analogous to atrial dissociation (discussed previously).

DOUBLE OR TRIPLE ATRIOVENTRICULAR JUNCTIONAL RHYTHMS OR TACHYCARDIAS

In a rare form of AV dissociation, the atria and ventricles are controlled by two different pacemakers in the AV junctional tissue. In this instance, the atria are activated in retrograde fashion. Occasionally, the atria may be intermittently activated by the sinus node in the presence of double AV JTs or JERs, resulting in triple rhythms. In this case, atrial fusion beats may be observed, placed between antegrade sinus and retrograde AV junctional impulses. Each pacemaker at the AV junction may produce an AV JT or JER.

Clinically, double or triple AV JTs or JERs are almost always observed in patients with far-advanced heart disease or severe digitalis intoxication.

FASCICULAR BEATS, RHYTHM, AND TACHYCARDIA

On rare occasions, ectopic impulses arise from one of the fascicles of the left bundle branch system. Thus, the ectopic impulses originating from one of the fascicles may produce isolated premature beats, slow escape rhythm, or tachycardia. The fascicular beats typically exhibit an incomplete right bundle branch block pattern with marked left or right axis deviation. Detailed diagnostic criteria of anterior and posterior fascicular beats and tachycardia are discussed later in this chapter.

In a broad sense, fascicular beats, rhythms, and tachycardia belong to ventricular arrhythmias. Clinically, the fascicular beats, rhythm, and tachycardia seem to be relatively benign arrhythmias. It has been shown that a fascicular tachycardia is observed not uncommonly during the first 24–72 hours of acute MI, but the arrhythmia is usually transient and self-limited.

RECIPROCAL BEATS AND RHYTHM

Definition

Reciprocal beats and rhythm result from the premature activation of the atria in a retrograde fashion after an AV junctional beat or Wenckebach AV or VA block (at times, after a marked first-degree AV block) due to a re-entry mechanism in the AV junction. The atrial echo beat (retrograde P wave) may be followed by a QRS complex, leading to a reciprocal beat.

Diagnostic Criteria (Fig. 13-3)

- Premature P wave that is conducted in a retrograde fashion (inverted P wave in leads II, III, and aVF, and upright P wave in lead aVR) after an AV junctional beat or Wenckebach VA or AV block (at times, after a marked first-degree AV block).
- The premature retrograde P wave may or may *not* be followed by a QRS complex.
- The R-P interval is usually longer than 0.20 second.
- The R-R interval, including a sandwiched retrograde P wave, is usually 0.50 second or less unless there is marked AV or VA conduction delay.
- The QRS complex following a retrograde premature P wave may show a bizarre configuration because of AVCs.
- The underlying rhythm is almost always sinus, but it may be atrial fibrillation.

Diagnostic Pearls

To accurately diagnose a reciprocal beat, a premature retrograde P wave that occurs after an AV junctional beat (either AV junctional premature beat, AV JT, or AV JER) or Wenckebach AV or VA block (rarely, after a marked first-degree AV block) must be identified. A reciprocal beat is usually *not* initiated by a sinus beat. A single reciprocal beat may lead to consecutive grouped reciprocal beats and even reciprocal (reciprocating) tachycardia.

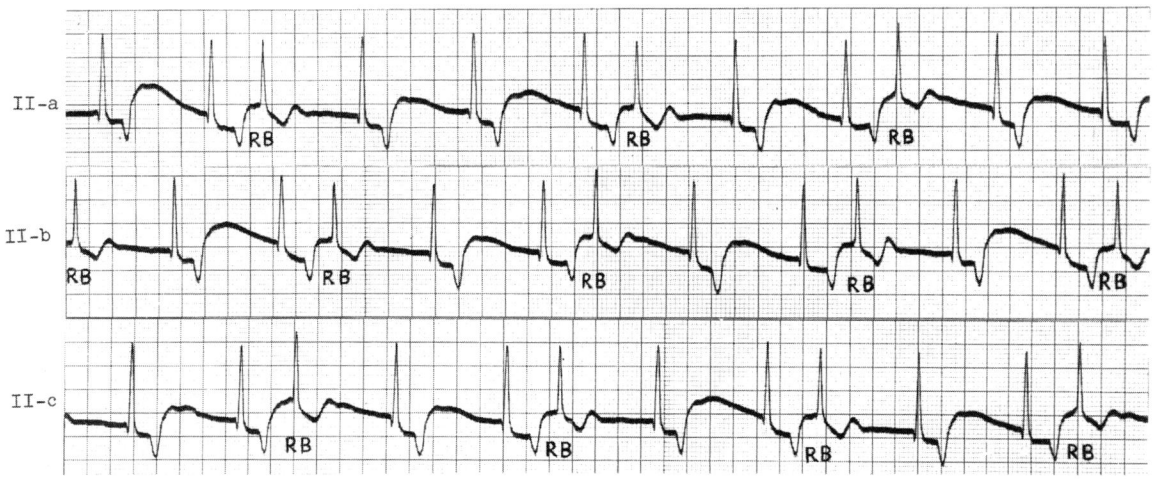

Figure 13-3
Atrioventricular junctional escape rhythm with retrograde Wenckebach ventriculoatrial block and frequent reciprocal beats occurring every third beat (marked RB). Leads II a–c are continuous.

VENTRICULAR PARASYSTOLE

Definition

A ventricular parasystole is a cardiac rhythm originating from any location in the ventricles independent of any underlying cardiac rhythm.

Diagnostic Criteria (Fig. 13-4)

- Ventricular rhythm independent of the basic rhythm.
- Varying coupling intervals.
- Constant shortest interectopic intervals.
- Long interectopic interval showing multiples of the shortest interectopic intervals.
- Frequent appearance of fusion beats.
- The usual rate ranges from 30 to 50 bpm.
- At times, the rate may be faster than the usual rate, resulting in parasystolic ventricular tachycardia.

Diagnostic Pearls

It is important to remember that the coupling intervals are constant in ordinary VPCs (see Fig. 10-1). In contrast, ventricular parasystole reveals varying coupling intervals. It can be said that parasystole is a unique cardiac arrhythmia that is benign in nature.

Figure 13-4
Sinus rhythm with ventricular parasystole. Note that the coupling intervals vary and the interectopic intervals remain constant. The Holter monitor electrocardiographic rhythm strips A–D are not continuous. The numbers represent hundredths of a second.

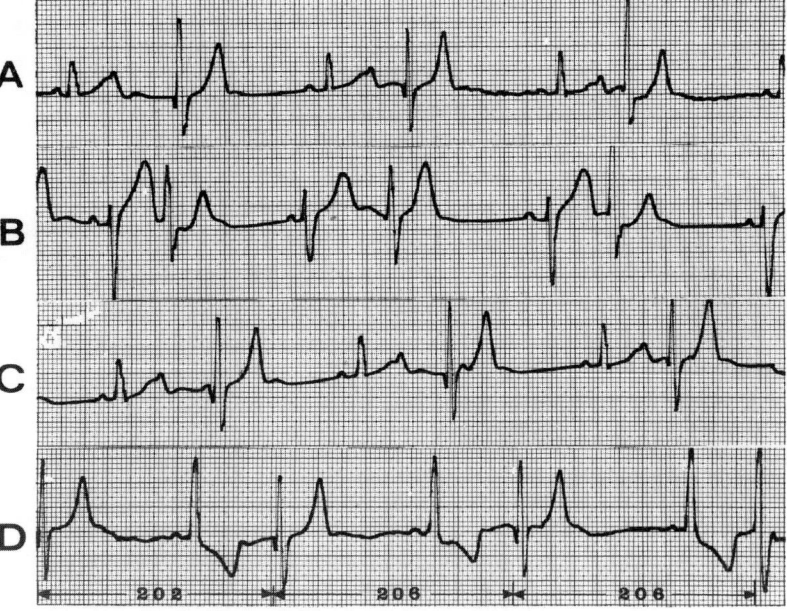

ATRIAL PARASYSTOLE

Definition

Atrial parasystole is a cardiac rhythm originating from any location in the atria independent of the basic sinus rhythm.

Diagnostic Criteria (Fig. 13-5)

- Atrial rhythm independent of the basic sinus rhythm.
- Varying coupling intervals.
- Constant shortest interectopic intervals.
- Long interectopic interval showing multiples of the shortest interectopic intervals.
- The usual rate ranges from 30 to 50 bpm.
- At times, the rate may be faster than the usual rate, resulting in parasystolic atrial tachycardia.

Diagnostic Pearls

It is important to emphasize that the coupling intervals are constant in ordinary APCs (see Fig. 8-1), whereas atrial parasystole reveals varying coupling intervals.

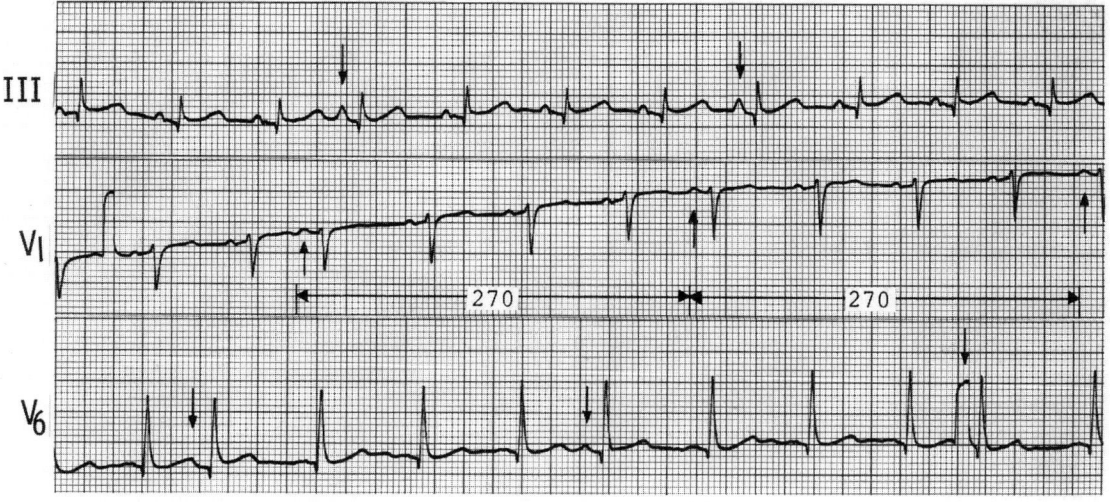

Figure 13-5
Sinus rhythm with atrial parasystole (indicated by arrows). The numbers represent hundredths of a second.

ATRIOVENTRICULAR JUNCTIONAL PARASYSTOLE

Definition

AV junctional parasystole is a cardiac rhythm originating from any location in the AV junction independent of the basic rhythm.

Diagnostic Criteria (Fig. 13-6)

- AV junctional rhythm independent of the basic rhythm.
- Varying coupling intervals.
- Constant shortest interectopic intervals.
- Long interectopic intervals showing multiples of the shortest interectopic intervals.
- The usual rate ranges from 30 to 50 bpm.
- At times, the rate may be faster than the usual rate, resulting in parasystolic AV JT.
- Retrograde P waves may be followed by or preceded by QRS complexes (at times, the retrograde P waves may be superimposed on the QRS complexes, leading to absent P waves).

Diagnostic Pearls

It is important to remember that the coupling intervals are constant in ordinary AV JPCs (see Fig. 9-1), whereas AV junctional parasystole shows varying coupling intervals.

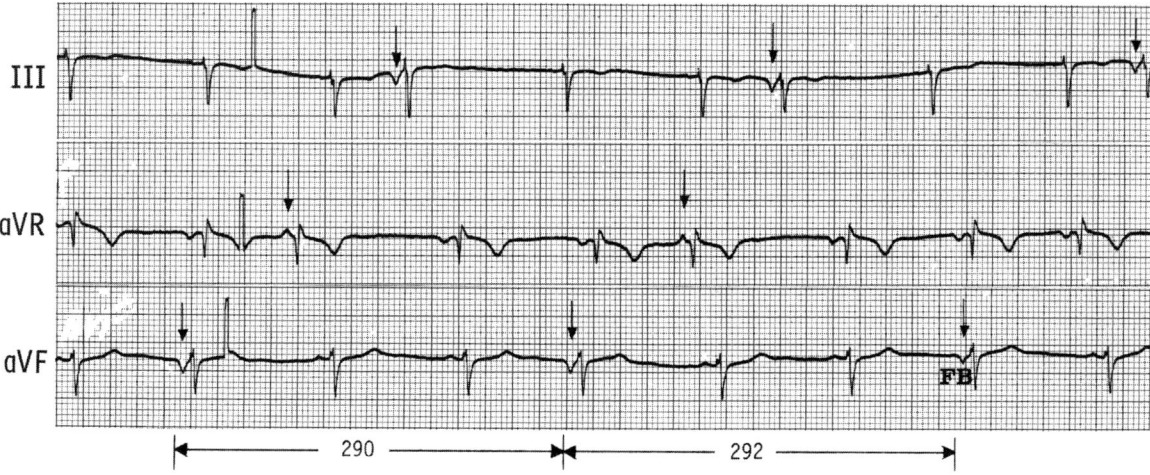

Figure 13-6
Sinus rhythm with atrioventricular junctional parasystole (indicated by arrows). The numbers represent hundredths of a second.

ATRIAL DISSOCIATION

Definition

Atrial dissociation is an independent unilateral atrial rhythm localized in a portion of the atria in which the ectopic atrial impulses are never conducted to the ventricles because of the intra-atrial block.

Diagnostic Criteria (Fig. 13-7)

The following are types of atrial dissociation:

- Unilateral slow atrial rhythm (most common)
- Unilateral atrial tachycardia
- Unilateral atrial fibrillation
- Unilateral atrial flutter

Diagnostic Pearls

Superficially, atrial dissociation resembles atrial parasystole. However, all ectopic P waves are usually conducted to the ventricles in atrial parasystole (see Fig. 13-5), whereas no ectopic P wave is followed by a QRS complex in atrial dissociation (unilateral atrial ectopic rhythm). Clinically, atrial dissociation is usually encountered in critically ill patients, whereas atrial parasystole is a benign cardiac arrhythmia.

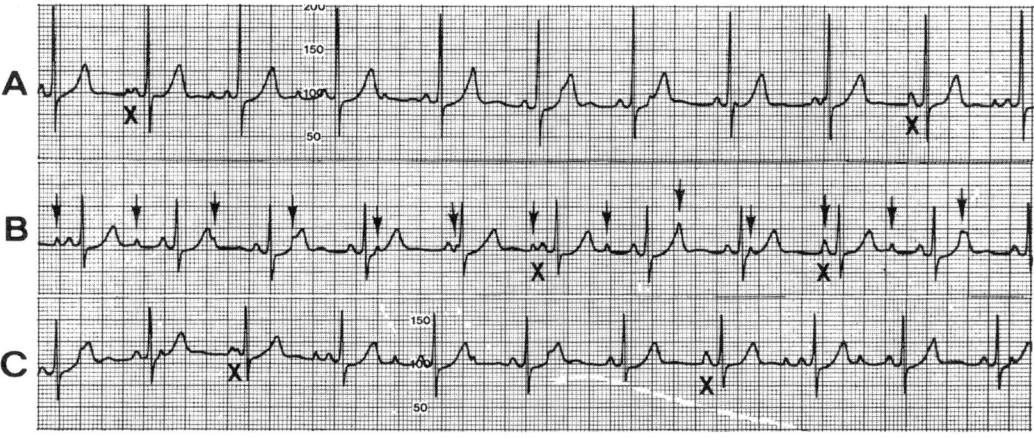

Figure 13-7
Unilateral slow atrial rhythm (indicated by arrows) in the presence of sinus rhythm producing atrial dissociation. Many ectopic P waves are superimposed on the sinus P waves (marked X). Note that none of the ectopic P waves (unilateral atrial rhythm) are conducted to the ventricles. The rhythm strips A–C are not continuous.

CORONARY SINUS RHYTHM

Definition

Coronary sinus rhythm is a regular cardiac rhythm originating from any portion of the coronary sinus region.

Diagnostic Criteria (Fig. 13-8)

- Inverted P waves in leads II, III, and aVF and upright in leads I and aVR (occasionally, P waves may be isoelectric or biphasic in lead I or aVR).
- P-R interval of 0.12–0.20 second.
- Constant P-R interval.
- Normal QRS complex (occasionally the QRS complex may be wide and bizarre, caused by either aberrant ventricular conduction or bundle branch block).

Diagnostic Pearls

Coronary sinus rhythm closely resembles AV JT or AV JER (see Figs. 9-4 and 9-6) because the P waves are conducted in a retrograde fashion in all of the above-mentioned arrhythmias. The P-R interval, however, is usually longer than 0.12 second in coronary sinus rhythm. In addition, coronary sinus rhythm mimics left atrial rhythm (discussed in the section on left atrial rhythm), but the characteristic features of left atrial rhythm distinguish it from coronary sinus rhythm. Remember that the P wave in left atrial rhythm shows only an upright (positive) component in lead V_1, whereas coronary sinus rhythm reveals a biphasic P wave in lead V_1.

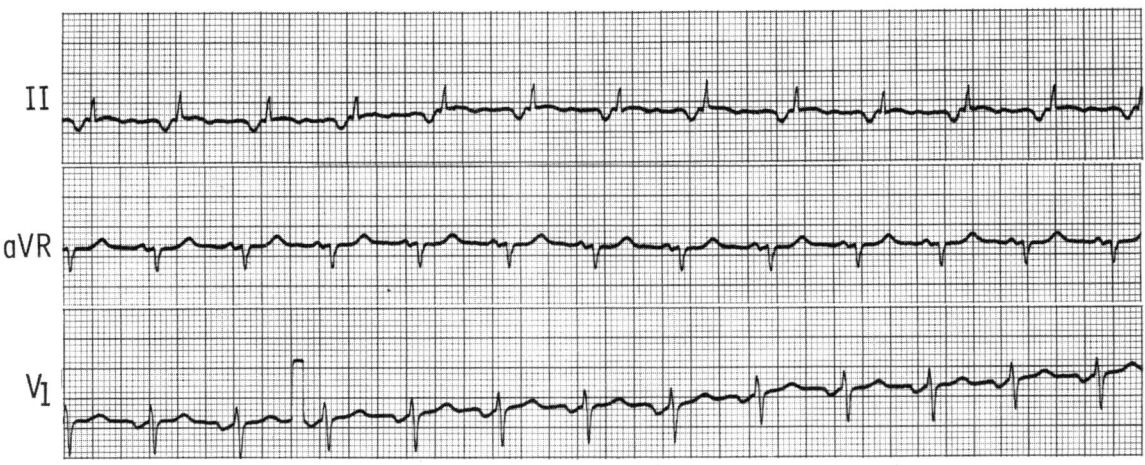

Figure 13-8
Coronary sinus rhythm with a rate of 98 bpm.

LEFT ATRIAL RHYTHM

Definition

Left atrial rhythm is a regular cardiac rhythm originating from any portion of the left atrium.

Diagnostic Criteria (Fig. 13-9)

- Inverted P waves in leads II and aVF (lead III also often shows inverted P waves) and upright P wave in lead aVR (rarely biphasic or isoelectric P wave).
- Inverted P wave in lead I (at times, biphasic or isoelectric P wave).
- Lead V_1 shows only a positive component of the P wave (a dome and dart P wave—pathognomonic feature).
- Inverted P waves in leads V_{4-6}.
- P-R interval of 0.12–0.20 second.

Diagnostic Pearls

Left atrial rhythm may closely mimic coronary sinus rhythm (see Fig. 13-8) and AV JER or JT (see Figs. 9-4 and 9-6). An upright P wave in lead V_1 (dome and dart P wave) with inverted P waves in leads I and V_{4-6}, however, are pathognomonic features of left atrial rhythm.

Figure 13-9
Left atrial rhythm with a rate of 76 bpm. Note that the P waves are inverted in leads I, II, III, aVF and V$_{4-6}$, whereas lead V$_1$ shows the P wave with only an upright (positive) component.

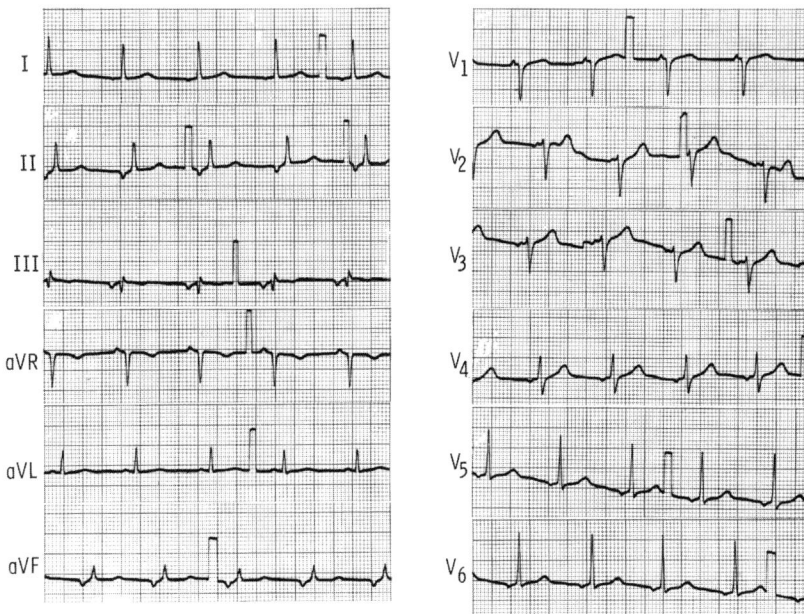

ABERRANT ATRIAL CONDUCTION (CHUNG'S PHENOMENON)

Definition

Aberrant atrial conduction (Chung's phenomenon) is an alteration of the P wave configuration of the sinus beat immediately following any ectopic beat (commonly following APCs).

Diagnostic Criteria (Fig. 13-10)

- Alteration of the P wave configuration of the sinus beat immediately following an APC (most common)
- Alteration of the P wave configuration of the sinus beat immediately following an AV JPC
- Alteration of the P wave configuration of the sinus beat immediately following a VPC
- Alteration of the P wave configuration of the sinus beat immediately following a parasystolic beat (rare)

Diagnostic Pearls

Aberrant atrial conduction (Chung's phenomenon) closely mimics an atrial or AV JEB. A full understanding of each arrhythmia is important to distinguish them. Remember that Chung's phenomenon occurs only following any ectopic beat (most commonly APC) and that two or more sinus beats may be involved. Chung's phenomenon is frequently observed following a blocked APC.

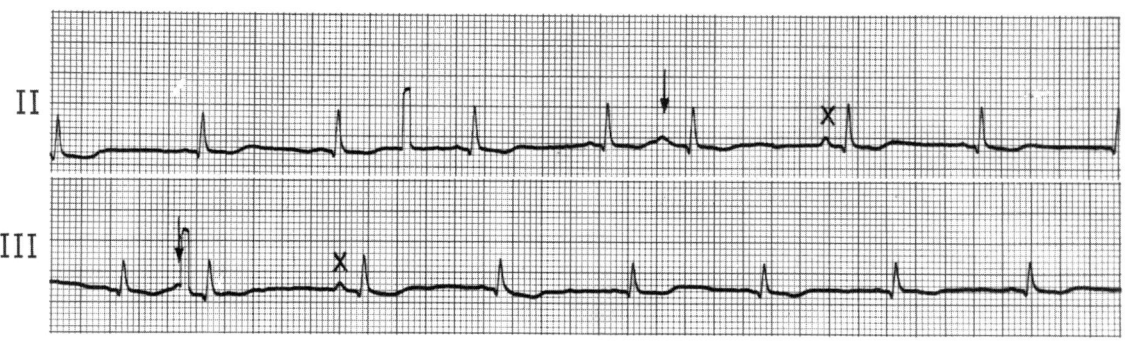

Figure 13-10
Sinus rhythm with atrial premature contractions (indicated by arrows) followed by aberrant atrial conduction (Chung's phenomenon, marked X).

VENTRICULAR ELECTRICAL ALTERNANS

Definition

Ventricular electrical alternans is an alteration of the QRS configuration on every other beat, every third beat, or every fourth beat, provided that the cardiac impulses originate from the same focus (most often from the sinus node).

Diagnostic Criteria (Fig. 13-11)

- Alteration of the QRS configuration on every other beat (most common ratio)
- Alteration of the QRS configuration on every third beat
- Alteration of the QRS configuration on every fourth beat

Diagnostic Pearls

It is essential that the electrocardiographic tracing shows that all QRS complexes originate from the same focus (most commonly the sinus node) in order to correctly diagnose ventricular electrical alternans. Superficially, ventricular bigeminy or trigeminy simulates ventricular electrical alternans. Similarly, intermittent left bundle branch block (LBBB) or right bundle branch block (RBBB) closely mimics ventricular electrical alternans. A full understanding of each electrocardiographic abnormality is essential to distinguish them (see Figs. 4-6 and 10-1).

Figure 13-11
*Sinus tachycardia with
2:1 ventricular electrical
alternans. Note that the
configuration of the
QRS complexes alter-
nate on every other beat.*

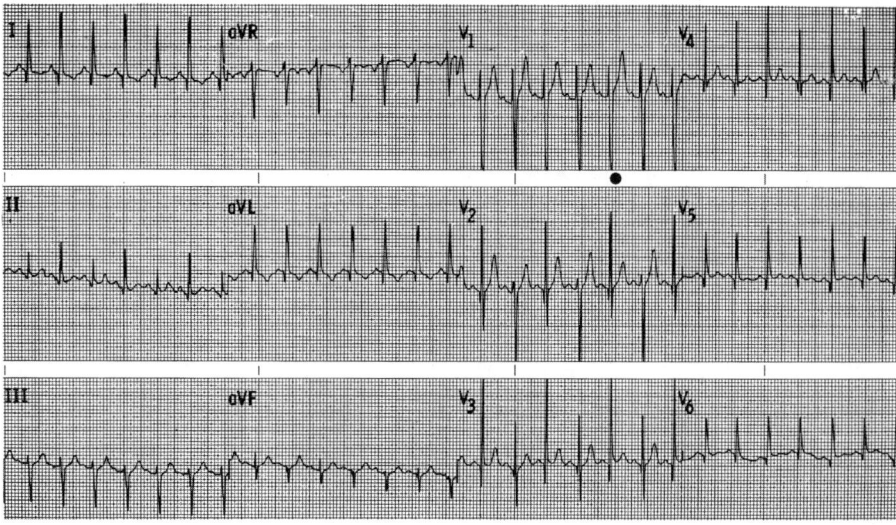

ATRIAL ELECTRICAL ALTERNANS

Definition

Atrial electrical alternans is an alteration of the P wave configuration on every other beat, every third beat, or every fourth beat, providing that all cardiac impulses are sinus in origin.

Diagnostic Criteria (Fig. 13-12)

- Alteration of the P wave configuration on every other beat (most common ratio)
- Alteration of the P wave configuration on every third beat
- Alteration of the P wave configuration on every fourth beat

Diagnostic Pearls

In atrial electrical alternans, every P wave must originate from the sinus node. Frequent APCs causing atrial bigeminy or trigeminy superficially resemble atrial electrical alternans. Remember that APCs mean prematurely occurring ectopic atrial beats (see Fig. 8-1 and 8-2), whereas atrial electrical alternans originate from the sinus node.

Figure 13-12
Sinus rhythm with 2:1 atrial electrical alternans. Note that the P wave configuration alternates on every other beat.

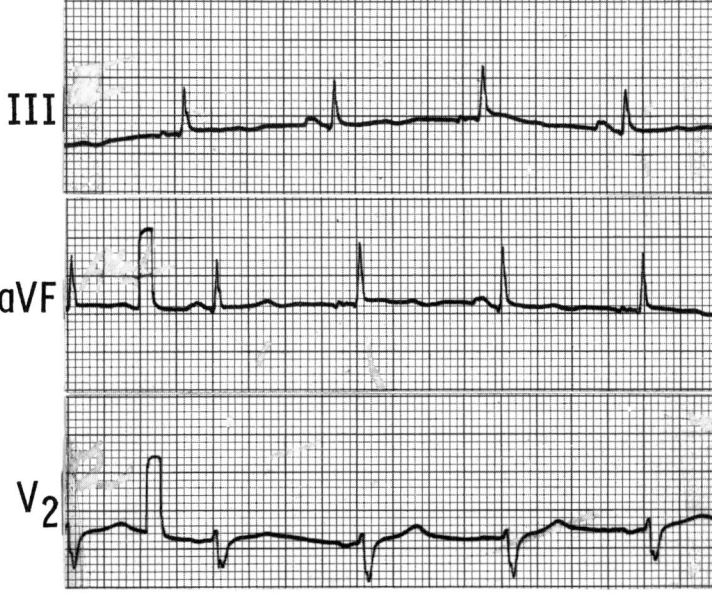

REPOLARIZATION ELECTRICAL ALTERNANS

Definition

Repolarization electrical alternans is an alteration of the S-T segment, T wave, or U wave (singly or with combination) on every other beat, every third beat, or every fourth beat, provided that all cardiac impulses originate from the same focus (most commonly the sinus node).

Diagnostic Criteria (Fig. 13-13)

- Alteration of the S-T segment on every other beat, every third beat, or every fourth beat
- Alteration of the T wave configuration on every other beat, every third beat, or every fourth beat
- Alteration of the U wave configuration on every other beat, every third beat, or every fourth beat
- Any combination of the above criteria

Diagnostic Pearls

In the diagnosis of the repolarization electrical alternans, one must be certain that every heartbeat originates from the same focus (commonly the sinus node). Various artifacts may resemble repolarization electrical alternans, but the differential diagnosis is usually made by careful inspection of a given electrocardiographic tracing.

Figure 13-13
Sinus arrhythmia (indicated by arrows) with 2:1 electrical alternans involving the S-T segment and T waves (repolarization electrical alternans). Advanced hyperkalemia is manifested by flat P waves with diffuse (nonspecific) intraventricular block due to severe renal failure.

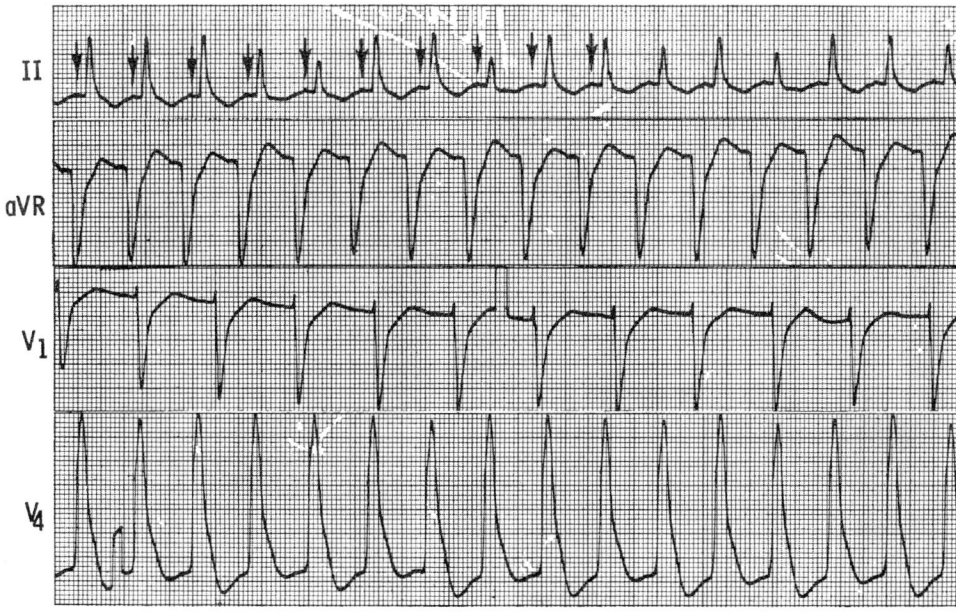

VENTRICULAR DISSOCIATION

Definition

Ventricular dissociation is the simultaneous occurrence of two or more independent ventricular rhythms or tachycardias that cause various forms of chaotic ventricular rhythms.

Diagnostic Criteria (Fig. 13-14)

- Ventricular tachycardia, fibrillation, or flutter in one portion of the ventricles and ventricular escape rhythm (idioventricular rhythm) in another portion of the ventricles, together causing two or more independent ventricular rhythms
- Two or more independent ventricular escape rhythms originating from different foci occurring simultaneously.

Diagnostic Pearls

Ventricular dissociation represents various forms of chaotic ventricular rhythm (see Chapter 10), which is usually observed in dying patients. Thus, it is rather difficult to make a precise diagnosis of ventricular dissociation in a practical sense, and often the broad term *chaotic ventricular rhythm* is used in this circumstance.

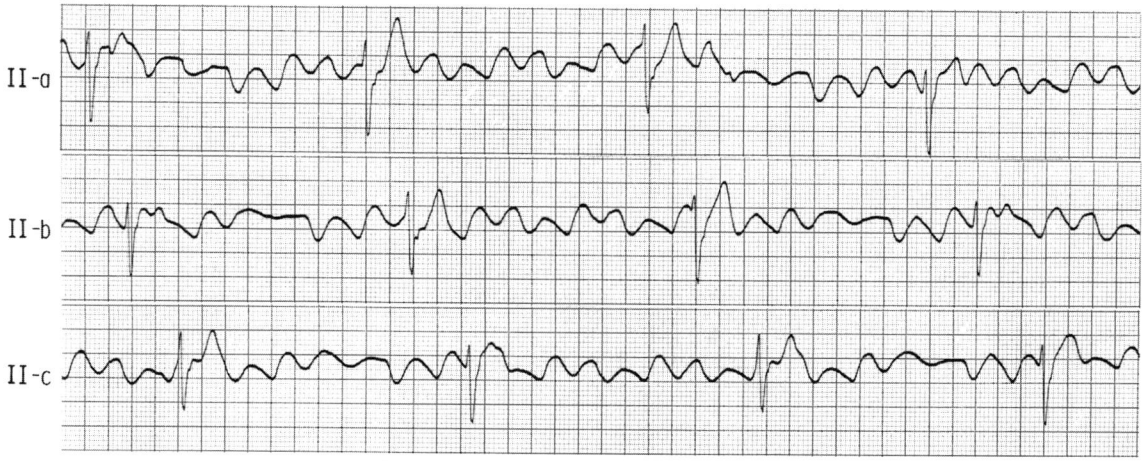

Figure 13-14

Ventricular flutter-fibrillation with independent ventricular escape rhythm (rate of 24 bpm) producing ventricular dissociation. Leads II a–c are continuous.

DOUBLE ATRIOVENTRICULAR JUNCTIONAL TACHYCARDIAS OR RHYTHMS

Definition

Double AV JTs or rhythms are two independent AV JTs or AV JERs that produce complete or incomplete AV dissociation.

Diagnostic Criteria (Fig. 13-15)

- One AV junctional pacemaker activates the atria in a retrograde fashion, causing AV JT, whereas another AV junctional pacemaker activates the ventricles, causing AV JER independently.
- One AV junctional pacemaker activates the atria in a retrograde fashion, causing AV JER, whereas another AV junctional pacemaker activates the ventricles, causing AV JT independently.
- Two independent AV JTs (one pacemaker activates the atria, while another pacemaker activates the ventricles independently).

- Two independent AV JERs (one pacemaker activates the atria, while another pacemaker activates the ventricles independently).

Diagnostic Pearls

Correct diagnosis of double AV JTs or AV JERs is rather difficult for inexperienced readers. Recognizing the retrograde P waves independent of the QRS complexes is a clue to diagnosing these complex arrhythmias.

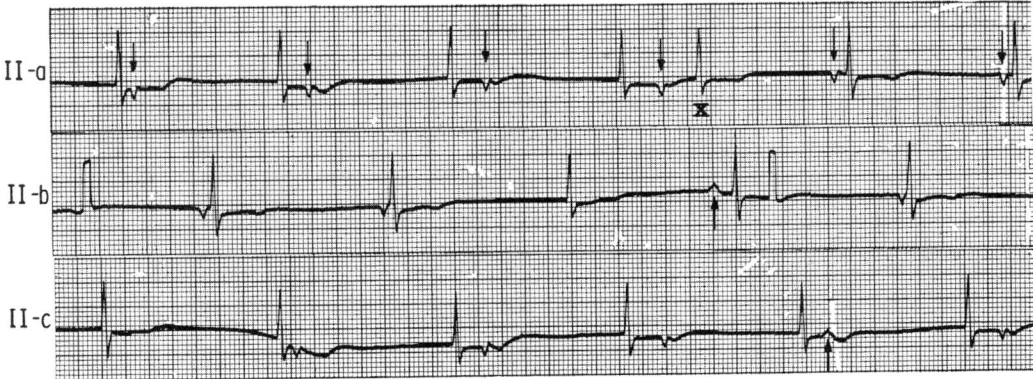

Figure 13-15
Double atrioventricular junctional escape rhythms with occasional sinus P waves (indicated by upward arrows) and a ventricular captured beat (marked X) producing incomplete atrioventricular dissociation. Downward arrows indicate retrograde P waves (one set of the atrioventricular junctional escape rhythm). Leads II a–c are continuous.

FASCICULAR TACHYCARDIA OR RHYTHM

Definition

Fascicular tachycardia or rhythm is tachycardia or rhythm that originates from one of the fascicles of the left bundle branch system.

Diagnostic Criteria (Fig. 13-16)

- The QRS complexes of tachycardia or rhythm showing an incomplete RBBB block pattern.
- Marked left axis deviation (–45 degrees or more) of the QRS complexes when the cardiac impulses originate from the left posterior fascicle.
- Marked right axis deviation (+105 degrees or more) of the QRS complexes when the cardiac impulses originate from the left anterior fascicle.
- The usual ventricular rate is 70–130 bpm.

Diagnostic Pearls

Fascicular tachycardia and rhythm are rare cardiac arrhythmias, and many readers are not familiar with them. Fascicular tachycardia or rhythm should be considered when dealing with a relatively slow tachycardia with an incomplete RBBB pattern with a marked left or right axis deviation, providing that bizarre QRS complexes are not preceded by premature P waves.

Figure 13-16
Sinus rhythm with intermittent fascicular tachycardia (marked X, rate of 93 bpm) producing incomplete atrioventricular dissociation. There is a ventricular fusion beat (marked FB). Note marked S-T segment elevation in leads V_1 and V_5 due to acute extensive anterior myocardial infarction (12-lead electrocardiogram shows S-T segment elevation in all precordial leads—not shown here).

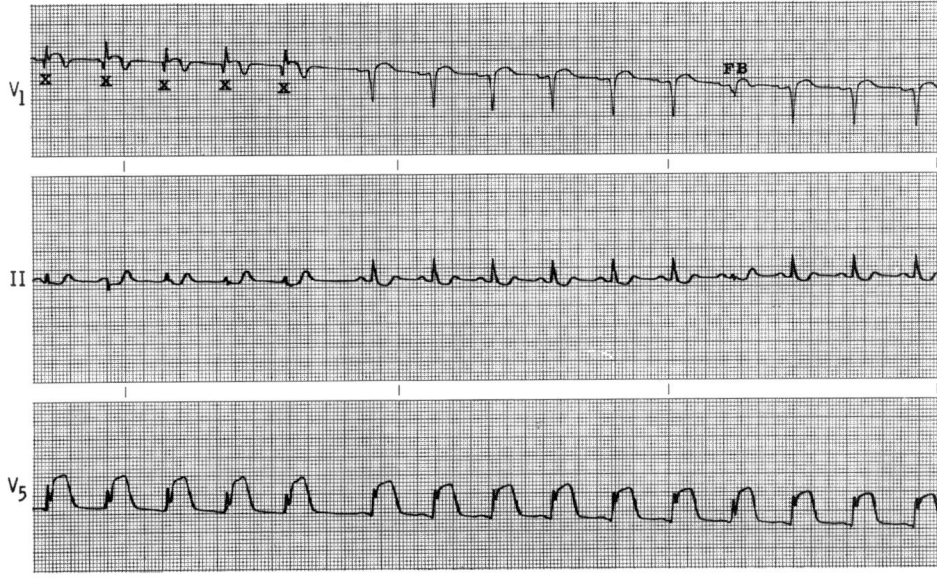

14

Artificial Pacemaker Rhythms

Various electrocardiographic findings are produced depending on the site and mode of artificial cardiac pacing. The ventricles may be paced in a fixed-rate mode or a demand mode. The atria or coronary sinus may be paced, and the atria and ventricles may be paced sequentially. Atrial-synchronized pacing uses the patient's own sinus P waves so that the artificial pacemaker functions as an electronic bundle of His. Although serious complications and malfunctions of artificial pacing are much less common when dealing with newer artificial pacemakers, a variety of problems (some major and some minor) related to artificial pacing may be observed from time to time in all types and models of artificial pacemakers. Serious complications and malfunctions are more commonly observed when fixed-rate ventricular pacing is used. In particular, ventricular fibrillation (VF), which is, of course, a life-threatening complication, is often provoked by the R-on-T phenomenon during fixed-rate ventricular pacing but is *not* due to any malfunction. "Runaway pacemaker," on the other hand, is nearly always a manifestation of malfunctioning fixed-rate ventricular pacing (discussed below).

In recent years, various malfunctions of artificial pacemakers have become very uncommon because of improved technology and more careful medical follow-up after pacemaker implantation. The life span of the newer pacemakers using a lithium battery is reported to be 10–12 years.

COMPLICATIONS AND MALFUNCTIONS OF ARTIFICIAL CARDIAC PACING

Pacemaker malfunction may be manifested by alterations of the preset pacing rate (acceleration or slowing), irregular pacing, failure of sensing, failure of cardiac capture, and any combination of the above (Table 14-1).

In addition, various complications other than malfunctions may be observed associated with artificial pacing (see Table 14-1).

VENTRICULAR FIBRILLATION

VF may occur in every patient during insertion or implantation of an artificial pacemaker, especially when the threshold of the VF is expected to be low, as in acute myocardial infarction (MI). It is also known that VF is frequently produced when the pacemaker artifact is superimposed during the vulnerable period of the ventricles as a result of the R-on-T phenomenon.

VF may also be produced as a result of far-advanced runaway pacemaker. It should also be noted that VF may occur entirely unrelated to the artificial pacemaker. In addition, VF may be associated with infectious complications after pacing.

PACEMAKER HYSTERESIS

Pacemaker hysteresis is a term that describes the difference between the rate at which a pacemaker initiates the pacing and the rate at which it discharges on a consecutive basis. The automatic interval is the time between two successive pacing spikes. A pacemaker escape interval is the length of the period from an intrinsic beat in the patient (sinus or ectopic) to the initial pacing impulse. In other words, the first pacemaker interval following the natural beat (either sinus or ectopic) is longer than the consecutively occurring ventricular cycle induced by the artificial pacemaker in pacemaker hysteresis. An example of 10-beat hysteresis is when a pacemaker does not "fire" until the patient's rate

Table 14-1. Complications and malfunctions of artificial cardiac pacing

Malfunctioning pacemakers	Miscellaneous
Acceleration of pacing ("runaway" pacemaker)	Electrode fracture
Slowing of pacing	Knotting of wire
Irregular pacing	Inhibition of pacemaker by noncardiac muscle potentials
Failure of sensing	Hypotension and cardiac failure
Failure of capture	Necrosis of bowels
Any combination of the above	Displacement of pulse generator
Ventricular fibrillation	Electromagnetic interferences
Perforation of the heart	Electrocardiographic interferences
Malposition of pacemaker electrode	Social and psychological problems
Infections	
Thromboembolic phenomena	
Pacemaker sounds	

drops to 60 beats per minute (bpm) or lower, at which time it starts pacing automatically at 70 bpm.

The only apparent advantage to pacemaker hysteresis appears to be its ability to preserve sinus rhythm. This is accomplished because the patient's own intrinsic rhythm can fall to lower levels (due to the longer escape intervals) before asynchronous pacing is initiated by the pacemaker. Thus, during rest or sleep when the intrinsic rate tends to be slow, a pacemaker with hysteresis would not fire asynchronously until the rate is slower than 60 bpm. This factor is important only when the patient is in normal sinus rhythm, which can occur intermittently in patients with atrioventricular (AV) block or with other forms of bradyarrhythmias.

There are several disadvantages to pacemaker hysteresis that should be emphasized. Many physicians may misinterpret the pacemaker hysteresis as a malfunction of the pacemaker because of the difference between the consecutive pacing intervals and the pacemaker escape interval.

Another disadvantage is related to the longer escape interval. After a sensed premature contraction, a longer-than-usual postectopic pause is produced that often leads to a long ineffective ventricular cycle. This is especially true after a ventricular premature contraction (VPC).

The effects of hysteresis on the pacemaker's battery life is still not clear. Although hysteresis does not appear to increase battery drain, the question of whether it increases battery life is unanswered.

FIXED-RATE VENTRICULAR PACEMAKER RHYTHM

Definition

Fixed-rate ventricular pacemaker rhythm is a regular ventricular rhythm initiated by an artificial pacemaker electrode placed in the right ventricular apex. Fixed-rate ventricular pacemaker rhythm is independent to and competes with the basic rhythm (the fixed-rate ventricular pacemaker rhythm does not sense the intrinsic heart rhythm).

Diagnostic Criteria (Fig. 14-1)

- Regular ventricular rhythm initiated by an artificial pacemaker that competes with the underlying cardiac rhythm (sinus or ectopic).
- The QRS complexes are broad, and they are negative in leads V_{1-2} and upright (positive) in leads I, aVL, and V_{4-6} (left bundle branch block [LBBB] pattern).
- The usual ventricular pacing rhythm rate is 60–70 bpm.
- VF may be provoked as a result of the R-on-T phenomenon because the fixed-rate ventricular rhythm competes with the underlying cardiac rhythm.

Diagnostic Pearls

Since the QRS configuration of the artificial pacemaker-induced ventricular rhythm closely simulates LBBB, some inexperienced readers may misdiagnose it as true LBBB. Remember that every QRS complex caused by an artificial pacemaker exhibits an artificial pacemaker spike. At present, the fixed-rate ventricular pacemaker is no longer used in most countries because of a danger of provoking VF.

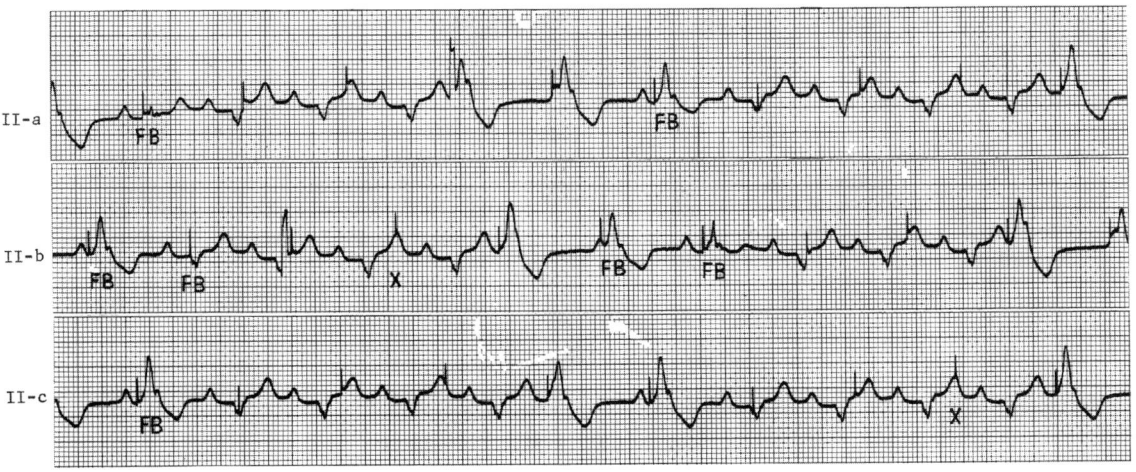

Figure 14-1
Sinus rhythm with first-degree atrioventricular block and intermittent fixed-rate ventricular pacemaker rhythm. Note frequent ventricular fusion beats (marked FB). Some pacemaker spikes are superimposed on the T waves (the R-on-T phenomenon). Leads II a–c are continuous.

DEMAND VENTRICULAR PACEMAKER RHYTHM

Definition

Demand ventricular pacemaker rhythm is a regular ventricular rhythm initiated by an artificial pacemaker electrode placed in the right ventricular apex. The pacemaker functions by sensing the intrinsic heartbeats (there is no competition between the intrinsic heart rhythm and the pacemaker rhythm).

Diagnostic Criteria (Fig. 14-2)

- A regular ventricular rhythm is initiated by an artificial pacemaker that senses the intrinsic heartbeats (sinus or ectopic).
- The QRS complexes are broad, and they are negative in leads V_{1-2} and upright (positive) in leads I, aVL, and V_{4-6} (LBBB pattern).
- The usual pacing rate is 60–70 bpm.

Diagnostic Pearls

Because the QRS configuration of the artificial pacemaker-induced ventricular rhythm closely resembles LBBB, inexperienced readers may misdiagnose it as true LBBB. Remember that all QRS complexes of the pacemaker rhythm are initiated by an artificial pacemaker spike. Demand ventricular pacemaker rhythm never competes with the intrinsic cardiac rhythm as long as the pacemaker functions normally.

Figure 14-2
*Sinus rhythm with intermittent
demand ventricular pacemaker
rhythm. Note frequent ventricular
fusion beats (marked FB). The
demand pacemaker was implanted
in this patient in the treatment of
sick sinus syndrome, manifested by
intermittent sinus arrest. The Holter
monitor rhythm strips A to D are
not continuous.*

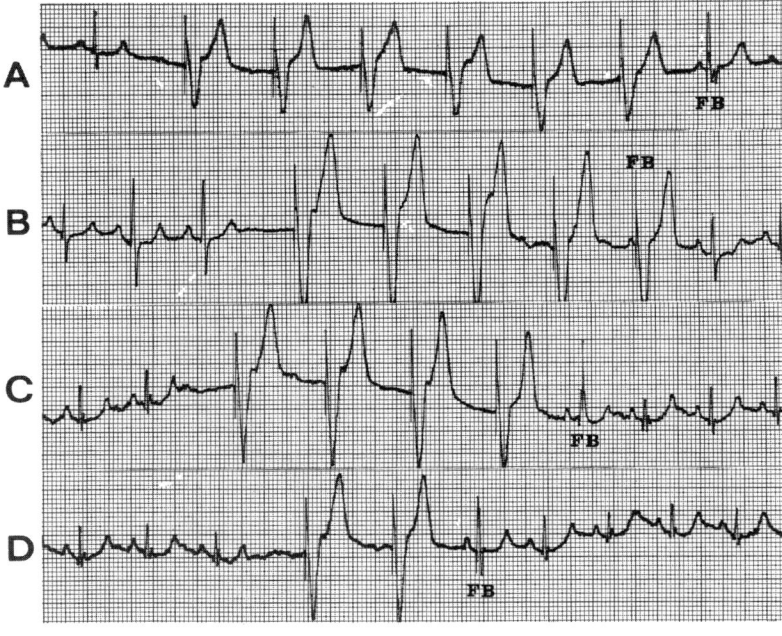

ATRIAL PACEMAKER RHYTHM

Definition

Atrial pacemaker rhythm is a regular atrial rhythm with normal QRS complexes initiated by an artificial pacemaker electrode placed in the right atrium. Each P wave is initiated by an artificial pacemaker spike.

Diagnostic Criteria (Fig. 14-3)

- There is a regular atrial rhythm with normal QRS complexes, and each P wave is initiated by an artificial pacemaker spike.
- The P waves are unusually upright in leads II, III, and aVF and inverted in lead aVR.
- The usual pacing rates range from 60 to 70 bpm.
- The QRS complexes may be broad and bizarre when there is preexisting LBBB or right bundle branch block (RBBB).

Diagnostic Pearls

Atrial pacemaker rhythm superficially mimics normal sinus rhythm, but each P wave is initiated by an artificial pacemaker spike in the former. Remember that atrial pacemaker rhythm uses the normal AV conduction system, just like sinus rhythm.

Figure 14-3
Atrial pacemaker rhythm with a rate of 120 bpm in a patient with recent diaphragmatic myocardial infarction. Note a ventricular premature contraction (the thirteenth beat). Each P wave is initiated by the pacemaker spike.

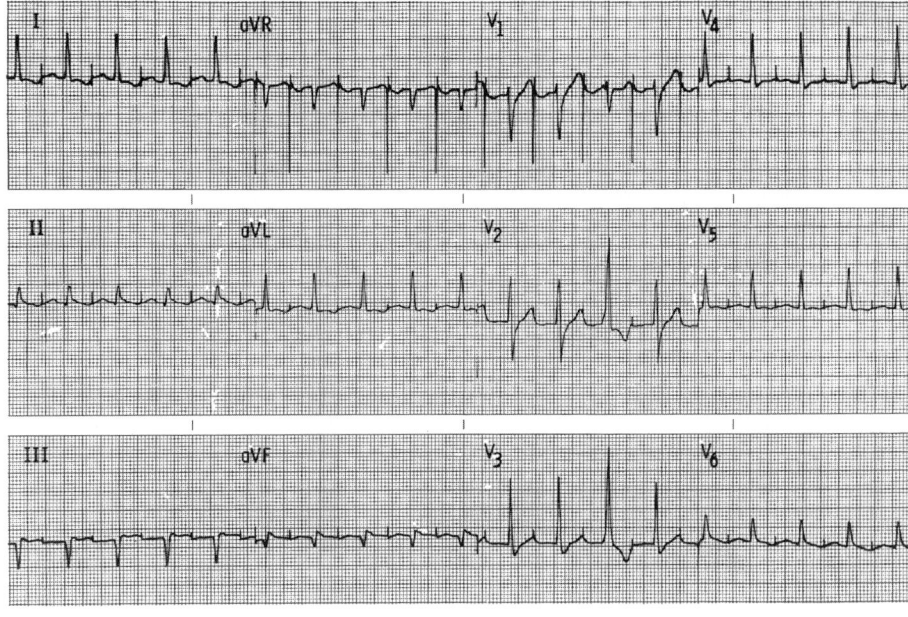

CORONARY SINUS PACEMAKER RHYTHM

Definition

Coronary sinus pacemaker rhythm is a regular atrial rhythm with normal (narrow) QRS complexes initiated by an artificial pacemaker electrode placed in the coronary sinus region.

Diagnostic Criteria (Fig. 14-4)

- Regular atrial rhythm with normal (narrow) QRS complexes initiated by an artificial pacemaker.
- The P waves initiated by artificial pacemaker spikes are inverted in leads II, III, and aVF and upright in lead aVR (retrograde P waves)
- The P-R intervals range from 0.12 to 0.20 second, depending on the preexisting AV conduction time.
- The usual artificial pacing rate is 60–70 bpm.
- The QRS complexes are broad and bizarre when there is preexisting LBBB or RBBB.

Diagnostic Pearls

When an artificial pacemaker spike is not recognized, some inexperienced readers may misdiagnose it as coronary sinus rhythm or AV junctional tachycardia. Coronary sinus pacemaker rhythm uses atrial kicking to improve cardiac output.

Figure 14-4
Coronary sinus pacemaker rhythm with a rate of 74 bpm. Note a ventricular premature contraction (marked O) and occasional atrioventricular junctional premature contractions (marked X). Each retrograde P wave is initiated by the artificial pacemaker spike.

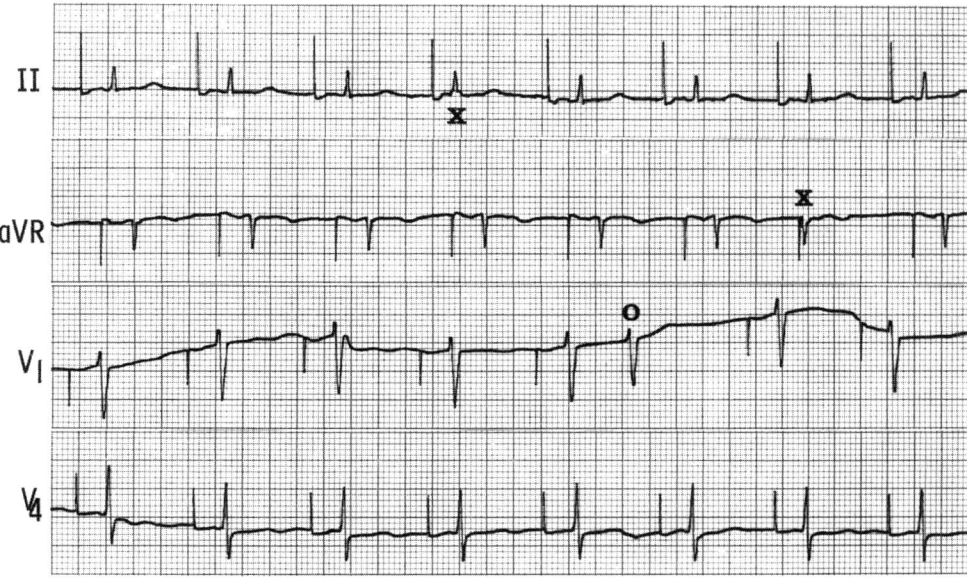

ATRIOVENTRICULAR SEQUENTIAL PACEMAKER RHYTHM

Definition

AV sequential pacemaker rhythm is a dual-chamber pacemaker rhythm initiated by two pacemaker electrodes so that the atria and the ventricles are paced sequentially.

Diagnostic Criteria (Fig. 14-5)

- The atria and ventricles are paced sequentially with the preset constant P-R interval.
- Each upright P wave is initiated by an artificial pacemaker spike, whereas each QRS complex is initiated by another pacemaker spike sequentially with the preset P-R interval.
- The paced QRS complex configuration exhibits a negative complex in lead V_1 and an upright (positive) complex in leads I, aVL, and V_{4-6} (LBBB pattern).
- The usual pacing rate is 60–70 bpm.
- There is no P wave when the underlying rhythm is AF or atrial flutter.

Diagnostic Pearls

When the artificial pacemaker spikes are not recognized, some inexperienced readers may misdiagnose it as a true LBBB with sinus rhythm. It should be noted that AV sequential pacing is the most commonly used pacing mode at the present time.

Figure 14-5
Atrioventricular sequential pacemaker rhythm with a rate of 100 bpm. Note that there are two sets of pacemaker spikes. One set of the spikes initiates P waves, whereas another set initiates the QRS complexes sequentially.

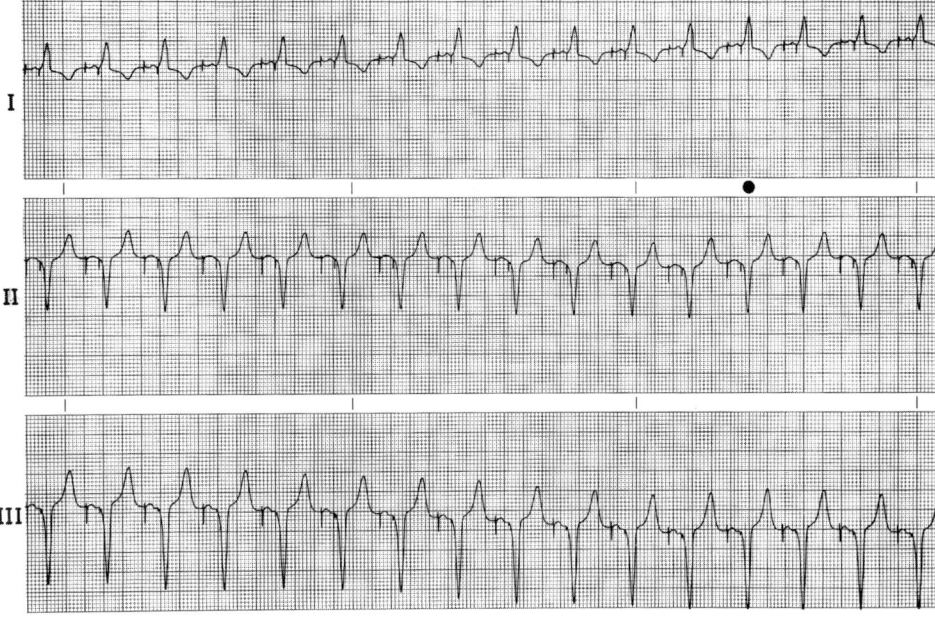

RUNAWAY PACEMAKER (ACCELERATION OF ARTIFICIAL PACING)

Definition

Runaway pacemaker (acceleration of artificial pacing) is the acceleration of artificial pacing at a rate faster than the preset pacing rate (ventricular fixed-rate mode in most cases).

Diagnostic Criteria (Fig. 14-6)

- Acceleration of the pacing rate is faster than the preset artificial pacing rate.
- The acceleration of the pacing rate may be as fast as 400–1,000 bpm.
- When the pacing rate exceeds 200 bpm, the pre-existing bradyarrhythmia often reappears.
- Other manifestations of artificial pacemaker (e.g., irregular pacing, failure of cardiac capture, failure of sensing, slowing of the pacing rate) may coexist with runaway pacemaker.

Diagnostic Pearls

Runaway pacemaker should be suspected even when the pacing rate is slightly faster than the preset pacing rate, providing that the equipment that recorded the electrocardiogram (ECG) is in good working order. Advanced runaway pacemaker is considered a medical emergency that requires immediate recognition and correction.

Figure 14-6
Malfunctioning pacemaker is manifested by "runaway pacemaker" (acceleration of the pacemaker rhythm, rate of 167 bpm). Malposition of the pacemaker electrode is considered in view of upright (positive) QRS complexes in lead V_1.

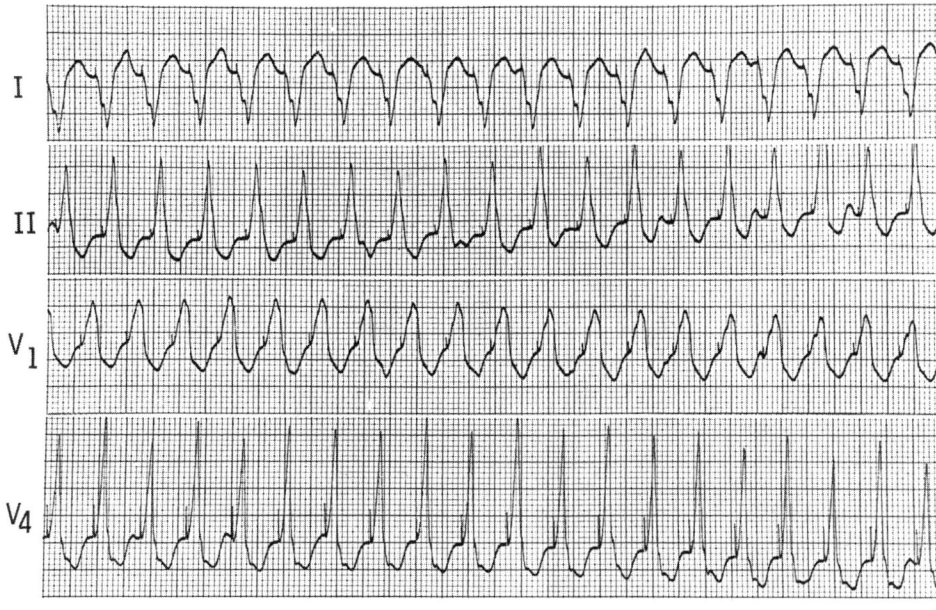

FAILURE OF CARDIAC CAPTURE BY PACING

Definition

Failure of cardiac capture by pacing is the failure of an artificial pacemaker to activate the atria, ventricles, or both (more commonly the ventricles).

Diagnostic Criteria (Fig. 14-7)

- Artificial pacemaker spikes fail to activate the atria, ventricles, or both (more commonly the ventricles).
- Other manifestations of artificial pacemaker malfunction (e.g., acceleration of pacing, slowing of pacing, irregular pacing, failure of sensing) may coexist.

Diagnostic Pearls

Failure of cardiac capture by artificial pacemaker is frequently observed in patients with advanced heart disease, quinidine or procainamide toxicity, and severe hyperkalemia. Thus, the possible underlying cause for the failure of cardiac capture should be corrected. Otherwise, relocating the pacemaker electrode may effectively establish cardiac capture.

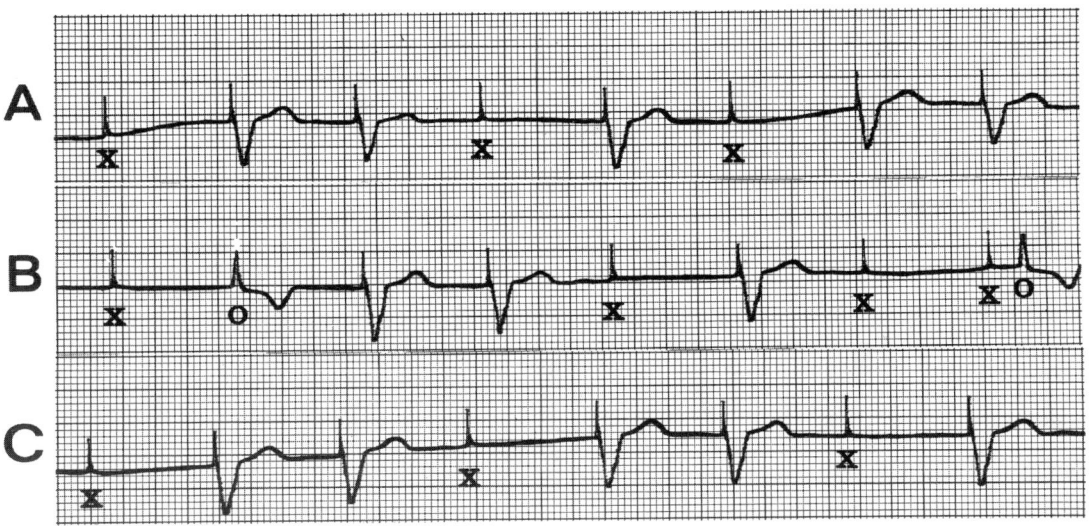

Figure 14-7
*Ventricular pacemaker rhythm (rate of 75 bpm) with intermittent failure of ventricular capture by the pacemaker spikes
(marked X). Note occasional intrinsic beats (marked O). The Holter monitor ECG rhythm strips A to C are not continuous.*

SLOWING OF ARTIFICIAL PACING

Definition

Slowing of artificial pacing is characterized by an artificial pacing rate that is slower than the preset pacing rate.

Diagnostic Criteria (Fig. 14-8)

- The artificial pacing rate is slower than the preset pacing rate.
- Irregular pacing often coexists with the slowing of artificial pacing.
- Other manifestations of pacemaker malfunction (e.g., failure of cardiac capture, failure of sensing) may coexist with slowing of artificial pacing.

Diagnostic Pearls

Malfunction of the artificial pacemaker should be suspected even when the pacing rate is slightly slower than the preset pacing rate, provided that the equipment that recorded the ECG is in good working condition. An extremely slow pacing rate, especially associated with irregular pacing, indicates a far-advanced malfunction of the pacemaker.

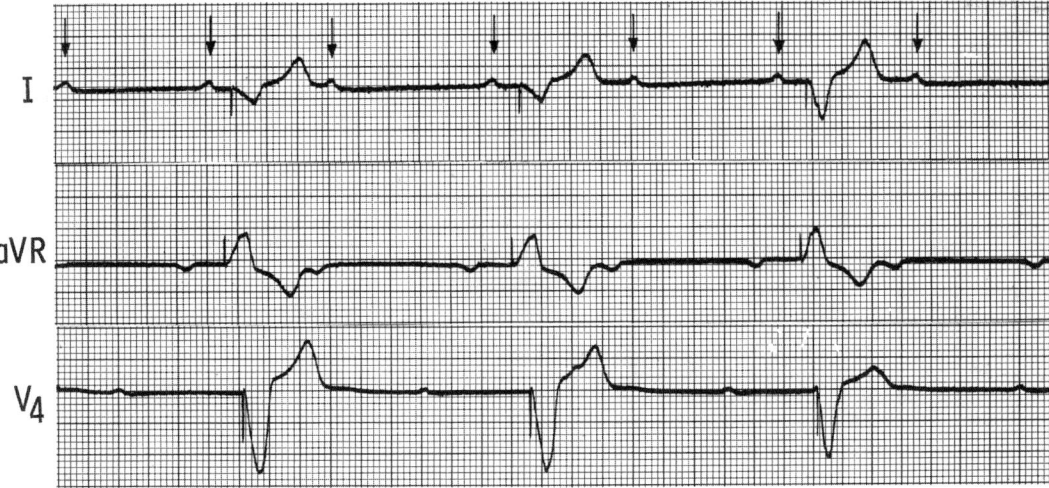

Figure 14-8
Malfunctioning pacemaker is manifested by markedly slow pacing rhythm (rate: 32 bpm). Arrows indicate sinus P waves.

IRREGULAR ARTIFICIAL PACING

Definition

Irregular artificial pacing is characterized by irregular cardiac cycles that are stimulated by the artificial pacemaker.

Diagnostic Criteria (Fig. 14-9)

- Irregular P-P cycles, R-R cycles, or both initiated by artificial pacemaker spikes.
- Slowing of artificial pacing often coexists with irregular artificial pacing.
- Other manifestations of artificial pacemaker malfunction (e.g., runaway pacemaker, failure of cardiac capture, failure of sensing) may coexist with irregular pacing.

Diagnostic Pearls

A malfunctioning pacemaker should be suspected even when the cardiac cycles initiated by artificial pacemaker exhibit slight irregularity, provided that the equipment that recorded the ECG is in good working order. Slowing of pacing often coexists with irregular pacing.

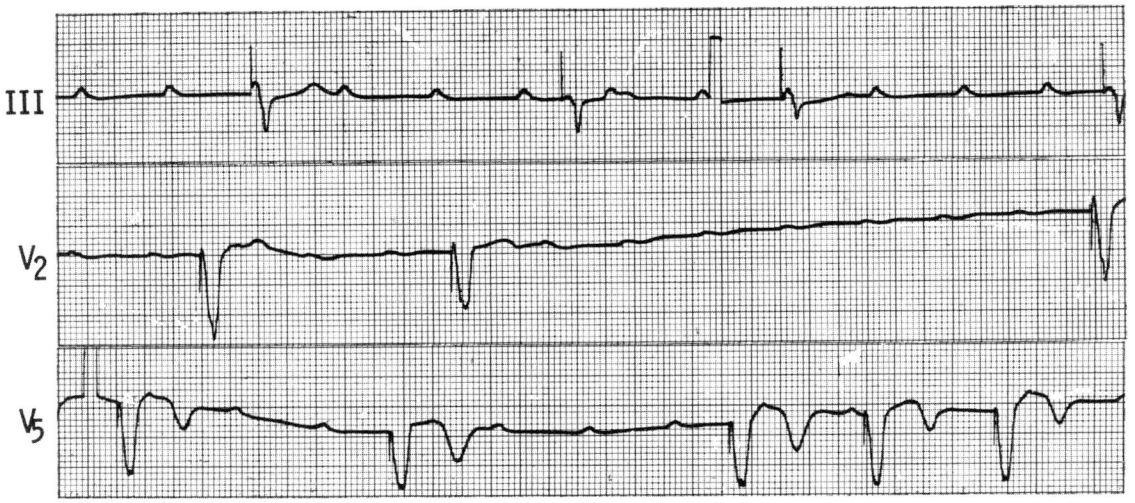

Figure 14-9
Malfunctioning pacemaker is manifested by a grossly irregular and slow pacemaker rhythm leading to an area of a long ventricular standstill (lead V$_2$).

PACEMAKER HYSTERESIS

Definition

Pacemaker hysteresis is characterized by a pacemaker escape interval (the length of the period from an intrinsic heartbeat to the initial pacemaker-induced beat) that is longer than the consecutively occurring pacing cycle (automatic interval).

Diagnostic Criteria (Fig. 14-10)

- The interval from the intrinsic beat (sinus or ectopic) to the next pacing beat (pacemaker escape interval) is longer than the cardiac cycle of consecutive pacing beats (automatic interval).
- The degree of the pacemaker hysteresis may vary, depending on the pacemaker model (minimum to marked hysteresis).

Diagnostic Pearls

It is important to understand the definition and diagnostic criteria of pacemaker hysteresis. Otherwise, an erroneous diagnosis of a malfunctioning pacemaker may be entertained. The practical value of pacemaker hysteresis is not fully established.

Figure 14-10
Sinus rhythm (marked S) and intermittent demand ventricular pacemaker rhythm with pacemaker hysteresis. Note occasional ventricular fusion beats (marked FB). The numbers represent hundredths of a second.

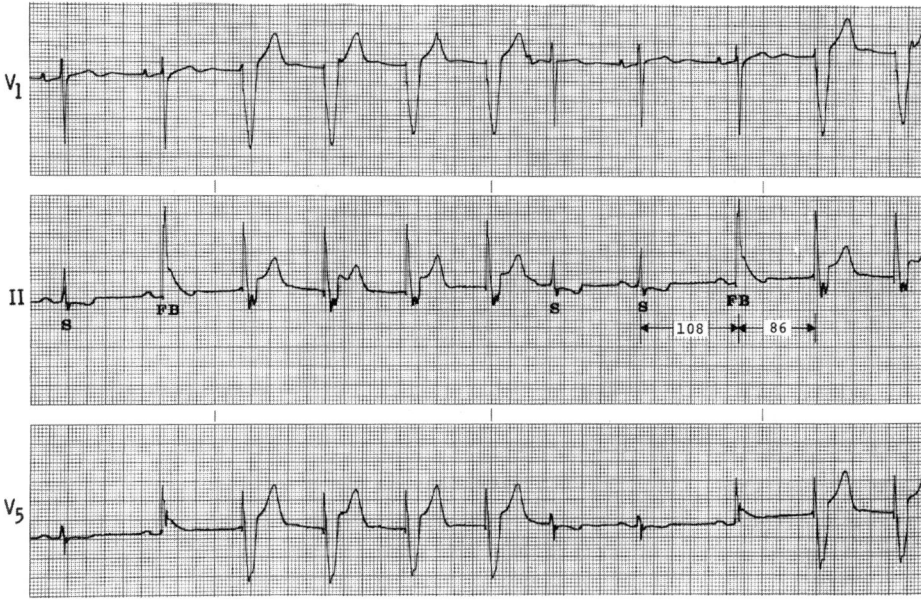

VENTRICULAR FIBRILLATION DURING ARTIFICIAL PACING

Definition

VF during artificial pacing is VF that occurs during artificial pacing that is either directly due to artificial pacing or to intrinsic heart disease.

Diagnostic Criteria (Fig. 14-11)

- VF is initiated by an artificial pacemaker stimulus as a result of the R-on-T phenomenon (usually during fixed-rate ventricular pacing).
- VF is provoked by advanced intrinsic heart disease (commonly acute MI or unstable angina) during artificial pacing (*not* directly due to pacing).

Diagnostic Pearls

Direct current shock should be applied immediately when VF develops during pacing regardless of whether VF is due to artificial pacemaker or to underlying heart disease.

Needless to say, it is important to be certain that the arrhythmia is a true VF and *not* various artifacts that may resemble VF (see Figs. 6-1 and 6-2).

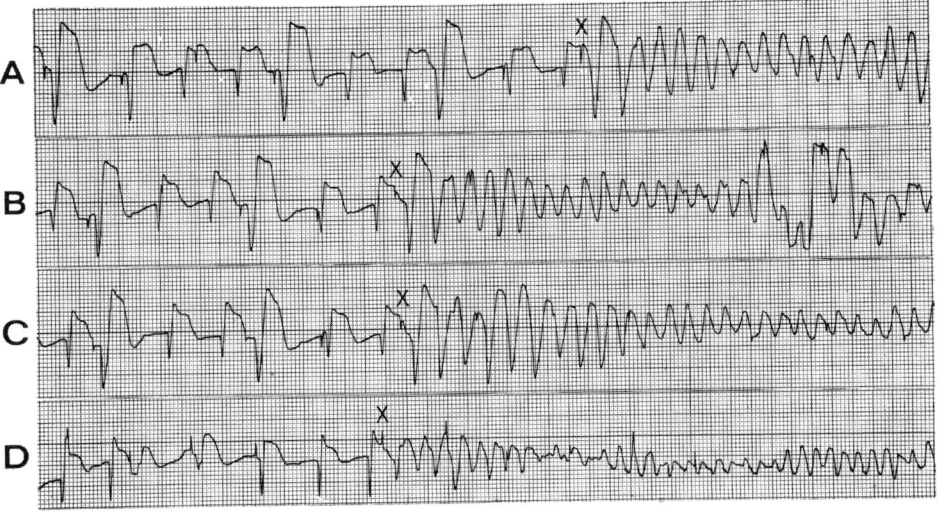

Figure 14-11   *Ventricular fibrillation initiated by artificial pacemaker spikes superimposed on the T waves (R-on-T phenomenon, marked X) in a patient with acute diaphragmatic myocardial infarction. The rhythm strips (lead II) A to D are not continuous.*

15

Congenital Heart Disease

The incidence of various congenital heart diseases varies significantly among different studies and varies markedly among different age groups. For instance, a small ventricular septal defect (VSD) is common in young children but rather uncommon in adults. In addition, the frequency of various cardiac anomalies has been altered recently because of the development of palliative and corrective procedures. For example, patent ductus arteriosus (PDA) is seldom seen in adults because a surgical corrective procedure is undertaken even in asymptomatic young children with the lesion.

Nevertheless, certain congenital cardiac lesions are considered to be very common, including VSD, atrial septal defect (ASD), PDA, pulmonic stenosis, tetralogy of Fallot, aortic stenosis, coarctation of the aorta, and transposition of the great vessels. This chapter deals primarily with the electrocardiographic findings of common congenital cardiac lesions.

As can be expected, the electrocardiogram (ECG) may be perfectly normal in various congenital heart diseases. This is particularly true in congenital cardiac lesions that produce stress primarily on the left ventricle. The best examples of these congenital cardiac lesions include coarctation of the aorta, aortic stenosis, PDA, and VSD. The ECG will less likely be normal in lesions such as ASD and pulmonic stenosis, which produce stress primarily on the right ventricle. The ECG will almost always be abnormal when two or more congenital defects coexist.

The electrocardiographic findings will vary markedly even in the same congenital lesion, depending on the severity of the defect. For example, the ECG may be completely normal in a small VSD or PDA, whereas the electrocardiographic tracing will likely show left ventricular hypertrophy (LVH) with a diastolic overloading pattern in more advanced cases. When there is significant *pulmonary hypertension*, there will be evidence of biventricular hypertrophy (BVH). In far-advanced cases, right ventricular hypertrophy (RVH) will be the dominant finding when marked pulmonary hypertension develops.

In *multiple congenital defects*, such as tetralogy of Fallot, the electrocardiographic findings will be greatly influenced by the dominant lesion. For example, the primary lesion in tetralogy of Fallot may be pulmonic stenosis, or it may be VSD. Therefore, markedly different electrocardiographic findings can be produced by the same clinical entity. From the above observation, the ECG should be interpreted in conjunction with a careful clinical history, detailed physical findings, and accurate X-ray findings in relation to the specific congenital cardiac anomaly.

The interpretation of the electrocardiographic findings in congenital heart diseases may be further complicated by the coexistence of other types of heart diseases, chest deformities, drug therapy, and electrolyte imbalance. Furthermore, coexisting electrocardiographic abnormalities, such as bundle branch block (particularly left bundle branch block [LBBB]) and Wolff-Parkinson-White (WPW) syndrome, often prevent the appearance of the expected electrocardiographic findings. The best example is that diagnosing an LVH pattern is usually impossible in the presence of LBBB. Another example is that LBBB and WPW syndrome frequently produce a *pseudo–myocardial infarction pattern (pseudo–MI pattern)*. The presence of bundle branch block or WPW syndrome itself, on the other hand, at times, is almost always diagnostic of certain congenital heart diseases. For instance, aortic stenosis should be strongly suspected when LBBB is present in children or young adults unless cardiomyopathy or severe hypertension is present. The presence of WPW syndrome often favors the diagnosis of *Ebstein's anomaly* and less commonly idiopathic hypertrophic subaortic stenosis (IHSS) when any form of congenital heart diseases is suspected.

Although no single electrocardiographic finding is specific for the diagnosis of any particular congenital cardiac anomaly, certain electrocardiographic patterns are almost diagnostic in many instances. For instance, right bundle branch block (RBBB) pattern associated with left axis deviation (left anterior hemiblock) is almost specific for the diagnosis of ASD of the ostium primum type in children and young adults. Another example is *dextrocardia* with situs inversus, which produces a unique electrocardiographic finding. Namely, all complexes including P, QRS, and T waves are inverted in lead I. In addition, certain electrocardiographic findings are extremely common in certain congenital heart diseases. RBBB pattern is encountered in nearly 90% of all types of ASD, and it is also almost uniformly present in Ebstein's anomaly. RBBB is less commonly observed in VSD, but the former is a frequent complication following surgical repair of VSD or tetralogy of Fallot.

The *Katz-Wachtel phenomenon* (an RS pattern with large amplitude in leads V_{2-4} and/or limb leads; see Chapter 3) tends to occur more commonly in advanced VSD, although BVH due to any congenital heart disease may produce a similar finding.

Pseudo–MI pattern (narrow and deep Q waves) is commonly encountered in IHSS and less commonly in VSD. On the other hand, marked chest deformity (especially pec-tus excavatum) without any cardiac anomaly may, at times, produce a pseudo–MI pattern.

Congenital heart diseases that may be associated with first-degree atrioventricular (AV) block include ASD, VSD, PDA, and Ebstein's anomaly. Among all congenital cardiac lesions, various cardiac arrhythmias, particularly paroxysmal atrial tachyarrhythmias, are most common in Ebstein's anomaly and ASD.

P-congenitale (tall and peaked P waves in leads II, III, and aVF and right precordial leads), which is due to right atrial enlargement (see Chapter 3), is commonly found in cyanotic congenital lesions and in pulmonic stenosis. Extremely tall P waves are frequently encountered in tricuspid valve diseases, including Ebstein's anomaly.

As emphasized previously, a normal ECG by no means excludes any congenital heart disease, and no particular electrocardiographic abnormality is pathognomonic of any particular congenital lesion. Electrocardiographic diagnosis certainly assists the clinical diagnosis to a significant degree, however, when interpreted intelligently in conjunction with all other available clinical and laboratory data.

Individual congenital heart diseases are discussed in their approximate order of frequency.

VENTRICULAR SEPTAL DEFECT

- VSD is the most common congenital heart disease in infants and children. Electrocardiographic findings as well as clinical manifestations vary markedly depending on the size of the defect, the pressure gradient between the two ventricles, and the direction and magnitude of the shunt. In addition, electrocardiographic findings will also be influenced by other coexisting congenital defects, such as those seen in tetralogy of Fallot, Eisenmenger's syndrome, and truncus arteriosus.
- The ECG is usually normal, but it may show LVH or even BVH in a small VSD. In VSD of moderate size, the electrocardiographic pattern of BVH is usually present (Fig. 15-1). When the defect is large, the ECG may show BVH, predominantly LVH with a diastolic overloading pattern, or RVH.
- The *Katz-Wachtel phenomenon* is very common in VSD (see Chapter 3) and is encountered in 50–75% of cases.
- RBBB pattern, more commonly incomplete, is also frequently found in VSD (20–30% of cases), although it is not as common as in ASD. RBBB following surgical repair for VSD is a common complication, however.

- The P waves may be tall and peaked in leads II, III, aVF, and V_{1-4} (P-congenitale).

Figure 15-1
Biventricular hypertrophy in a patient with ventricular septal defect.

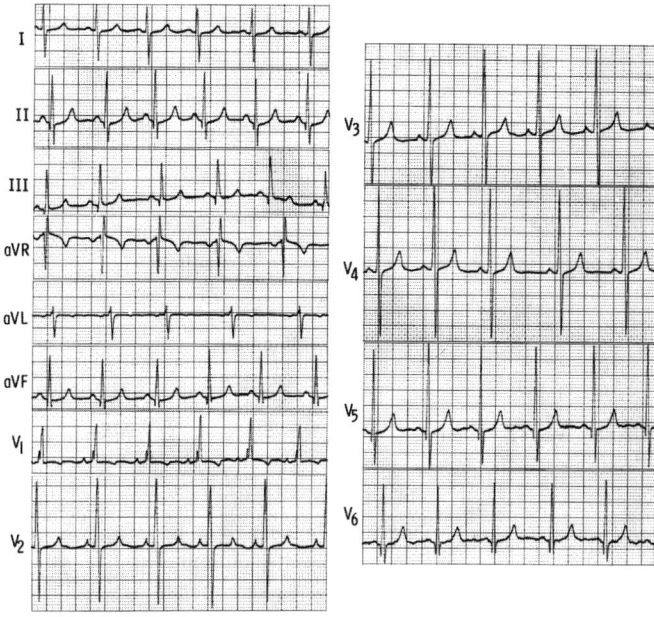

ATRIAL SEPTAL DEFECT

- ASD is the most common congenital heart disease in older children and adults.
- An ostium secundum defect is a defect in the region of the fossa ovalis and is associated with normal AV valves. The defects have been reported to be multiple in some cases.
- An ostium primum defect is located in the lower portion of the atrial septum and overlies the mitral and tricuspid valves. A cleft in the anterior leaflet of the mitral valve is found in the majority of patients. The tricuspid valve is usually normal, although some thickening of the septal leaflet may occur. The ventricular septum is usually intact from a functional viewpoint, although its proximal part is deficient anatomically.
- Common AV canal consists of an interatrial and an interventricular septal defect. An AV valve is common to both ventricles and consists of an anterior and a posterior leaflet related to the ventricular septum, with a lateral leaflet in each ventricle. This congenital lesion is common in children with Down's syndrome.
- RBBB (either complete or incomplete) pattern is almost always found in cases of all types of ASD (in up to 90% of cases) (Fig. 15-2). The incomplete RBBB pattern is more common than the complete form. RBBB pattern has been attributed to hypertrophy of the crista supraventricularis rather than to a true RBBB.
- The QRS axis in secundum type ASD is frequently right axis deviation because of RVH with a diastolic overloading pattern, but the QRS axis may be normal (see Fig. 15-2). On the other hand, an ostium primum defect usually produces left axis deviation in the presence of RBBB. Under these circumstances, left axis deviation is considered to represent congenital left anterior hemiblock (see Chapter 4).
- Less common electrocardiographic abnormalities include P-congenitale and first-degree AV block. Rarely, ASD may be associated with WPW syndrome (see Chapter 12). In far-advanced cases of ASD, particularly in ostium primum defect, BVH is often encountered.
- Atrial tachyarrhythmias, especially atrial fibrillation, is common in the end stage of the disease. Second-degree AV block or complete AV block is extremely unusual in ASD. The electrocardiographic tracing may be normal in some cases of ASD, but an absence of RBBB pattern makes the diagnosis of ASD extremely unlikely in most instances.

Figure 15-2
Sinus rhythm with incomplete right bundle branch block in a patient with atrial septal defect.

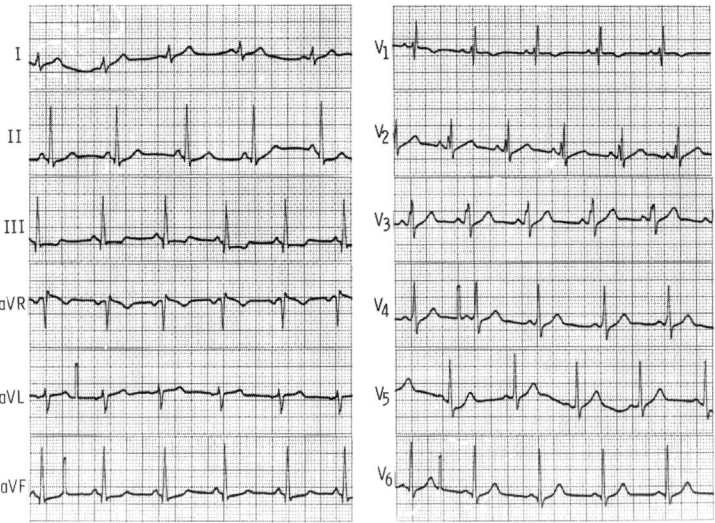

- ASD is the most common congenital cardiac anomaly associated with an RBBB pattern, and it is also one of the most common congenital lesions to produce cardiac arrhythmias.

- It has been shown recently that some patients develop sick sinus syndrome 10–15 years following successful surgical repair of ASD.

PATENT DUCTUS ARTERIOSUS

- PDA is the second most common congenital heart disease in all age groups, especially in infants and young children. PDA is encountered approximately two times more frequently in females than in males. This congenital lesion has been reported to be frequently associated with maternal rubella during early pregnancy.
- The ECG is often normal in mild cases of PDA. LVH with a diastolic overloading pattern is usually produced with a large defect (Fig. 15-3).
- In severe cases, especially those associated with significant pulmonary hypertension, BVH may develop.
- Left atrial enlargement and first-degree AV block are not uncommon.
- RBBB may be occasionally encountered in PDA.

Figure 15-3
Sinus rhythm and left ventricular hypertrophy with diastolic overloading pattern in a patient with patent ductus arteriosus.

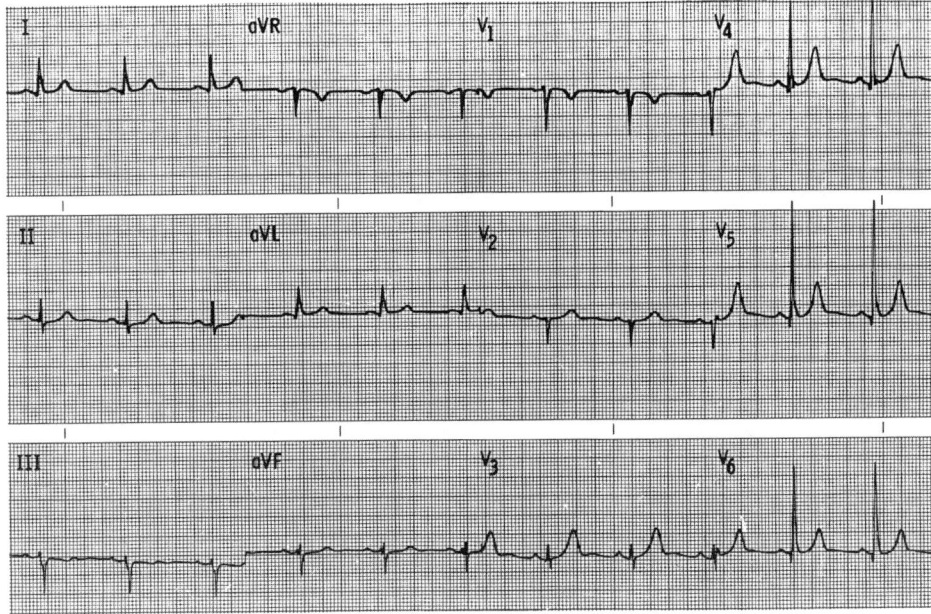

PULMONIC STENOSIS

- Pulmonic stenosis is one of the relatively common congenital cardiac lesions in children and adults. Pulmonic stenosis may be an isolated lesion; however, it may be associated with ASD or VSD.
- In mild cases, the ECG is often normal; however, slight RVH may be produced.
- In advanced cases, when right ventricular pressure is equal to or higher than left ventricular pressure, RVH with a systolic overloading pattern is present (Fig. 15-4).
- The configuration of the QRS complex shows characteristically a tall R wave or qR complex in lead V_1, with secondary T wave changes in leads V_{1-3} (occasionally up to leads V_4 and V_5).
- In addition, P-congenitale is also a common finding in advanced cases of pulmonic stenosis.

Figure 15-4
Right ventricular hypertrophy with right atrial enlargement in a patient with pulmonic stenosis. Note an atrial premature contraction (indicated by the arrow).

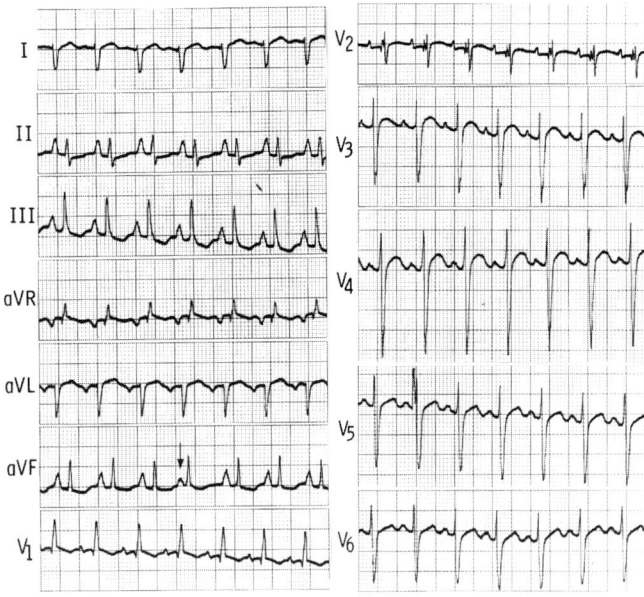

AORTIC STENOSIS

- Aortic stenosis is also not uncommon, accounting for approximately 3% of all congenital cardiac lesions.
- Aortic stenosis has been found to be three times more common in males. The stenosis is valvular in the majority of cases.
- The ECG is usually normal in mild cases, and it may be normal in even some cases of severe aortic obstruction.
- In most of the severe cases, the ECG shows LVH with a systolic overloading pattern (Fig. 15-5).
- In extremely advanced cases of aortic stenosis, LBBB may develop in a late stage of the disease.

Figure 15-5
Sinus rhythm with marked left ventricular hypertrophy due to severe aortic stenosis.

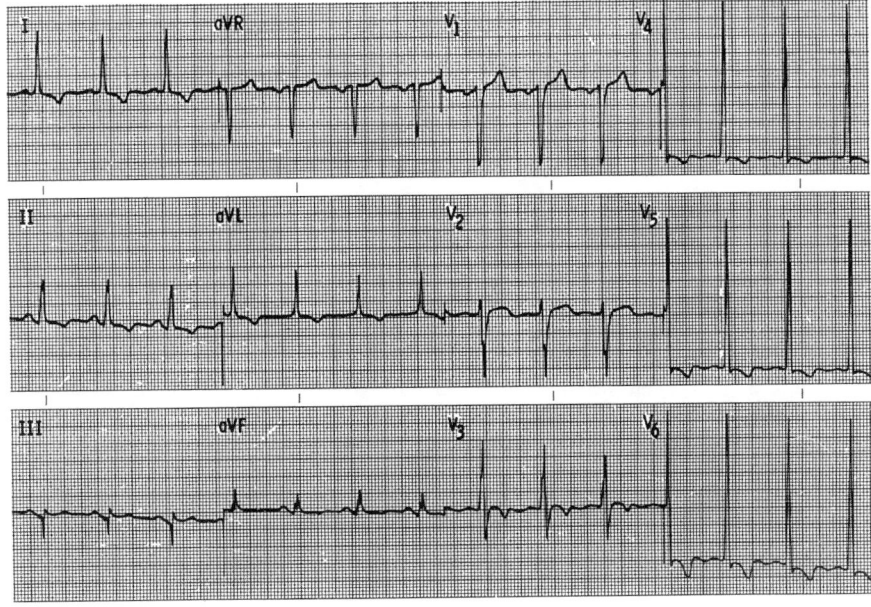

TETRALOGY OF FALLOT

- Tetralogy of Fallot consists of pulmonic stenosis, VSD, dextroposition of the aorta, and RVH. The clinical picture as well as the electrocardiographic findings vary markedly. There may be predominantly pulmonic stenosis or VSD.
- In many cases of tetralogy of Fallot, RBBB is present, and the QRS complexes are very broad (Fig. 15-6).
- RBBB often develops postoperatively, but it may be present at birth in patients with tetralogy of Fallot.
- Tetralogy of Fallot may coexist with dextrocardia.
- There may be evidence of P-congenitale.
- Tetralogy of Fallot should be considered strongly when children or young adults demonstrate RBBB with marked right axis deviation.

Figure 15-6
Right bundle branch block in a patient with tetralogy of Fallot associated with dextrocardia (see Figs. 15-8 and 15-9).

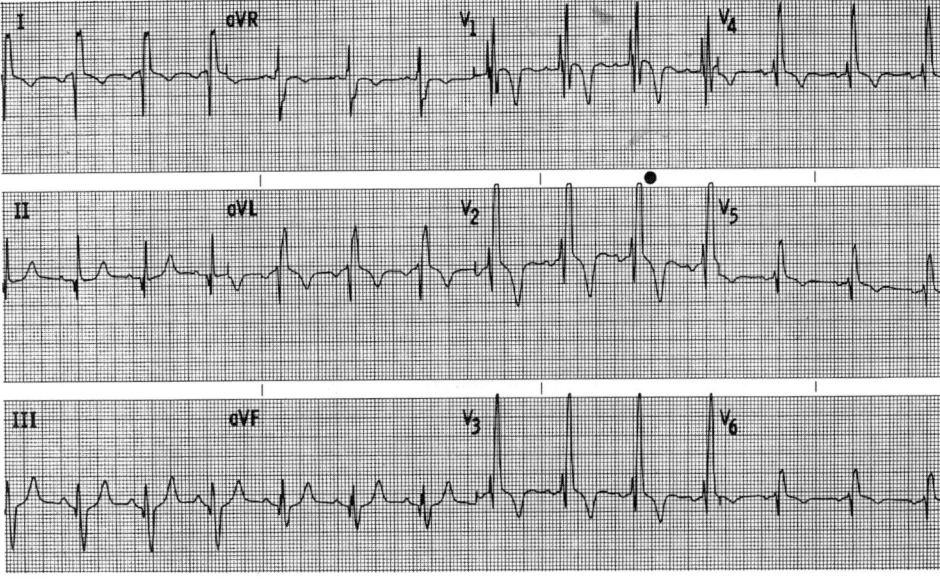

EBSTEIN'S ANOMALY

- Ebstein's anomaly is characterized by downward displacement of an abnormal tricuspid valve into the right ventricle. Tricuspid regurgitation is commonly present, but the valve is not stenotic.
- The most common electrocardiographic finding in Ebstein's anomaly is most likely an RBBB pattern with a bizarre QRS configuration. In addition, a characteristic electrocardiographic abnormality is an extremely tall and peaked P wave in leads II, III, and aVF (Fig. 15-7).
- Ebstein's anomaly is the most common congenital heart disease associated with WPW syndrome (see Fig. 15-7).
- Various cardiac arrhythmias, including atrial tachy-arrhythmia, premature beats, and first-degree AV block (rarely second-degree or complete AV block), are also frequently associated with this anomaly.
- Ebstein's anomaly and ASD are the most common congenital cardiac lesions that produce various arrhythmias.

Figure 15-7
Marked right atrial enlargement in a patient with Ebstein's anomaly associated with Wolff-Parkinson-White syndrome.

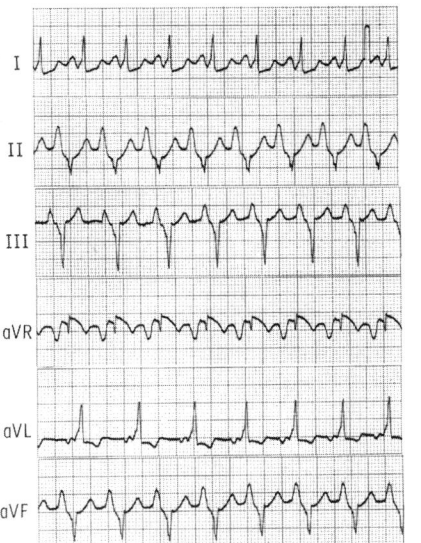

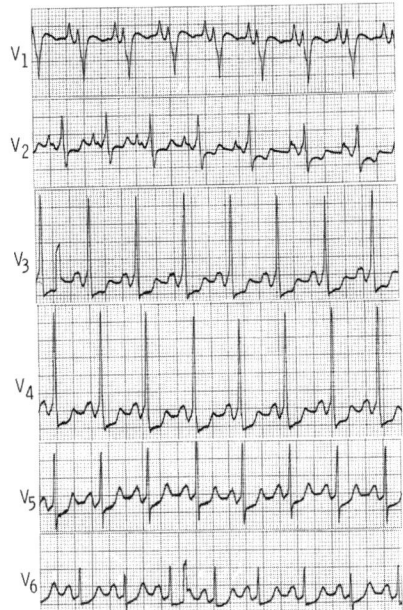

DEXTROCARDIA

- Dextrocardia with situs inversus (mirror-image dextrocardia with total transposition of the abdominal viscera) may be present in a perfectly normal heart functionally; however, other congenital cardiac defects coexist in approximately 50% of cases.
- When dextrocardia is without any congenital lesion, the electrocardiographic findings are characteristically a mirror-image pattern (Figs. 15-8 and 15-9). In other words, extremity leads will show the electrocardiographic findings identical to the tracing taken with reversed limb lead electrodes between the left and right arms in normal individuals. Specifically, the P, QRS, and T complexes in lead I are inverted; leads II and III are reversed, as are leads aVR and aVL (see Figs. 15-8 and 15-9). The electrocardiographic pattern, of course, will be altered when there is another coexisting congenital cardiac lesion.
- Isolated dextrocardia is usually associated with other congenital cardiac defects, including single ventricle, transposition of the great vessels, pulmonic stenosis, VSD, tetralogy of Fallot, ASD, or truncus arteriosus. Therefore, the electrocardiographic abnormalities in isolated dextrocardia depend greatly on the severity of the coexisting congenital anomaly. An inverted P wave in lead I is indicative of atrial inversion. The characteristic mirror-image pattern is unusual in isolated dextrocardia.

Figure 15-8
*Electrocardiographic
tracing of a patient with
dextrocardia recorded
with the usual 12-lead
placement. Note that all
P, QRS, and T complex-
es are inverted (negative)
in lead I. In the precor-
dial leads, the QRS
amplitude becomes pro-
gressively smaller from
lead V_1 to lead V_6.
Figures 15-8 and 15-9
were obtained from the
same patient with
dextrocardia.*

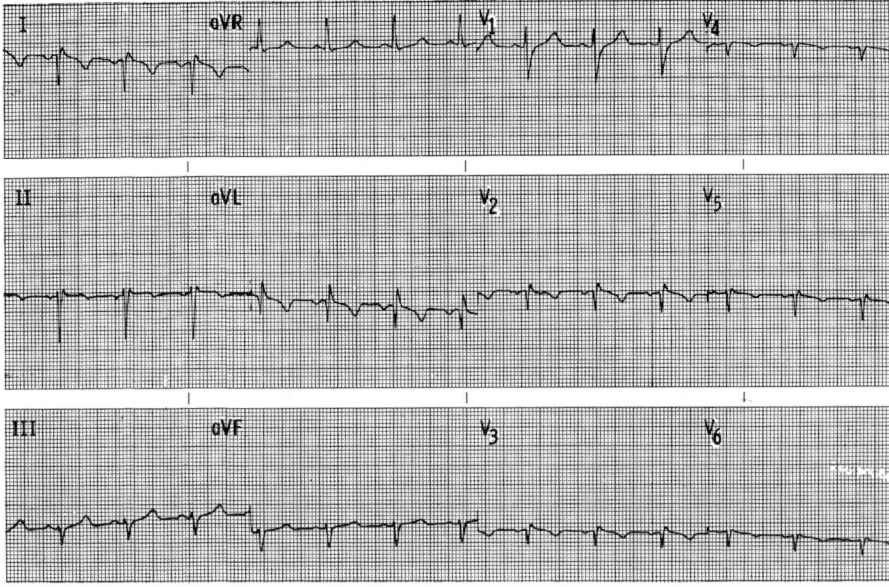

Figure 15-9
This electrocardiographic tracing was recorded using the right chest lead placement in the same patient with dextrocardia. Figures 15-8 and 15-9 were obtained from the same patient with dextrocardia.

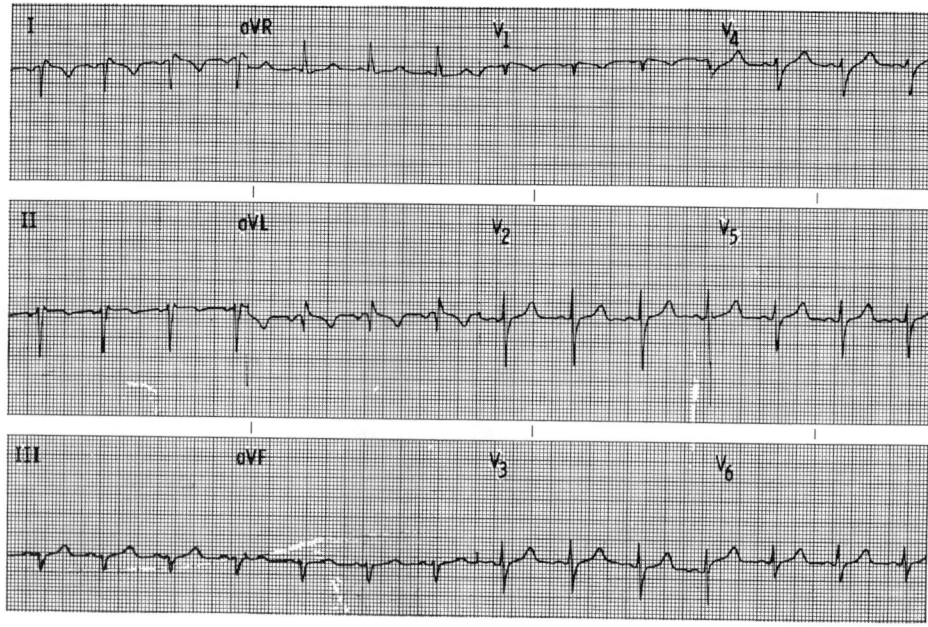

IDIOPATHIC HYPERTROPHIC SUBAORTIC STENOSIS

- IHSS often produces characteristic electrocardiographic findings.
- Common electrocardiographic findings may include deep Q or QS waves in leads II, III, and aVF and in the left precordial leads that closely resemble diaphragmatic lateral MI.
- In addition, the R wave in lead V_1 is often tall, simulating posterior MI or RVH.
- IHSS often produces a tall R wave in lead V_1 and deep Q waves in leads V_{4-6} so that posterolateral MI is closely simulated.
- These electrocardiographic findings are considered to be due to ventricular septal hypertrophy.
- Occasionally, WPW syndrome coexists with IHSS.
- The recognition of IHSS is important because a pseudo–MI pattern is frequently encountered (Fig. 15-10; see Chapter 5).

Figure 15-10
Pseudo–posterolateral myocardial infarction pattern in a patient with idiopathic hypertrophic subaortic disease.

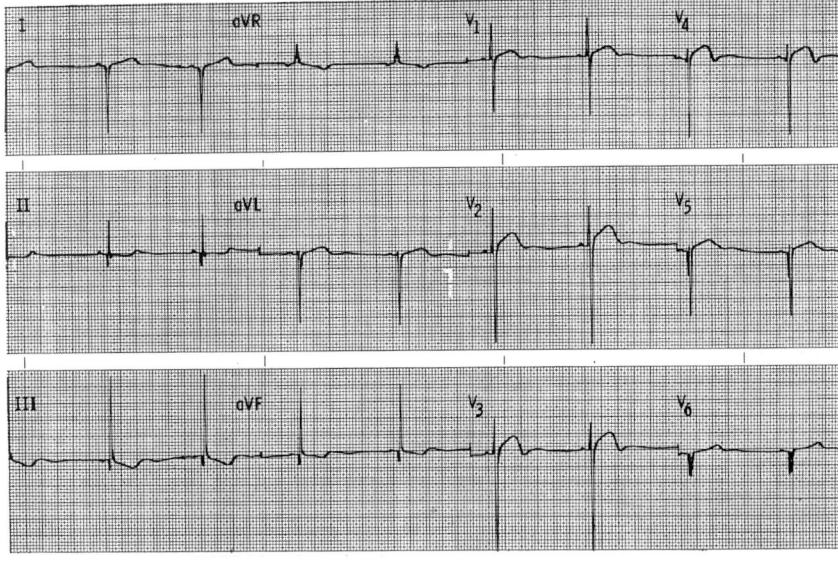

WOLFF-PARKINSON-WHITE SYNDROME

- WPW syndrome is considered to be a congenital conduction system anomaly.
- A very high incidence of various supraventricular tachyarrhythmias in this syndrome has been stressed previously (see Chapter 12).
- The fundamental mechanism responsible for the production of various tachyarrhythmias is considered to be due to the fact that the ectopic impulses are conducted very rapidly via a congenital accessory bypass that connects the atria and ventricles.
- A detailed description of WPW syndrome is found in Chapter 12.

16

Electrolyte Imbalances

Various *electrolyte imbalances* influence cardiac function, impulse formation, and conduction. This is especially true of abnormalities of *potassium* and *calcium* levels. The role of the potassium ion in maintaining normal cardiac function was demonstrated as early as 1883 by Ringer, and later, extensive experimental and clinical studies confirmed its role. It has been shown that the degree of hyperkalemia correlates well with the severity of cardiac arrhythmias, but there is a much weaker correlation between the degree of hypokalemia and the alteration of cardiac impulse formation and conduction.

It is known that electrolyte imbalances that influence cardiac arrhythmias in humans are much more complex than the experimental results obtained in intact animals or in isolated preparations. This is because various factors in humans other than electrolyte imbalances influence cardiac impulse formation and conduction, including the nature and severity of the heart disease, vagal and sympathetic systems, digitalis and various antiarrhythmic drugs, various noncardiac diseases (e.g., renal disease), and acid-base balance. For example, the fact that hypokalemia frequently predisposes to the development of various digitalis-induced cardiac arrhythmias is well documented. In addition, electrolyte imbalance of a single ion is relatively uncommon, and combined electrolyte imbalance makes the clinical picture more complex. It is interesting to note that the combined effects of multiple electrolyte imbalances may have a synergistic or antagonistic action in producing cardiac arrhythmias. For instance, calcium and, to a lesser degree, sodium have actions that are pharmacologically antagonistic to those of potassium. Clinically, hyperkalemia and hypocalcemia frequently coexist in patients with renal insufficiency. Recently, the important role of magnesium in the production of cardiac arrhythmias has been emphasized. Furthermore, hypomagnesemia is known to predispose to the development of digitalis-induced cardiac arrhythmias.

In general, the production of cardiac arrhythmias is closely related to the extracellular and intracellular concentrations of various electrolytes. However, the correlation between cardiac arrhythmias and electrolyte imbalance in humans is primarily made with the extracellular concentrations of ions, since the intracellular component cannot be measured. Nevertheless, it is known that intracardiac hypokalemia, manifested by electrocardiographic findings, is closely related to the production of cardiac arrhythmias in which a serum potassium determination may be within normal limits or even higher than normal.

Various electrocardiographic changes in potassium and calcium imbalances are summarized in Table 16-1.

POTASSIUM

The electrolyte that most commonly produces electrocardiographic alterations and various cardiac arrhythmias is, without doubt, potassium. It has been said that the correlation is much more accurate in hyperkalemia than in hypokalemia. Electrocardiographic abnormalities and cardiac arrhythmias due to hypokalemia may be observed even when the serum potassium level is normal, especially during digitalis therapy. This paradoxical phenomenon represents a definite discrepancy between the serum and cellular levels of potassium.

Electrocardiographic abnormalities due to altered potassium were first noted by Wiggens in 1930 and later by McLean et al. in 1933. Subsequently, Winkler et al. described in detail the new changes correlated with the level of potassium.

Table 16-1. Electrocardiographic changes in electrolyte imbalances

ECG findings in hyperkalemia
    Tent-shaped and tall T waves (narrow base)
    Flat P waves
    Atrioventricular blocks (varying degrees)
    Intraventricular blocks (various types)
    Ventricular arrhythmias
    Ventricular standstill
ECG findings in hypokalemia
    Prominent U waves
    Peaking and tall P waves (II, III, and aVF)
        (pseudo P-pulmonale)
    Atrioventricular block (rare)
    Predisposes to digitalis toxicity
ECG findings in hypercalcemia
    Shortening of Q-T interval (shortening or even
        absence of S-T segment)
ECG findings in hypocalcemia
    Prolongation of Q-T interval (lengthening of
        S-T segment)

HYPERKALEMIA

- Hyperkalemia may be observed in various clinical conditions, particularly those associated with renal insufficiency, acidosis, shock-like state, and overadministration of potassium. The development of cardiac arrhythmias in patients with moderate hyperkalemia (potassium concentrations of 5.5–7.5 mEq/liter) is rare.
- It is generally agreed that the earliest and most common electrocardiographic finding of hyperkalemia is a tall, tent-shaped, peaked T wave that is often symmetric and often has a narrow base (potassium concentration of 5.5–7.5 mEq/liter). In some cases of hyperkalemia, the amplitude of the T wave may be within normal limits; therefore, a narrow and tent-shaped appearance is a more characteristic feature.
- In hyperkalemia, the direction of the T wave may be altered. For instance, the physiologically inverted T waves, seen in leads V_{1-3} in children or young adults (*juvenile T wave pattern*) may become upright; the inverted T wave of left ventricular hypertrophy (LVH) (secondary T wave change) may also become upright.
- The T wave change is best seen in leads II, III, and V_{2-5} in most cases.

- When hyperkalemia is more advanced (potassium concentrations of 7.5–10.0 mEq/liter), the T wave change may be followed by flattening and widening of the P wave, a prolonged P-R interval, depression (occasionally elevation) of the S-T segment, and, later, the disappearance of the P wave, a decrease in amplitude of the R wave, and increased depth of the S wave.
- In far-advanced hyperkalemia (potassium concentrations ≥10 mEq/liter), the QRS complex becomes definitely widened and is followed by the development of ventricular tachycardia (VT) or ventricular fibrillation (VF), slow ventricular escape rhythm, and finally, ventricular standstill as the potassium level rises further.
- Diffuse intraventricular block with flat P waves due to advanced hyperkalemia may closely resemble VT. Diffuse or nonspecific intraventricular block is relatively common in advanced hyperkalemia.
- Occasionally, however, a true hemiblock, right bundle branch block (RBBB), left bundle branch block (LBBB), bifascicular block (BFB), or trifascicular block (TFB) may be produced acutely by severe hyperkalemia.
- Clinically, hyperkalemia and hypocalcemia often coexist, and the electrocardiographic findings in this circumstance are manifested by a prolonged Q-T interval (due to lengthening of the S-T segment) and a tent-shaped T wave. In this case, the T wave may be upright or inverted in certain leads (particularly in leads I, aVL, and V_{4-6}), depending on the pre-existing electrocardiographic abnormalities.
- Advanced hyperkalemia with marked hypocalcemia produces diffuse intraventricular block, a flat P wave, first-degree atrioventricular (AV) block, and a tent-shaped T wave associated with a markedly prolonged Q-T interval.
- Severe hyperkalemia-induced intraventricular disturbances are often followed by VT or VF and ventricular standstill, leading to death unless proper management is provided immediately.
- Progressive normalization of intraventricular conduction has been observed in a patient with advanced hyperkalemia-induced intraventricular block due to chronic renal failure during hemodialysis.
- The effect of hyperkalemia on the sinus node varies. The sinus rate may be accelerated or reduced in experimental as well as in clinical studies. In general, the degree of change in the sinus rate due to hyperkalemia is insignificant.
- Experimental and clinical investigative studies have demonstrated that hyperkalemia has a dual effect on AV

conduction time. Shortening of the P-R interval occurs initially during mild hyperkalemia; later, the P-R interval becomes prolonged as hyperkalemia is further advanced. The prolongation of the P-R interval in hyperkalemia may be due to a widened P wave, the prolonged P-R segment, or both.

- When marked hyperkalemia is induced experimentally in both animals and human subjects, second-degree or complete AV block may occur. However, second-degree or higher AV block in spontaneous hyperkalemia in humans is extremely uncommon. One of the reasons for this is that the P wave often disappears before advanced AV block is recognized. Needless to say, the diagnosis of second-degree or complete AV block is difficult or even impossible to make when there are no discernible P waves.

- When hyperkalemia is markedly advanced (≥ 10 mEq/liter), death may be caused by VF or ventricular standstill. Ventricular standstill may be due to a failure of the conduction of the sinus impulse to the ventricles and failure of the AV junction or ventricles to produce escape impulses. VT or VF, on the other hand, may be induced by a re-entry phenomenon due to uneven recovery. This is considered to occur when intraventricular conduction becomes so slow that some ventricular fibers, depolarized earlier, recover their excitability before some other fibers complete depolarization. VF is believed to be a more common mechanism of death than is ventricular standstill in uremic patients with hyperkalemia.

- The production of ventricular standstill and VF is considered to be related not only to the degree of hyperkalemia but also to the mode of the progression of the hyperkalemia. In experimental animal studies, slow administration of potassium, as a rule, results in ventricular standstill, whereas rapid injection leads to VF. In general, VF is often preceded by isolated or coupled ventricular premature contractions (VPCs) or VT, whereas ventricular standstill is preceded by a slow idioventricular rhythm with a very wide QRS complex as a terminal event. Not uncommonly, VF may be preceded by a slow ventricular rhythm or vice versa in terminal hyperkalemia.

- Recent clinical observations indicate that the ventricular excitability threshold may be increased by hyperkalemia in the presence of an implanted artificial pacemaker.

- Hyperkalemia affords relative protection against the development of digitalis-induced arrhythmias, whereas digitalization lowers the threshold for potassium toxicity.

- In practice, combined electrolyte imbalance is more common than the disturbance in the level of a single ion. For example, hyperkalemia and hypocalcemia frequently coexist in patients with renal insufficiency.
- Clinically, hyperkalemia and hypercalcemia may coexist in patients with renal insufficiency because of hyperparathyroidism or other treatment with calcium salts. In this case, hypercalcemia and hyperkalemia are expected to counteract each other so that the production of AV conduction disturbances, intraventricular conduction disturbances, or VF may be delayed or even prevented.
- Similarly, hypernatremia may be expected to counteract the effects of hyperkalemia, whereas hyponatremia may be expected to augment the effect of hyperkalemia on AV and intraventricular conduction disturbances.
- Hypermagnesemia may also augment the effect of hyperkalemia on AV and intraventricular conduction disturbances.

MODERATE HYPERKALEMIA

Definition

Moderate hyperkalemia is characterized by electrocardiographic changes that are due to a moderately elevated serum potassium level (5.5–7.5 mEq/liter).

Diagnostic Criteria (Fig. 16-1)

- Tall, tent-shaped, peaked T wave with a narrow base.
- The amplitude of the T wave may be within normal limits (in some cases).
- The direction of the T wave may be altered (e.g., LVH).
- The T wave change is best seen in leads V_{2-5} (next best seen in leads II, III, and aVF).

Diagnostic Pearls

The T wave change in hyperkalemia may resemble the T wave change in myocardial ischemia, myocarditis, pericarditis, or CNS disorders, but a tent-shaped T wave with a narrow base is the key to identifying hyperkalemia. It should be noted that the T wave tends to be peaked in healthy children and young adults as a normal variant.

Figure 16-1
Moderate hyperkalemia is manifested by tall and peaked T waves with a narrow base in many leads.

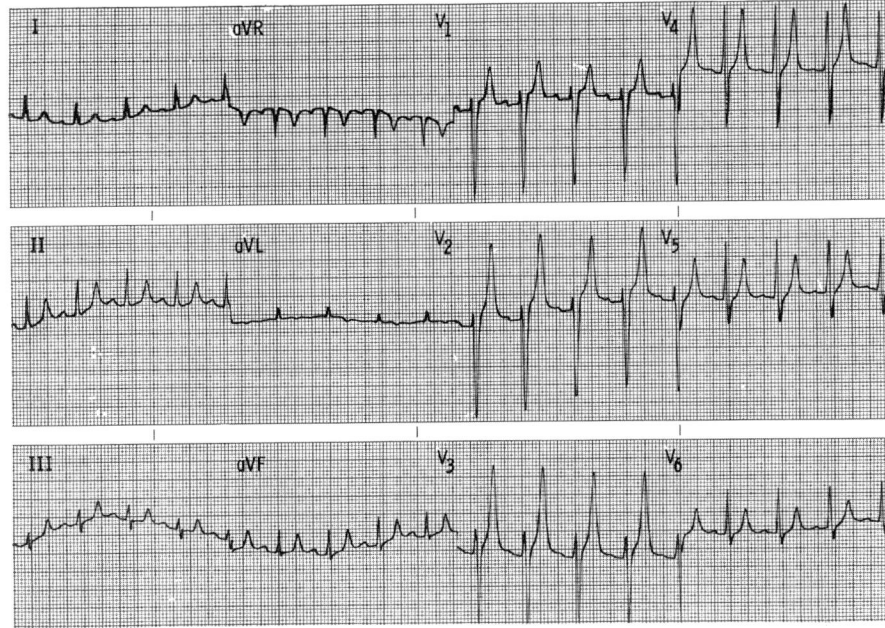

ADVANCED HYPERKALEMIA

Definition

Advanced hyperkalemia is characterized by electrocardiographic changes that are due to a serum potassium level of 7.5–10.0 mEq/liter.

Diagnostic Criteria (Fig. 16-2)

- Tall, tent-shaped, peaked T wave with a narrow base
- Flattening and widening of the P wave (no obvious P wave in some cases)
- Prolonged P-R interval (first-degree AV block)
- Depression (occasionally elevation) of the S-T segment
- Reduction of the R wave amplitude with increased depth of the S wave

Diagnostic Pearls

Again, a peaked T wave with a narrow base is the essential electrocardiographic finding to diagnose hyperkalemia.

Figure 16-2
Advanced hyperkalemia is manifested by peaked and tall T waves associated with flat P waves and nonspecific intra-ventricular block.

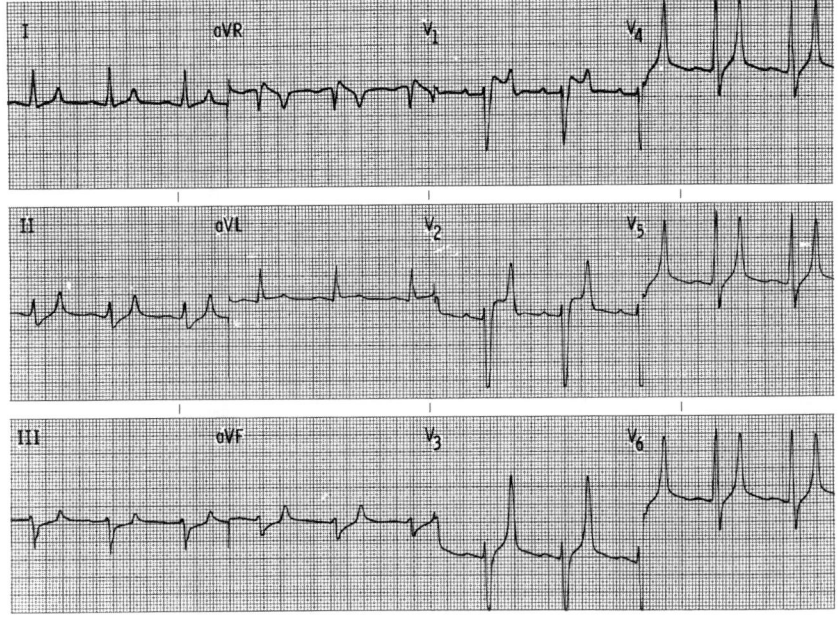

FAR-ADVANCED HYPERKALEMIA

Definition

Far-advanced hyperkalemia is characterized by electrocardiographic changes due to a serum potassium level of more than 10 mEq/liter.

Diagnostic Criteria (Fig. 16-3)

- Peaked T wave may no longer be present.
- Diffuse intraventricular block.
- RBBB, LBBB, hemiblock, BFB, and TFB (in some cases).
- VT or VF followed by ventricular escape rhythm and finally ventricular standstill.
- Flat or no clear P wave even during sinus rhythm.

Diagnostic Pearls

In far-advanced hyperkalemia, the QRS complex is usually broad and bizarre, even during sinus rhythm; finally, VT or VF and ventricular standstill follow. It should be emphasized that the peaked T wave is no longer present in far-advanced hyperkalemia.

Figure 16-3
Far-advanced hyperkalemia is manifested by a bifascicular block consisting of a right bundle branch block and a left anterior hemiblock and associated with intermittent ventricular flutter-fibrillation. Note that the QRS complexes are extremely broad in this patient with advanced renal failure because of the diffuse intraventricular block in addition to a bifascicular block. Peaked T waves are no longer present.

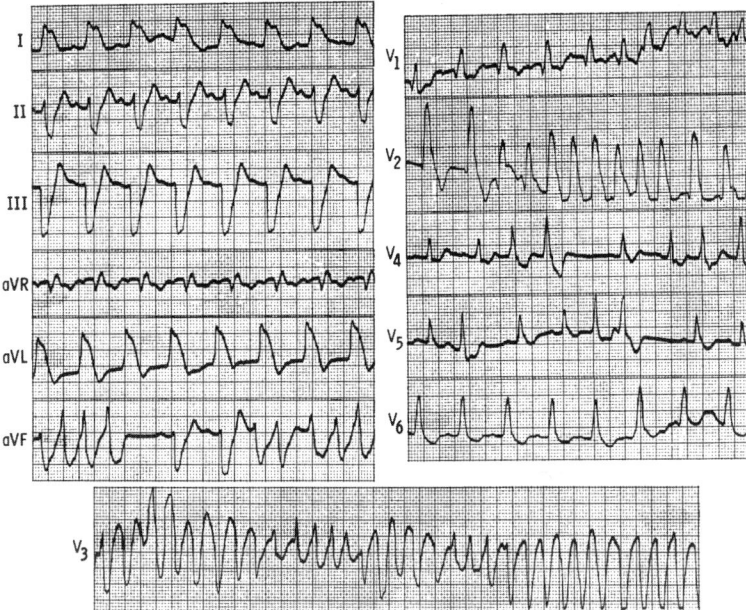

HYPOKALEMIA

- Hypokalemia is much more frequently encountered in medical practice than hyperkalemia. Various clinical situations may be associated with hypokalemia, including insufficient intake of potassium (i.e., starvation or malnutrition), gastrointestinal loss (e.g., vomiting, diarrhea, ileostomy, biliary fistula, gastric suction, ulcerative colitis), large amounts of intravenous fluid administration without potassium supplement, salt-losing nephritis, steroid therapy, diuretic therapy (especially with thiazides), hemodialysis, aldosteronism, diabetic acidosis, hypokalemic periodic paralysis, and administration of alkalinizing agents such as sodium bicarbonate or molar sodium lactate.
- Electrocardiographic abnormalities correlate poorly with low serum potassium levels as compared with their correlation with hyperkalemia.
- Electrocardiographic abnormalities, including various cardiac arrhythmias, frequently occur when the serum potassium level is less than 3 mEq/liter.
- The most common and perhaps the earliest electrocardiographic finding in hypokalemia is a prominent U wave. It should be noted that the prominent U wave is usually not associated with prolongation of the Q-T interval.
- The depression of the S-T segment, lowering or inversion of the T wave, or both may fuse with the prominent U wave in hypokalemia. This finding may resemble the electrocardiographic change encountered in myocardial ischemia, myocarditis, pericarditis, and various cerebrovascular accidents.
- The term *prominent U wave* should be used when the U wave is equal to or taller than the T wave in the same lead, especially in leads V_{2-4}, regardless of its actual amplitude.
- Since S-T segment depression occurs in various conditions other than hypokalemia (e.g., digitalis effect, myocardial injury, other electrolyte imbalances), it should not be considered strongly in the diagnosis of hypokalemia.
- In addition to a prominent U wave, one of the most important electrocardiographic changes in hypokalemia is the prominent P wave, which is usually evident in leads II, III, and aVF. The prominent P wave is a manifestation of advanced hypokalemia. This P wave change may closely resemble P-pulmonale (*pseudo–P-pulmonale*).

- Cardiac arrhythmias occur much more frequently when hypokalemia is found in advanced heart disease, digitalis intoxication (DI), or both. The most common cardiac arrhythmias are atrial premature contractions (APCs), atrial tachycardia (AT) with or without AV block, and supraventricular tachycardia. Less commonly, AV junctional tachycardia (JT) or junctional escape beats (JER) and reciprocal beats or rhythm may occur. VPCs are usually found in marked hypokalemia, but VT or VF is rather uncommon.
- In clinical hypokalemia, AV block other than a prolonged P-R interval is only rarely observed, although AV block of varying degrees can be produced easily by experimentally induced hypokalemia.
- It has been said that hypocalcemia counteracts the effect of hypokalemia, whereas hypercalcemia may augment hypokalemia-induced cardiac arrhythmias.
- Hypokalemia predisposes to the development of DI. For the same reason, various digitalis-induced tachyarrhythmias are often best treated with potassium.

HYPOKALEMIA

Definition

Hypokalemia is characterized by electrocardiographic abnormalities and cardiac arrhythmias due to a serum potassium of less than 3.2 mEq/liter.

Diagnostic Criteria (Fig. 16-4)

- The earliest electrocardiographic finding is a prominent U wave (pronounced in leads V_{3-6}).
- In advanced hypokalemia, a peaked P wave is pronounced in leads II, III, and aVF.
- Common cardiac arrhythmias are APCs, AT with or without AV block, and supraventricular tachycardia.
- Less common arrhythmias are AV JT or JER.
- In far-advanced hypokalemia, VPCs are common (VT or VF is rather uncommon).
- First-degree AV block may occur, but more advanced AV block is rather uncommon.
- Hypokalemia predisposes to digitalis-induced arrhythmias.

Diagnostic Pearls

When the prominent U wave is fused with the T wave, the electrocardiographic finding may closely resemble a prolonged Q-T interval. A peaked P wave due to advanced hypokalemia (pseudo–P-pulmonale) may mimic true P-pulmonale due to chronic obstructive pulmonary disease. Remember that the peaked P wave due to hypokalemia is always associated with a prominent U wave.

Figure 16-4
Hypokalemia is manifested by prominent U waves (marked U).

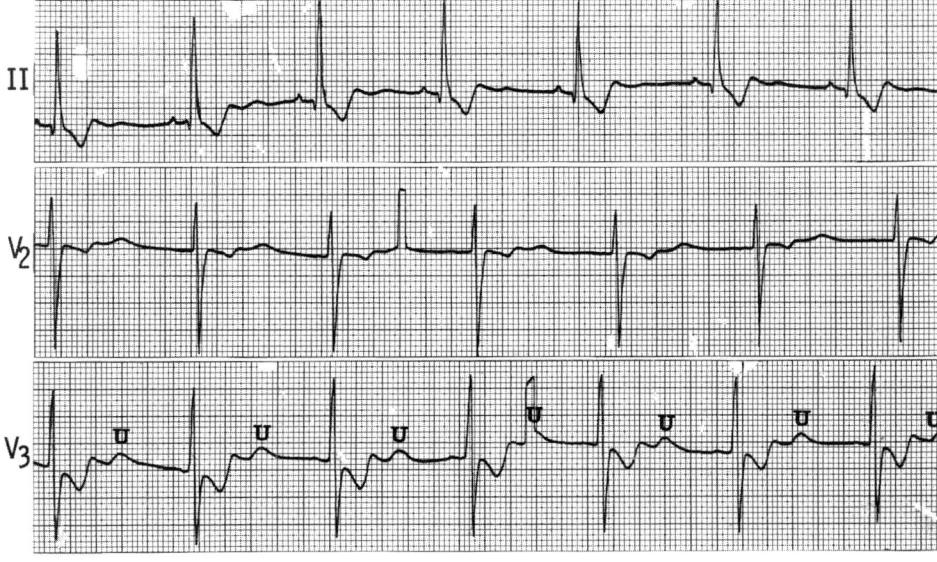

CALCIUM

- Calcium ion disturbances are much less common than potassium ion disturbances.
- Hypercalcemia may be encountered clinically in primary hyperparathyroidism, vitamin D intoxication, malignant neoplasm with osseous metastasis, milk alkali syndrome, sarcoidosis, acute bone atrophy, and overadministration of calcium. In addition, hypercalcemia may be observed in multiple myeloma, Paget's disease, and hyperthyroidism.
- The earliest and probably the most common electrocardiographic abnormality in hypercalcemia is shortening of the Q-T interval.
- Less commonly, the P-R interval, the QRS duration, or both may be prolonged.
- Cardiac arrhythmias are relatively uncommon in hypercalcemia, but VPCs, VT, and VF have been reported. Sudden death in patients with hypercalcemia is often attributed to VF, as is seen in hyperparathyroidism and DI.

- A synergetic action between digitalis and calcium has been repeatedly emphasized.
- The reason for the production of ventricular tachyarrhythmias in hypercalcemia is considered to be due to a re-entry phenomenon resulting from the combined effects of decreased conduction velocity and a shortened refractory period in the ventricles.
- Hypocalcemia may be observed in several clinical situations, including chronic renal insufficiency, insufficient intake of calcium, loss of calcium (e.g., diarrhea, essential hypercalciuria, renal tubular acidosis), vitamin D deficiency, idiopathic hypoparathyroidism, partial or total parathyroidectomy, osteomalacia, and respiratory or metabolic alkalosis.
- The most common and earliest electrocardiographic change in hypocalcemia is prolongation of the Q-T interval, primarily due to lengthening of the S-T segment.
- Less commonly, flattening or inversion of the T wave may be observed in hypocalcemia.
- Significant cardiac arrhythmias due to hypocalcemia are extremely rare, except for premature beats.
- The fact that hypocalcemia and hyperkalemia commonly coexist has been stressed above.

HYPERCALCEMIA

Definition

Hypercalcemia is characterized by electrocardiographic abnormalities and cardiac arrhythmias due to excessive amounts of calcium in the body.

Diagnostic Criteria (Fig. 16-5)

- The earliest and the most common electrocardiographic abnormality is shortening of the Q-T interval due to the shortening or even the absence of the S-T segment.
- Less common electrocardiographic findings include prolongation of the P-R interval (first-degree AV block) and QRS duration (intraventricular block).
- VPCs and VT or VF may occur in advanced cases.
- There is synergetic action between digitalis and calcium.

Diagnostic Pearls

It should be noted that the Q-T interval tends to be short in healthy children and young adults as a normal variant. Thus, the diagnosis of hypercalcemia should be made with special care in this circumstance.

Figure 16-5
Short Q-T interval due to hypercalcemia.

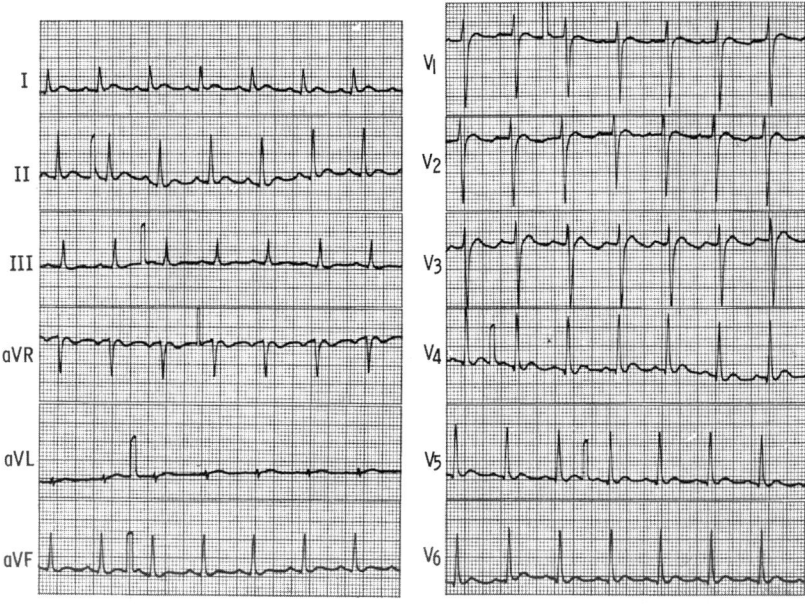

HYPOCALCEMIA

Definition

Hypocalcemia is characterized by electrocardiographic abnormalities and cardiac arrhythmias due to depleted levels of calcium in the blood.

Diagnostic Criteria (Fig. 16-6).

- The earliest and the most common electrocardiographic finding is prolongation of the Q-T interval due to a lengthening of the S-T segment.
- A less common electrocardiographic finding is flattening or inversion of the T wave.
- Significant cardiac arrhythmias other than premature beats are extremely rare.
- Hypocalcemia commonly coexists with hyperkalemia.

Diagnostic Pearls

The Q-T interval may be prolonged in many clinical conditions, including quinidine or procainamide toxicity, congenital Q-T syndrome, and CNS disorders. In addition, many elderly individuals show a prolonged Q-T interval without any clear-cut reason. Remember that hypocalcemia produces the prolonged Q-T interval as a result of the lengthening of the S-T segment, a unique electrocardiographic abnormality.

Figure 16-6
Hyperkalemia associated with hypocalcemia in a patient with renal failure. Hyperkalemia is manifested by peaking T waves, whereas hypocalcemia is manifested by the prolongation of the Q-T interval secondary to the lengthening of the S-T segment.

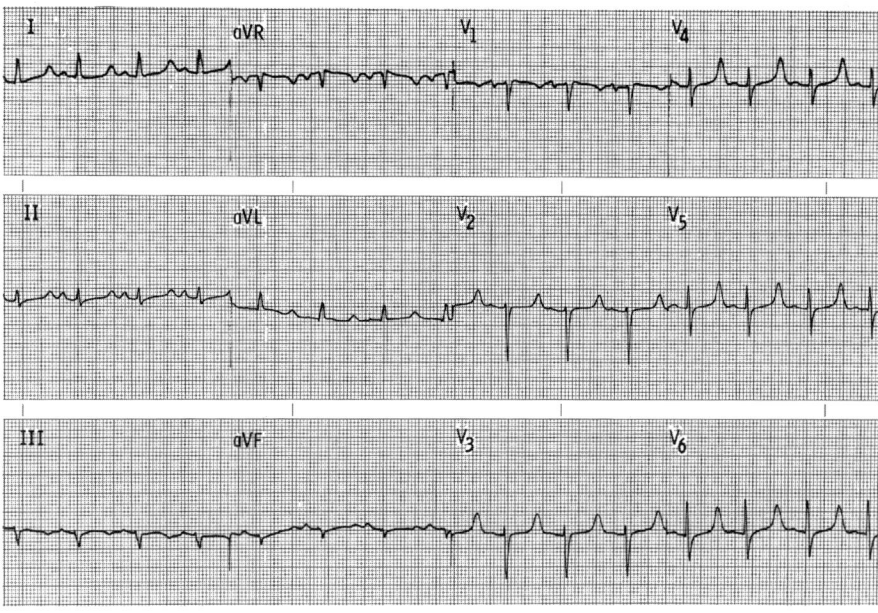

MAGNESIUM

- The importance of recognizing hypomagnesemia has been emphasized recently because magnesium deficiency alone may produce cardiac arrhythmias and may predispose to DI. It has been shown that hypomagnesemia results in a secondary loss of intracellular potassium. Thus, DI may be directly related to magnesium deficiency itself, due to intracellular hypokalemia, or both. It is well-documented that monkeys and dogs with hypomagnesemia are prone to develop digitalis toxicity.
- VF associated with hypomagnesemia in humans has been reported recently.
- Electrocardiographic abnormalities produced by hypermagnesemia are similar to those found in hyperkalemia. Thus, the early change in hypermagnesemia is often a prolonged P-R interval followed by a widened QRS complex when the magnesium concentration rises.

SODIUM

The relationship between the development of cardiac arrhythmias and abnormal serum sodium concentrations has not been studied in depth. It has been said that marked hyponatremia may cause an effect similar to that observed in hyperkalemia.

17

Miscellaneous Electrocardiographic Findings

PULMONARY EMBOLISM

- Various electrocardiographic abnormalities may be observed in pulmonary embolism, infarction, or both (Fig. 17-1).
- Common electrocardiographic findings include P-pulmonale, inverted T waves in leads V_{1-3} (*right ventricular strain pattern*), and right axis deviation with or without posterior axis deviation.
- S_1, Q_3 pattern; S_1, S_2, S_3 patterns; and Q waves in leads II, III, and aVF with inverted T waves (pseudo–diaphragmatic myocardial infarction [MI]) are not uncommon.

- Less commonly, transient right bundle branch block (RBBB) (often associated with right axis deviation and/or S_1, Q_3 patterns) and paroxysmal atrial tachyarrhythmias, particularly atrial fibrillation (AF) or multifocal atrial tachycardia, may be observed in pulmonary embolism.
- These electrocardiographic abnormalities tend to occur during the first 24–48 hours of the disease and are usually transient in nature.
- Sinus tachycardia is almost always present in pulmonary embolism unless atrial tachyarrhythmias are produced.

Figure 17-1
Acute pulmonary embolism is manifested by a very rapid sinus tachycardia (rate of 148 bpm), atrial premature contractions, right axis deviation of the QRS complexes, and right bundle branch block. In addition, there is a nonspecific S-T segment and T wave abnormality involving many leads diffusely.

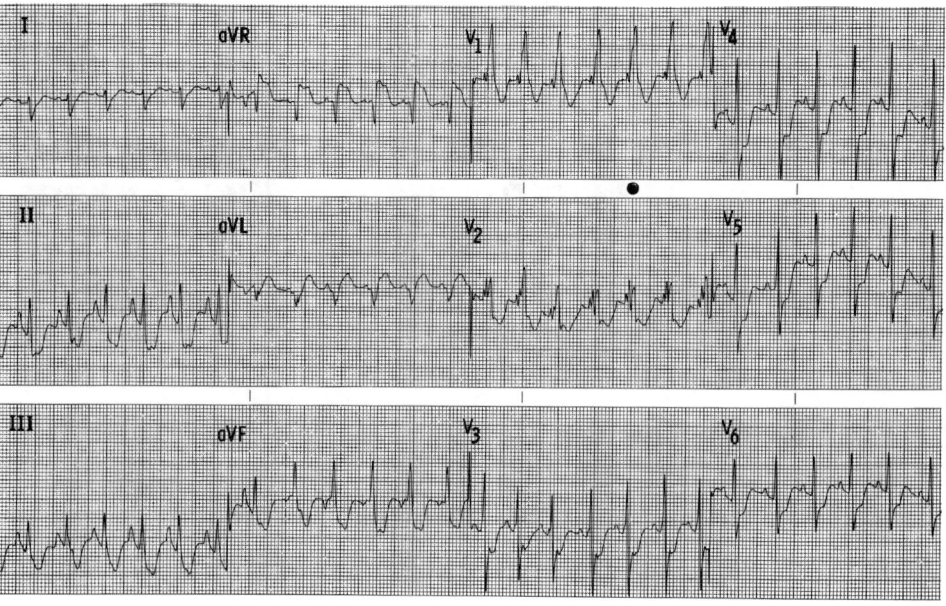

MYOCARDITIS

- There is no specific electrocardiographic abnormality diagnostic of myocarditis.
- It is common to observe that myocarditis and pericarditis often coexist.
- The most common electrocardiographic finding in acute myocarditis is probably diffuse T wave changes, particularly inverted T waves involving practically every lead (Fig. 17-2).
- Other electrocardiographic abnormalities may include atrioventricular (AV) blocks of varying degrees, left bundle branch block (LBBB) or RBBB, bilateral bundle branch block (BBBB), diffuse (nonspecific) intraventricular conduction defect, and extrasystoles of various origins.
- First-degree AV block is one of the most reliable signs in diagnosing rheumatic carditis in children.
- Uncommon electrocardiographic findings in myocarditis include a nonspecific abnormality of the S-T segment (usually sagging or depression), notched and broad P waves, a prolongation of the Q-T interval, and various ectopic tachyarrhythmias.

Figure 17-2
Myocarditis is manifested by T wave inversion involving many leads diffusely associated with low voltage of the QRS complexes.

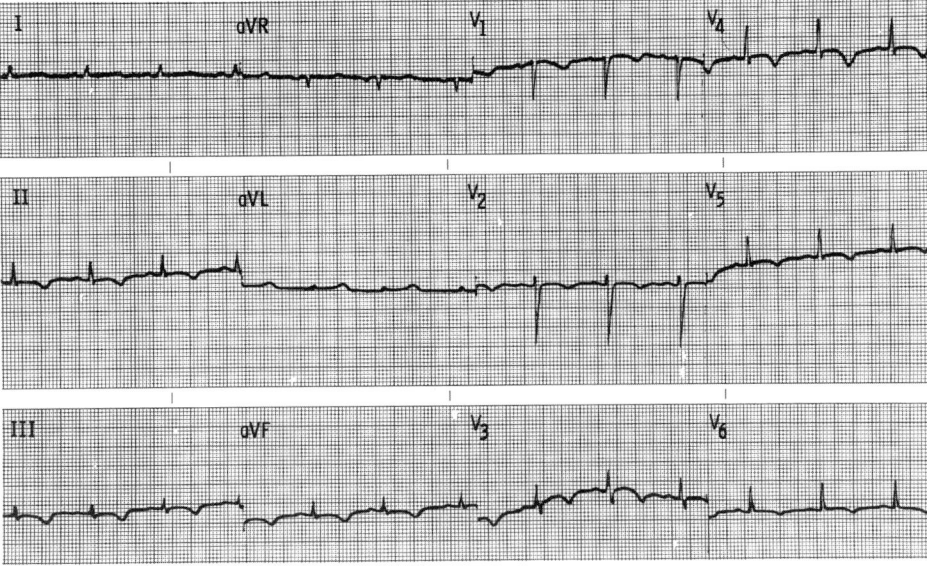

PERICARDITIS

- Since pericarditis is also diffuse in nature, the electrocardiographic abnormalities usually involve many leads.
- During the early phase of acute pericarditis, upward elevation of the concave S-T segment occurs diffusely in practically all leads except lead aVR (Fig. 17-3). Because of the diffuse process in pericarditis, no reciprocal depression of the S-T segment is observed.
- During the late stage (i.e., the subacute and chronic phases) of pericarditis, the S-T segment elevation returns to the isoelectric line and the T waves begin to be inverted.
- The T wave inversion in pericarditis may last for weeks or months.
- Low voltage of the QRS complexes is very common in chronic pericarditis, particularly in constrictive pericarditis and massive pericardial effusion.
- In myxedematous pericardial effusion, the QRS amplitude becomes so low that the electrocardiographic tracing appears to be the isoelectric line in many leads.
- The terms *postcardiotomy syndrome* and *postpericardiotomy syndrome* are commonly used to describe pericarditis resulting from any trauma, including cardiac surgery. In fact, the most common cause of postcardiotomy syndrome at the present time is coronary artery bypass surgery.
- The term *post-MI syndrome* (Dressler's syndrome), on the other hand, is used to designate pericarditis that follows acute MI. Post-MI syndrome is considered to be due to an autoimmune mechanism and is relatively benign in most cases.

Figure 17-3
Acute pericarditis is manifested by S-T segment elevation involving practically every electrocardiographic lead diffusely.

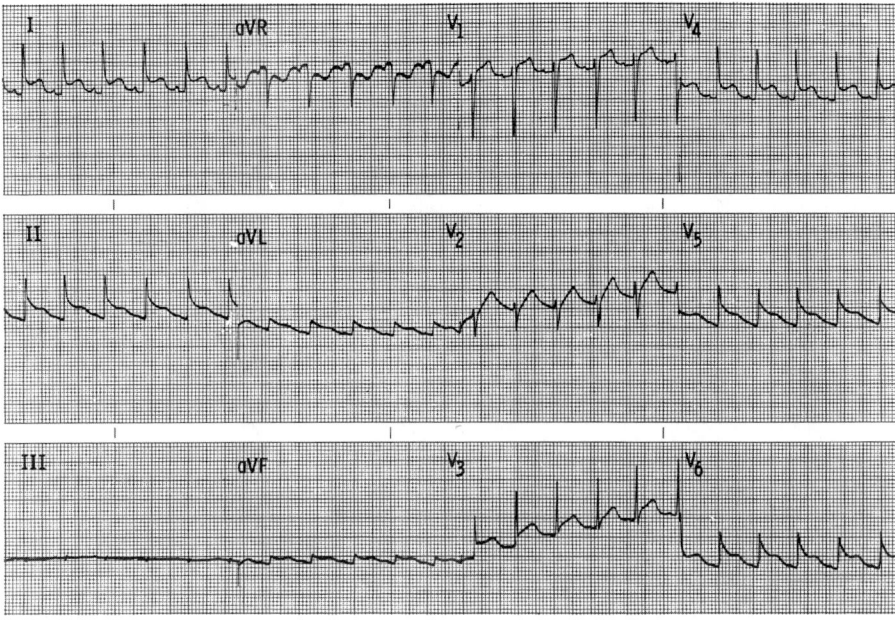

CARDIOMYOPATHY

- Cardiomyopathies of various causes may produce many different electrocardiographic abnormalities and cardiac arrhythmias. In particular, idiopathic cardiomyopathy is nearly always associated with various electrocardiographic abnormalities.
- Common electrocardiographic abnormalities (Fig. 17-4) may include enlargement of various cardiac chambers, LBBB or RBBB, BBBB, diffuse intraventricular conduction defects, multifocal ventricular premature contractions (VPCs), and various ectopic tachyarrhythmias.
- Often, all cardiac chambers are hypertrophied, especially toward the end stage of the disease.
- In idiopathic cardiomyopathy, bundle branch block (either left or right) is frequently atypical in that the QRS configuration is extremely bizarre and very broad.
- In addition, more than one fascicle of the intraventricular conduction system are commonly involved (bifascicular block or trifascicular block), so that various degrees and forms of BBBB are observed (see Chapter 4).
- RBBB has been reported to be the most common electrocardiographic abnormality associated with Chagas' heart disease in South and Central America.
- Among various cardiac arrhythmias, idiopathic cardiomyopathy seems to be specifically related to the production of unilateral atrial tachyarrhythmias resulting in atrial dissociation (see Chapter 13).
- The diagnosis of cardiomyopathy is extremely doubtful when there is no significant electrocardiographic abnormality or cardiac arrhythmia.

Figure 17-4
Nonspecific intraventricular block with very broad and bizarre QRS complexes in a patient with idiopathic cardiomyopathy. Left bundle branch block is superficially simulated.

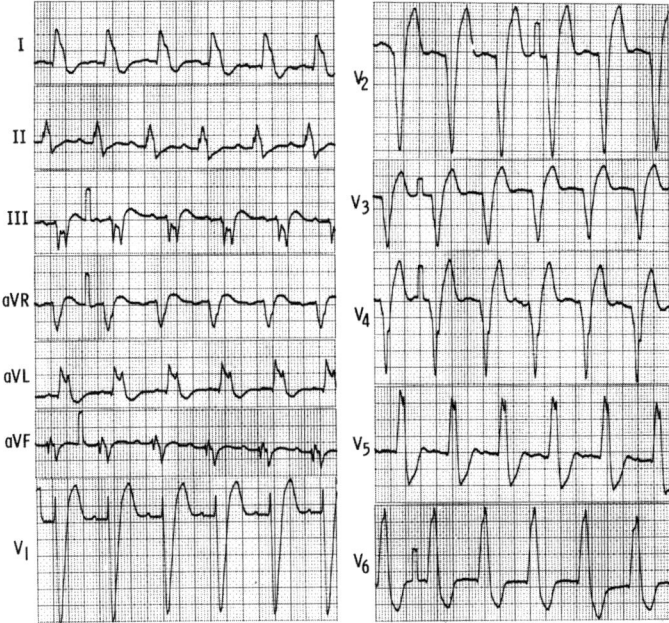

VENTRICULAR ANEURYSM

- Ventricular aneurysm is not an uncommon complication of acute MI, particularly when the anterior wall is involved and when the patient fails to limit his or her activity during the acute phase.
- Ventricular aneurysm is strongly suspected when the S-T segment elevation reappears during the subacute or old phase of MI or the S-T segment elevation persists (>1 week), provided that there is no evidence of superimposed acute MI.
- A ventricular aneurysm is prone to follow an extensive anterior MI (Fig. 17-5).
- The exact mechanism responsible for the production of this electrocardiographic finding in ventricular aneurysm is still not clearly understood. Nevertheless, subepicardial injury caused by pressure from the ventricular aneurysm is considered to be responsible for this electrocardiographic abnormality, although a transmission of the ventricular cavity potential through a thin ventricular aneurysmal wall is an alternative explanation.

Figure 17-5
Left ventricular aneurysm is manifested by a persisting S-T segment elevation in all of the precordial leads following extensive (massive) anterior myocardial infarction.

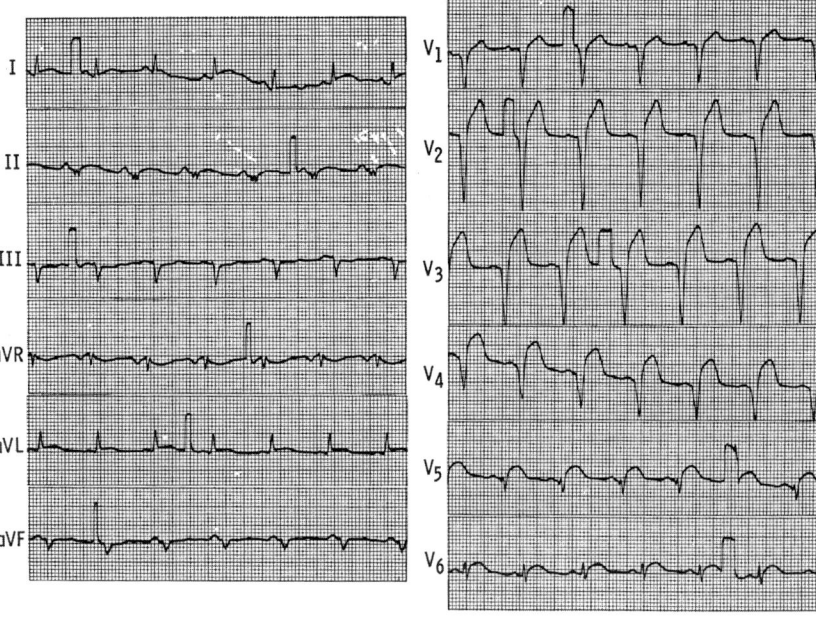

CENTRAL NERVOUS SYSTEM DISORDERS

- Various central nervous system (CNS) disorders, including cerebrovascular accidents, brain tumors, heat stroke, head trauma, delirium tremens, and coma due to various causes (e.g., hepatic or diabetic coma), may produce various electrocardiographic abnormalities.
- Among CNS disorders, subarachnoid hemorrhage is prone to produce electrocardiographic abnormalities more frequently.
- Common electrocardiographic findings in CNS disorders include elevation of the S-T segment, T wave changes, a prolongation of the Q-T interval, prominent U waves, and various supraventricular tachyarrhythmias.
- Diffusely inverted broad T waves with a prolonged Q-T interval are often considered to be a unique feature of subarachnoid hemorrhage (Fig. 17-6), but in an early stage, the S-T segment elevation is often a pronounced change.
- The S-T and T wave changes in CNS disorders often closely resemble the electrocardiographic findings in acute myocardial ischemia, acute MI, and acute pericarditis.

Figure 17-6
Inverted T wave with a markedly prolonged Q-T interval due to a very broad T wave in a patient with subarachnoid hemorrhage. In addition, a possibility of anteroseptal myocardial infarction is considered.

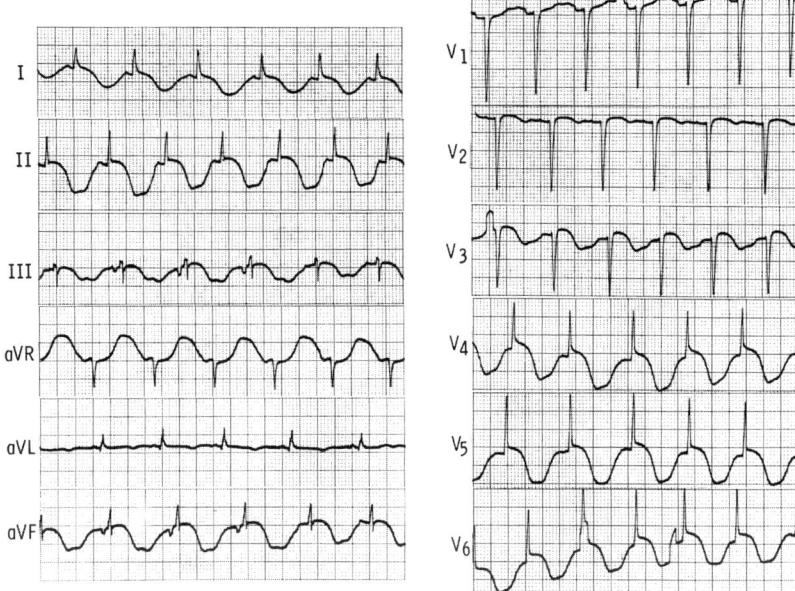

HYPOTHERMIA

- In significant hypothermia, characteristic electrocardiographic changes are often observed.
- The electrocardiographic abnormalities may include marked bradycardia (usually sinus) associated with prolongation of all intervals (P-R, QRS, and Q-T intervals) and junctional elevation of the S-T segment, especially in the precordial leads (Fig. 17-7).
- Atrial tachyarrhythmias, particularly AF, may be encountered in hypothermia.
- Hypothermia-induced electrocardiographic changes may resemble an early repolarization pattern (a form of normal variant), acute pericarditis, an early phase of acute MI, and various intraventricular conduction disturbances.

Figure 17-7
Atrial fibrillation with advanced atrioventricular block and grouped ventricular premature contractions (in lead aVF) associated with nonspecific (diffuse) intraventricular block in a patient with hypothermia following an auto accident on an extremely cold day.

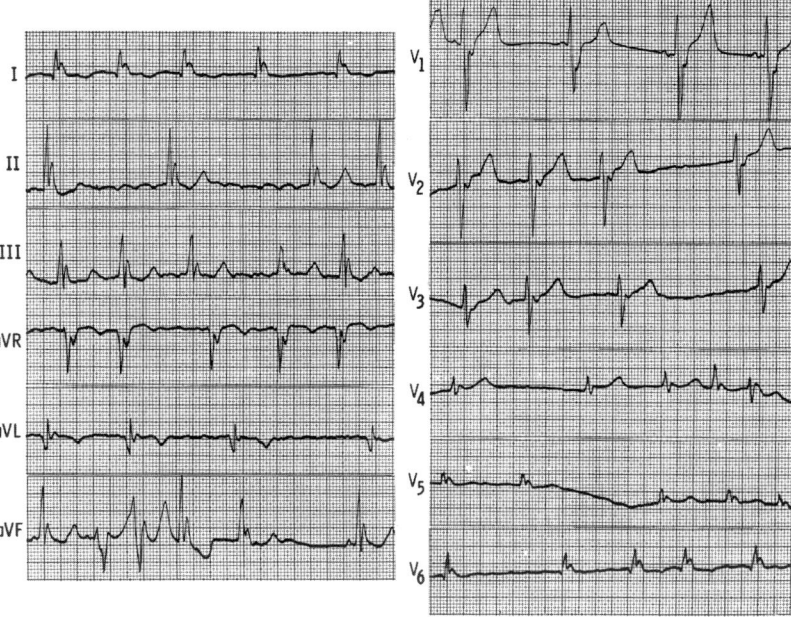

SICK SINUS SYNDROME

- We have become increasingly aware of the entity *sick sinus syndrome* (SSS) in the past decade because the syndrome is found to be relatively common in our practice, particularly among elderly individuals. It can be successfully treated with artificial cardiac pacing in most cases.
- The term *sick sinus syndrome* has been used to describe a broad spectrum of clinical manifestations (e.g., syncope or near-syncope, dizziness, increased congestive heart failure [CHF] and/or angina, and palpitations) as a result of dysfunction of the sinus node.
- Electrocardiographic manifestations in SSS (Fig. 17-8) may include (1) persistent and marked sinus bradycardia, (2) sinoatrial block, (3) sinus arrest, (4) long pause following an atrial premature contraction, (5) chronic AF or atrial flutter with slow ventricular rate, (6) carotid sinus hypersensitivity, (7) no stable sinus rhythm after cardioversion, (8) AV junctional escape rhythm with or without slow and unstable sinus activity, and (9) brady-tachyarrhythmia syndrome. These electrocardiographic findings in SSS are *not* drug-induced.

- The degree of the sinus node dysfunction may be so minimal that the SSS may be manifested only by slight sinus bradycardia. In this case, the patient is usually asymptomatic.
- On the other hand, the sinus node may be severely diseased, leading to complete generator failure so that prolonged sinus arrest or AF with slow ventricular rate will be produced.
- Various symptoms in SSS are usually related to either cardiac or cerebral dysfunction. Namely, the perfusion deficit in these organs is responsible for the production of various symptoms in the SSS. Syncope or near-syncope is the most common clinical manifestation of the SSS. Advanced SSS is nearly always symptomatic.

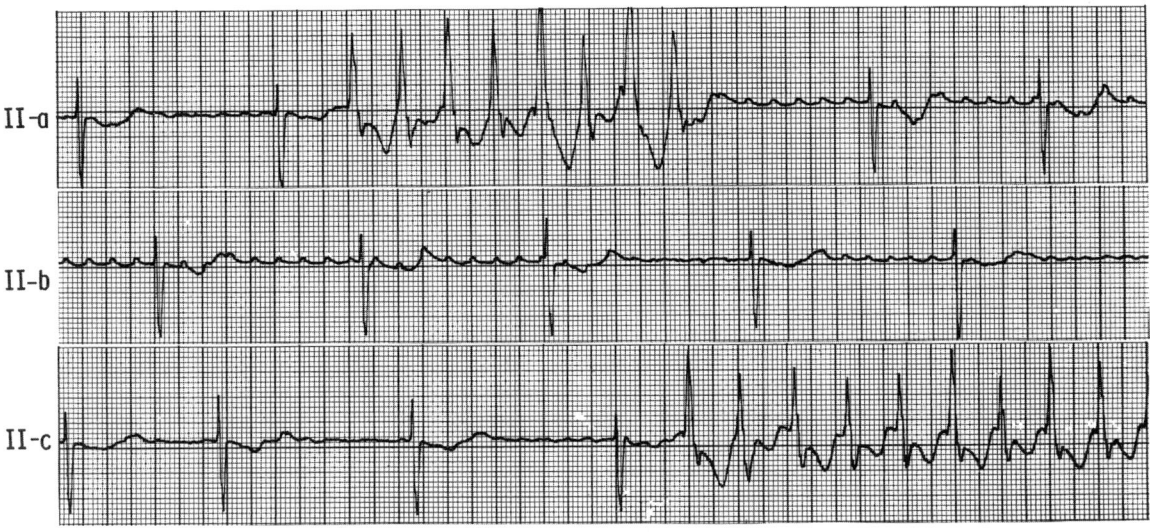

Figure 17-8
Far-advanced sick sinus syndrome is manifested by atrial flutter-fibrillation with advanced atrioventricular block associated with intermittent ventricular tachycardia leading to brady-tachyarrhythmia syndrome. Leads II a–c are continuous.

LOW VOLTAGE

- By definition, the term *low voltage* is used when the total sum of the QRS amplitudes (positive as well as negative component) in leads I, II, and III is 15 mm or less (Fig. 17-9).
- Low voltage may be observed in various clinical circumstances, including severe obesity, pericardial effusion, constrictive pericarditis, chronic obstructive pulmonary disease, advanced CHF, myxedema, and massive MI.
- Low voltage is relatively common among elderly people.

Figure 17-9
Extensive anterior myocardial infarction associated with low voltage of QRS complexes.

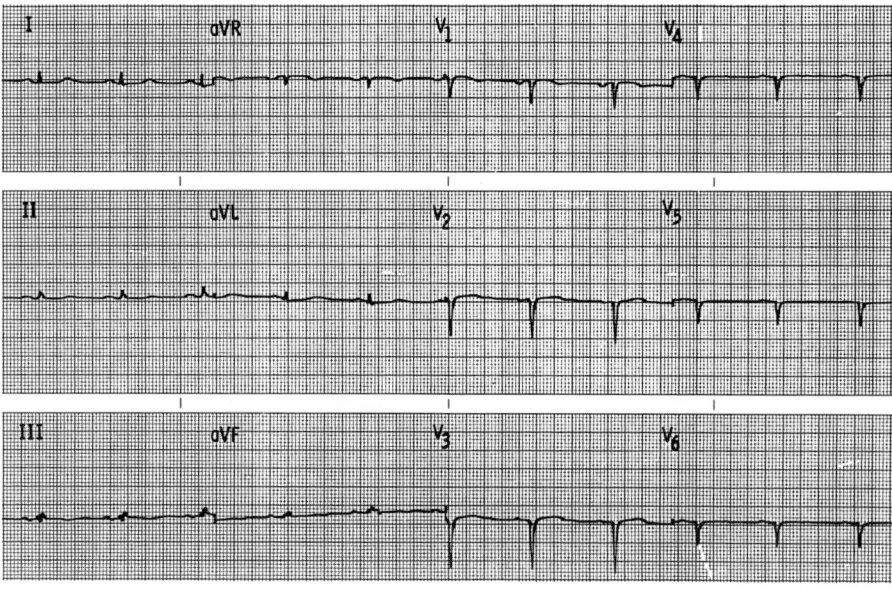

Index

*The page numbers with **bold** letters indicate major discussion.*